T0323453

The Grey Zone of
Health and Illness

The Grey Zone
of Health and Illness

by Alan Blum

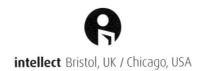

intellect Bristol, UK / Chicago, USA

First published in the UK in 2011 by Intellect,
The Mill, Parnall Road, Fishponds, Bristol, BS16 3JG, UK

First published in the USA in 2011 by Intellect, The University of Chicago Press,
1427 E. 60th Street, Chicago, IL 60637, USA

A catalogue record for this book is available from the British Library.

Front cover image: Antonin Artaud, *La Bouillabaisse de formes dans la tour de Babel*,
ca. February 1948 © Estate of Antonin Artaud / SODRAC (2010).

Cover design: Jenny Scott
Copy-editor: Jennifer Alluisi
Typesetting: John Teehan

ISBN 978-1-84150-364-6
Culture, disease, and well-being (Print) ISSN 2042-177X
Culture, disease, and well-being (Online) ISSN 2042-1788

Printed and bound by Gutenberg Press, Malta.

Contents

ACKNOWLEDGMENTS

This book reflects influences developed from my collaboration with Peter McHugh and the different generations of graduate students we worked with over the years at universities in New York, Toronto, London, England and at workshops, seminars, and meetings in other places. The support of the Canadian Institutes of Health Research made possible our research project *The City and Well-Being: The Grey Zone of Health and Illness*, giving me an opportunity to make this approach palpable through application to the area of health and illness and to the historic study of medicine and the place of doctoring from Plato's *Republic* through those such as Freud, Parsons, Foucault, and Lacan. The generous support of the administration of the University of Waterloo, particularly Amit Chakma who was then Provost, and Dean of Arts Ken Coates, contributed to the perpetuity of our Culture of Cities Centre in Toronto as an intellectual and civic centre, recognizing the import of providing a place for students and researchers to meet and discuss their work in a vital urban environment. Despite the signature of this university as a centre of scientific research, their creativity in relation to our research astonished me in comparison to the relations I had endured with previous university administrations. My colleagues, the principle investigators on the project, have always engaged me in valuable ways over its course, and here I mention Kieran Bonner, Tristanne Connolly, Kevin Dowler, and Sholom Glouberman, never appearing too impatient, sometimes nurturing, often civil but not bureaucratic, invariably ready to engage me intellectually. Our project workshops over this period have centered a continuous and vital exchange of ideas, reflecting a collective willingness to participate critically and to give trouble where it was assumed to be needed, trouble only in the way of inviting rethinking of what had been treated as secure. The Grey Zone research collective includes: J. C. Cloutier, John Faichney, Elke Grenzer, Amelia Ruby Howard, Saeed Hydralli, Diego Llovet, Jan Plecash, Stephen Svenson, Gord Thompson, and Morgan Tunzelmann. The workshops benefited from the intermittent participation of visitors and from the regular attendance of other colleagues, especially Steve Bailey, and Marta-Marin Domine. Amanda Delong was an indispensible member of our project, not only working on my various manuscripts and files, but in lightening the mood at our Centre in many ways through her social and intellectual fluency. I must especially record my gratitude to Nashia Prcic for her diligent work on this manuscript.

My three daughters Paula, Beth, and Hannah in order of seniority, stimulated me in different ways over the course of this writing, provocatively providing different generational views of my representation of the paternal function, sending up in their ways the Grey Zone of the symbolic order as a continuous challenge and opportunity for me to live with. Elke of course, made sure that none of these influences would destroy me or escape my attention, bringing home the Grey Zone of intimacy in ways that remain unforgettable. Elke's presence has not been taken lightly, challenging me in enumerable ways to measure up in work and play and to resist using the Grey Zone as a pretext for inaction.

If the Grey Zone is a figure standing for the fundamental ambiguity intrinsic to the relation of speech to action (word to deed), then this book might be said to be inspired by the Greek conception of *en medias res*, of the mark of human mortality as intermediate (in the formula) between the divine and the animal. This formula is not empirical, that is, an attack on theology or animal rights, but a formulation of the imaginary by and for the human as an intrinsic condition of subjectivity, making the need to heal rather than cure circularity the problem of the subject. This resonates with Lacan's slogan that the body is a paradigm of resemblance (1991, pp. 54, 165–168). I orchestrate an inquiry intended to be dialectical in relation to the overtones of this formula and to rethink it in relation to the collective discourse on health and illness. We can understand the formula as a way of expressing how mortality is a condition of representation that cannot be exceeded, that is, how life can only fantasize what is other or unlike it

The Grey Zone as a canon

This book has enabled me to imagine the Grey Zone as forming something of a canon, or at least what anthropologists might call a culture, and I have used such a notion as an important resource for this work. The convention of a literature review has been provisionally redefined as the discourse evoked by such a collective interest and the concern to formulate ambiguity that appears as the symptom most visible throughout its various speeches and positions. Borrowing from what Bruce Fink (2004, pp. 111–128) in his discussion of Lacan calls a "graph of desire," we will locate the primordial source of such a figure in Plato's (1945) Divided Line in the *Republic*, and in the derivatives taken up in Hegel's (1968) *Logic* as the three stages evolving through the course of objectification as development, explication and actuality, and incarnated in Lacan's triad of imaginary-symbolic-real. Nothing more should be taken from this image of continuity than its status as a figure needed to make intelligible the trajectory of an ideal speaker for formulating any problem whatsoever as a course of narrative action. Similarly,

Baudrillard's important works describing the movement of inquiry through exigencies of waste, calculation and the remainder (1983a, 1983b, 1990, 1993, 2006), along with Arendt's (1958) vision of labor, work and action, have been useful tools for helping me to imagine theorizing not as simple problem solving, but as a way of meeting, enduring and having to redefine the problem of ambiguity that inhabits any topic and that assumes a different shape at various points in any situation of inquiry. In this respect, besides figures developed by Kenneth Burke (1957, 1965) in his rich repertoire of strategies of inquiry, most helpful is the implicit graph of desire Žižek (1997) lays out in his *Plague of Fantasies* that depicts the ideal speaker engaging the problem of distinguishing the ideological posture of social construction from theorizing, thus resurrecting Plato's task of distinguishing philosophy from sophistry as a problem of mistaken identity.

Such talk as this is intended to dramatize for an academic audience the problem of the Grey Zone as that nascent moment originating in the Greek enlightenment of Plato and in contrast to a typical contemporary conceit, not to be thought of as an unprecedented modern invention signaling the historic advance of theorizing over the bones of an antiquated essentialism. If this is one conventional consequence of this book, I will be pleased if it registers the value of an improvisational relationship to influences meant to enliven our capacities for a more refined literacy and a more subtle sense of tradition and dissemination than is usually shown.

In a way similar to this book's use of the figure of the graph of desire, it will also implicitly use the figure of the totem developed by Durkheim (1961) as an image of how the signifier and the problem of signification, even in the case of ambiguity, remains a focus of collectivization that establishes a relatedness in the collective in the shape of a discourse for any topic picked up. Here the work of Eric Gans (1982) on the relation of centre and periphery and the writings of Simmel (1956, 1959, 1971, 1991) and Weber (1930, 1947, 1958) become indispensable resources for overcoming academic fragmentation in order to show the necessity of a sociological vision of the collective representation for research in the arts and humanities. This is another important conventional function of my work.

If it has to be reemphasized that this is not intended as an autobiographical inventory of influences; the reader must take action for herself to see how matters stand and what is important, essential and stimulating and how many influences could and should be seen to play upon a writing such as this, if such a play of forces is worth noting. Yet I am the mediator and it remains my signature, even in speaking of a collective interest as such and of diagnosing its artifice as a canon. My citation of such influences is only designed to show how I cannot think of myself as an unmoved mover and of the Grey Zone as an eccentric and peculiar intuition, but as part of a corpus of influences that emerges in response to automated speech and to the apparent rule today of a mechanical vision of inquiry that authorizes palpable and convenient representations and associations that are governed by procedures for ensuring unambiguous conclusions and findings as if the law of the land. In response to such an atmosphere, my objective is not simply to note the fact of ambiguity but to show how its necessity as an aspect of symbolization creates irreconcilable problems that can be seen as researchable and so, as important moments for inquiry into health and illness.

These figures enable us to conceive of the practice of theorizing, first as originating in a kind of tribal moment of fascination created by signification and the signifier as if a totemic spectacle (the collective representation); then as the desire of one, both together with the collective and apart (the subject of desire, the ideal speaker), to engage this spectacle as if a collective enigma that intimates a problematic situation; and finally, in the practice or course of action that aspires to make this problem actual in a narrative in order to demonstrate how its very irresolute character makes demands upon the collective to come to terms with the specific and singular nature of a problem (such as health and illness) while yet preserving the status of demonstration itself as inconclusive, as a remainder (and as good by virtue of its comic awareness of knowing this and of going on at the same time as if unaware).

Popular versions of the Grey Zone

We cannot be unmindful of the power of the notion of the Grey Zone as what Baudelaire might call a "philosophical worry" in everyday life (1972). This worry is treated as a conundrum in a variety of ways that have come to influence the public culture and the prosaic usages that have developed around projects that either try to resolve indeterminacy or to pass judgment on its appearance and constancy as if an exception to the rule, or if unexceptional, possibly too paralyzing to be acted upon reflectively, remaining an object of respect that can only elicit awe or consternation. Such versions are often tempted to treat the very condition of symbolization and the symbolic order as a source that might be removed (or cured) rather than acted upon with irony (healed), making ambiguity itself into an implicit curse. We can more fruitfully convert such figures into aspects of the discourse that we will have occasion to explore, but now must treat as akin to proverbial formats that we might name as formulae: interdisciplinary studies, transference, reasonable doubt and limitlessness.

Interdisciplinary studies. In this case, what is identified as crucial to ambiguity is a sense of Other seen as withdrawn, abandoning actors to interaction without apparent recourse to a sense of a whole that can mediate their differences. The imaginary ground of this standard is its belief that specialization frees people from absolutism, enabling them to be experimental and yet, anxiety-ridden in the absence of such security. This is a situation in which any sense of Other seems to be based not only upon a vision of the whole as inhibitory but as capricious and inaccessible, and at worst as a pretext for those in positions of advantage to hold on to their power. The idea of a division of labor is imagined along the model of Durkheim's (1938a) organic solidarity as a paragon of togetherness, equating dialogue with cooperation. This emancipatory vision might be contrasted with the vulgarity of Richard Florida's (2002) notion of a creative city. Thus, in response to such "progress" and its applicability to the sciences, the recurrent idea emphasized by Gadamer (1996, pp. 31–45) and others treats this withdrawal as correlative with a sense of loss in which knowledge is fragmented into a series of specialties that have no sense of anything that exceeds the limits of their partial perspectives.

The Grey Zone, visible as a worry generated by such a division of labor that (in medical science) models its knowledge on the view of bodily parts, not only creates disciplines as specialties, but as lacking any sense of the ideal of health against which such specialized disturbances offend. Girard's (1977) notion of sacrificial crisis was meant to describe the limited and rancorous exchanges in a fragmented environment that lacks collective resources for mediating such a commitment to shared being or common purpose (the transcendental), making the referee, umpire, tribunal and such figures of sovereignty intended solutions to such differentiation. In sociology, Parsons (1937) discussed this worry as the social order problem in an exemplary study emanating from Hobbes, and it persists today as one of the most immediate ways in which the Grey Zone is registered in academic circles. The loss of the whole expressed in this vision of the Grey Zone is reflected in the experience of the parts as failing to live up to the whole and so is based upon a fundamental experience of division between part and whole as a division that is never addressed, because the whole is only accessible through its image, and so it is fated to be derivative and inconclusive. What seems clear is that this worry can only be healed by rethinking the conception of Being as both partial and necessary, making the objectification of speech a task for theorizing.

Transference. The literature derived from the Holocaust, and specifically Primo Levi's (1988) testimony, names the Grey Zone as a fundamental problem, especially in Levi's citation of ambiguity as an irresolute problem that plagued inmates in their everyday life as a condition of captivity, as a confusing aspect of the total institution and indeed of any organization or relationship, but dramatized as a condition in the concentration camp. Many commentators exploit recognition of this condition by imagining ambiguity as creating a problem in decision-making that makes accountability either inevitable or impossible as another vision of the either/or, and so, as a problem to cure through the invention of criteria for differentiating the perpetrator from the victim. Much crisscrossing in the camp experience exploits the cliché of identification with the aggressor in this way to develop implications suggesting that any such distinction must remain indistinct. Thus, Levi's subtleties in identifying the equivocal relations in the camp, instead of being joined to a discussion of the relationships of total institutions (or indeed, of any organization, family, relation) between freedom and determination in which agency becomes problematic through the quandary of complicity, responsibility, autonomy and dependence, often seems to gives interpreters criteria for conclusive determination of an action as one thing rather than another, instead of treating the inevitable ambiguity as topical and provocative, confusing analysis with judgment (also see Ruth Leys [2007], *From Guilt to Shame*, for a discussion of these issues). The indistinction between victim and perpetrator is an operating feature of the Grey Zone, perhaps heightened and exacerbated under such horrible conditions, but still a parameter of a relationship as such (imagine a condemnation of the figure of the master-slave relation in Hegel [1977,pp. 1–46, 104–136] rather than a formulation of the figure as a reflective move, as if we assign guilt to any party who passes analytically through these positions rather than see such a passage as a move in the economy of any relationship). The Grey Zone must inhabit any transference relationship. For example, the idea that the child could be a victim or a perpetrator, or the judge, or the criminal or the parent, means that the Grey Zone appears as a phenomenon in many areas of life, inviting theorizing rather than either/or declarations of responsibility. Indeed, Levi's discussion of indistinction and his examples point to the irrevocable and irresolute problem of identification and of overcoming the transference as the problem to be explored, as the phenomenon, not only in the concentration camp but in teaching and learning (who is the victim and who is the perpetrator?) and in the discourse of mastery. It is this sense of the Grey Zone as a phenomenon and not as a fait accompli that we need to pursue and will, through the work of Freud and in a way that has relevance for health and illness. Thus, if the prosaic understanding is that it is the relation of doctor to patient that seems to raise this question, it is actually the relation of body to mind that arouses us to ask if the body is the victim or the perpetrator in ways that will become important in the following chapters.

Reasonable doubt. Much like the derivative discussion of the transference, the Grey Zone appears as a worry in works of philosophers who try to calculate, impossibly, how guilt and responsibility is to be allocated and assigned in situations that remain essentially ambiguous and so, resistant to propositional declarations of guilt and innocence. Here the Grey Zone follows from the inevitable separation of judgment from what it judges, from the hole in the signifier that licensed Clinton to say, "It depends on what *is* is," and that makes any act of signification essentially opaque. Thus, Bennett (1995) discusses the difficulty of deciding responsibility for actions (wrong actions) when an unequivocal line cannot be drawn between doing an action, making it happen, influencing an action, contributing to it in other ways such as witnessing and the like, as if the notion of an action being done has so many senses that the question of reasonable doubt can always be raised. This kind of juridical approach, implicitly using an either/or model of artificial language as a standard against which speaking always must offend, identifies life as a Grey Zone, but only by treating language as a perversion. What is perverse about language is that the irrevocable transparency of the word means that a fundamental division between signifier and signified, amounting to a gap between what is seen for oneself and what is "inferred" (or between seen and unseen, visible and invisible) must haunt any declaration by stamping it as probable rather than certain. Because the relation of cause to effect can only be imaginary as Hume said (1956), any proposition is essentially revisable. Yet the inconclusive nature of any such conclusion only confirms the Grey Zone as the truth of skepticism embodied in the liar's paradox as philosophers have long recognized. The perversity in such a recognition appears when the paradox is faced with the test of licensing a course of action or way of life under such auspices. Such a strategy is often used as grounds for denying responsibility for actions, for example in excusing mistakes, in evading accusation of corruption or participation in nefarious activities, but it also can and needs to be employed in any act of disavowal in ways that make ambiguity always appear evasive.

For example, Wolin (1990) uses Heidegger's theorizing as grounds for a critique of his conception of ambiguity as a pretext: saying that such theorizing exempts itself from accountability by treating the engagement with detail and decision-making as essentially ontic and so in this way, always potentially incidental as a mere material condition of speaking. Here, Heidegger is treated as an example of one who tries to live according to the paradox and in a way that can only show the perverse limits of any vital relation to ambiguity.

What reasonable doubt discloses as a phenomenon are the multiple ways in which negotiating guilt, innocence and responsibility pervade everyday life as irresolute situations in which members of society, including doctors and patients, try to calculate where the causal force of action should be located, how and why, and on what grounds. This book will take up many of these attempts to calculate and arrest ambiguity as a demonstration of the invasion of the Grey Zone into every area of life as an influential worry and problem to be solved.

Limitlessness. Kant's genius in identifying the Grey Zone as the division between human capacity and incapacity (in itself-for itself, accessible-inaccessible) makes it interior as a division intrinsic to the human self engaging the limits of what can be determined. As the surfeit or remainder exceeding determination, the Grey Zone becomes the heir of the experience of sublimity that can only defer to the immensity (the greatness) of what is unknown in relation to its limitation, that still grows and prospers in our knowledge of this as we gain power by the implication of being powerless (what Nietzsche [1956, pp. 170–173] might call the song of a slave). That is, if what seems greatest is the unknown as such, it appears that it is our capacity to see this as great that might be greatest, that it might be our imaginary that makes this possible even as it seems to sacrifice our stature in relation to such greatness.

Thus, the division in the human is seen to be inversely related to the unknown insofar as the ineffable indivisibility of what we cannot know serves as a standard against which the human cannot measure up, and in such a failure, measures up to what the human is at best, showing the human as both large and small, divided against herself in this way, guilty about her smallness, and yet proud of her singularity by virtue of this. In his essay on the world picture, Heidegger (1982) developed this sense of the impossibility of mastery, modeled after the relation of *dasein* to his own death, as that sense of the incalculable as the possibility of impossibility.

As in the idea of the withdrawal of the whole, or of the erosion of the aura, and particularly Weber's discussion of how science is driven by a sense of the whole being knowable "in principle," the Grey Zone becomes viewed as a visible worry exercising collective fascination around the object and, in particular, the advance of technology. As Heidegger says (pp. 115–155), the annihilation of great distances by technology and its achievements means that the intractable distance between humans and nature is overcome without the fluency expected as a consequence of such reconciliation. The "reconciliation" always remains fundamentally irresolute because of the alienation implicit in any application. For example, if technology brings the body to view, opening its interior from concealment, such accessibility accentuates that very distance by virtue of the division between the façade of potential mastery evoked by this relation to the body and its visibility, and the reality of the limits of human perspective as of every here-and-now.

As we shall eventually come to note, the advances of technology tend to make transparent the enigmatic character of what Lacan (1992) calls *das Ding*, where what is external seems intimate and what is near seems distant in ways that mix proximity and remoteness in any experience. For example, mass media bring events close (e.g., a ferry accident in Asia) but without a degree of intimacy, that is, as information that leaves the exposed actor affected but untouched since receiving the image does not guarantee how it is applied or integrated. In these ways, it might be said (as an aspect of the Grey Zone to consider) that the abundance of objects and images in circulation give us opportunity to take a perspective on events and to have experiences (to be literate and informed with respect to "what happened") but not necessarily to be able to take possession of the experience, that is, to integrate images and objects into trajectories of self-formation and self-knowledge. This also applies to relations to suffering that are abundant in the world in ways that make them appear immense and complex and, at the same time, incalculable by virtue of the aura of sublimity with respect to means and methods for alleviation that always seem as if scarce (Boltanski, 1999). Thus, technology and the power it seems to release for picturing and representing progress as an overcoming of our limits, making possible the experience of division between our greatness and impotence in any such moment of "advance," accentuates the paradox of the Grey Zone as a sense of having the resources and yet lacking the means for integrating them, giving the spurious appearance that the only hindrance here is knowledge "translation" whereas the enigma resides in the problematic relationship to any object. Again, as in the other cases, these various notations on the Grey Zone in the public discussion will be addressed at various points in what follows.

Of course Derrida is significant not simply for noting the Grey Zone but for pursuing the question of how to inhabit the Grey Zone in speech and action, a problem (in the most prosaic sense) of needing to disavow essentialism essentially, or of taking exception to sovereignty in what can only be a sovereign gesture. I try to show that the format of *en medias res*, of the absolute in Hegel, of Lacan's *das Ding*, are primordial initiatives in this quest if these figures are read as imaginary gestures and not as signs of an unironic submission to essentialism(or derided as literalism). Derrida translates such canonical usage through distinctions such as sovereignty, the unconditioned, ipseity, as a complicated exchange of signifiers that both makes possible(as the unconditioned) and qualifies(as sovereignty) any resolution, inducing the actor to suffer this irresolution in ways that(as Derrida recognizes) can be aporetic or paralyzing. I treat this project also as fated to work within the horizon of the Greeks despite its various disavowals. I provide grounds for this in the book. Plato described ipseity as a relationship, a course of social action that mixes and matches impossibly but necessarily the Same and the Other as what Kenneth Burke came to call "equipment for living." Note that this very question of reading, misrecognizing or translating the works of the past are themselves features of the discourse on sovereignty that seems to reflect the corporeal drive to say "no but" to past works that are comparable rather than "yes and," perhaps as signs of the aspiration of contemporaries at any historical moment to mark their departure from the past or to position themselves unforgettably as singular in relation to an inheritance (conditions that must also influence my relation to the question of the Grey Zone as a canon).

The primordial character of the formula en medias res in this work serves me well for the way it brings the division in subjectivity to view. The formula that places humans between gods and animals is meant to stipulate that gods are not mortal, and animals do not reflect upon mortality, making humans intermediate by virtue of needing to engage in such a reflection. This means that what humans suffer is the ambiguity of (what Derrida calls) ipseity. *En medias res* translates this as the need and desire to orient to mortality (unlike Gods and beasts) in the absence of certain knowledge of what are gods and animals, that is without knowing the truth of this distinction. Thus, what humans suffer is their relation to the unknown, that they have to act knowingly about what they cannot know(what today is taken as the sign of the sovereign exception) while knowing full well that they are ignorant. This is the Grey Zone in a nutshell. That is, humans must distinguish, and given the conventionality of any distinction, must both do it and know that it can be otherwise (as Peter McHugh put it). This is not a choice, a decision, happy or sad, reasonable or not, but an example of drive, almost corporeal, showing (in the words of Kenneth Burke) how the handicap (in this case, of mortality)is converted into a virtue. Thinking about humans is not a reflection upon suffering per se(because animals are assumed to suffer), but the practice of enacting in enumerable concrete ways, a reflection upon the human way of suffering, taking the risk of distinguishing between suffering that is human and suffering that is (imagined as) other than human, and so, necessarily reviving the sovereign notion of form.

The interpenetration of culture and health and illness is often thought of as a zone of ambiguity in which the necessity for clear-cut actions and decision-making of practitioners and clients involved in relationships to modern medicine is always haunted by unspoken assumptions, understandings and equivocations that cannot be completely mastered and made explicit. We call this region of ambiguity the Grey Zone because it is the space of indeterminacy upon which all determination ultimately depends. Yet this "zone of ambiguity" is linked to human conduct much more fundamentally than it is connected to medical decision-making, specifically through its spacing in speech itself in ways that have pervasive ramifications. In what follows, we shall inquire in part into the ways in which our knowledge of health and illness is conceptualized in practice and linked to collective values regarding life in complex modern times and in particular to notions of the way urbanity functions in such relationships; yet, on a primordial level, this narrative on the collective representation of health and illness in modern life and as inflected in the city must be grounded in a more elemental vision of the place of health and illness in collective life, a vision that enables us to conceive of one subject to ambiguity in a more fundamental way, a way that expresses dialectically nuanced relationships.

The Grey Zone is a figure of speech meant to collect the essential ambiguity intrinsic to all social phenomena as it becomes topical in mundane ways (perhaps through the ideas of uncertainty or "noise" in communication theory, or conventionally in clichés about the limits of totality, or supposed "gaps" between subjective and objective, ideal and actual) or on critical occasions or crises when our inability to completely master events becomes apparent. The Grey Zone is based upon a proverbial sense of the distinction between "black and white" dualistic thinking that posits unambiguous alternatives as if choosing between them is the fundamental ambiguity (either/or) and a more pervasive sense of irresolution that haunts all words and deeds.

Of course the "positive" sense of the either/or derived from Kierkegaard's (1955) notion of commitment contrasts with the "negative" notion of its status as an impediment to Hegel's *aufheben* (Birchall, 1981) that is assumed to overcome opposition through a reflective move that preserves the difference between what was initially opposed (reflected in the slogan to cancel the opposition and preserve the difference). In the sense that Kierkegaard focuses upon the necessity for any action to be as unambiguous as the conclusion is, his notion of the either/or makes an essentialism of action inescapable; even and insofar as ambiguity must inhere in the consequences of any such act, its fate as an inheritance is to be oriented to in ways forever inconclusive. This suggests that the either/or *and* ambiguity must coexist because the *aufheben* as a demonstrable practice can only be this rather than that. Both Kierkegaard and Hegel seem right in identifying the fundamental ambiguity of the relation of ambiguity to the either/or as another way of approaching the relation of the symbolic order (and its lawfulness) to the Real (the Lacanian hole in Being) that exceeds symbolization, identifying what Baudrillard (1983a, pp. 75–78) calls the remainder.

These comments are meant to recommend that the Grey Zone is not a feature of medical practice alone (as if *it* is ambiguous and everything else is perfectly clear), nor a critical judgment on the practice as if it shows a fault or deficiency (of domineering, test-crazed doctors, or of gabby, self-absorbed delusional clients, or even of its so-called biomedical reductionism, though each and all of such conditions can and do enter into our relations to health and illness as troubles and content), nor is the Grey Zone a result of the so-called subjectivity of medical practice or of the uncertainty and equivocal nature of any medical decision or of medicine being, as they say, an art, or even an "ideology." These images of ambiguity are external to the Grey Zone (in the way choosing between signing or not signing an informed consent form in the hospital prior to a crucial decision about a medical intervention is less a feature of the Grey Zone than is the question of whether the choice is a choice at all). In other words, choosing one option over another does not show this as a real choice just as shopping for different brands of the same product or deciding between classes at university, or subjects to major in, or items on a menu, might certainly create ambivalence for the subject, whereas in contrast, what is fundamentally ambiguous is the notion of the choice *as a* choice. For example, think of deciding between political candidates here or any situation in which we are tempted to treat a difference of degree as a difference in kind. The idea that choices we are forced to make are real choices is designed to create the impression that we participate in the situation as a decision-maker where the parameters of the situation as offering decisive alternatives has already been decided or chosen for us without our participation. What we are deciding upon has already been decided for us in ways that equate our having the possibility of accepting or rejecting the alternatives offered with the idea that the choice reflects an offer of alternatives that makes a difference and is a real choice of options different in kind rather than degree.

In this vein, we must reiterate the many views suggesting that the cultural element of health and illness and of medical practice lies not simply in science but in the ideas and beliefs that include relationships to objects, and particularly, the imaginary relationship to the "object" that is the body, and the contested judgment that always needs to be applied to any particular case about what seems best here and now (Raffel, 1985). As Gadamer (1996) suggests, the great achievements of medicine and its advances in technology and informatics that mark the development of objective knowledge come unencumbered by a science (or art) of interpretation, and judgment that still remains necessary for using and deciding among the options provided by such accomplishments an art, necessary for informing and grounding the decision-making that must invariably be worked out as part of the application of such knowledge. If Gadamer shows in his discussion of *phronesis* and craftsmanship how knowledge cannot provide for its unambiguous application, making "application" invariably problematic, then this is because an action (as Kierkegaard says) is unequivocal as *this* rather than *that* and must always make an exception to ambiguity, must "ban" it in the contemporary vernacular.

For example, the myriad links imagined between health, illness and medicine seem to be mediated by a totemic relationship to the body that establishes the relatedness of all concerned, but a relatedness that cannot be anything but divisible. Despite its repeatedly great advances, theorizing the body has succeeded in establishing an indivisible corpus of knowledge only when the authority of some particular beliefs (science, medicine, fundamentalism) is accepted without further ado. Without such trust or incredulity, equivalent to what Agamben (1998) calls the state of exception or the ban on ambiguity, the body, as any signifier, must be a beginning, an open question, in terms of which truthful speech always remains undeveloped, implicit and abstract. It is not medicine that errs here, for this provisional character of the object such as the body is a feature of the split in the signifier itself, the ambiguity of the body as a notion being "interior" to it and not a result of a crime committed by medicine. On the other hand, the crime committed by any practice of inquiry, such as medicine, does lie in its denial of such a split and its adoption of a dogmatic conception of the indivisibility of the notion of the body and in a practiced disregard of anything other.

Imagining the body as our "object," is it fair to suggest that at any point in time, all of the information imaginable could not enable us to live with the body and its irrationality unambiguously, and that an unknowable excess invariably remains as a trace of the object's inaccessibility for us? It is not farfetched to suggest that the gap between advances in objective knowledge of the body and our aspiration to develop ourselves (our well-being) in relation to the body remains the irremediable problem of our life *while yet* a fertile source for discovering occasions when this gap comes to view as a discrepancy both "produced" in collective life and worked out in various ways and at various sites.

Yet, we must proceed with caution here on any number of grounds, first because the instabilities in the human relation to the body and its incoherence might be a symptom of elemental problems that reflect the status of the body as an image of more fundamental relationships, and secondly, because such a fundamental process might only be differentiated historically in the way one elemental problem is disseminated and displaced in many particular manifestations much as a repetitious recurrence that takes on different shapes, assuming diverse disguises (which we then mark after the fact as historical transformations that seem to make what is different in degree different in kind); and finally, that the Grey Zone, as a phenomenon of desire and not as a historical incremental process materializing as modern progress (or in the debate between enlightenment and its critics), is the variant of a problem medicine inherits and disguises in its diversity of approaches to health and illness. This remains the problem of desire, its limits and prospects for refashioning the conditions that materialize in any present and so, the problem of giving form to material conditions in ways that can be just towards its irresolution *hic et nunc*. In an elemental sense, the problem of the body (as any term, signifier, object) is implicated in the problem of the image, promising (or threatening) to absorb the history of medicine into the history of art (Didi-Huberman, 2005, pp. 138–228). By this is meant that notions such as health, illness, disease, medicine and the body are animated as objects of desire, and in this sense, as collective representations. As an image, any signifier begins in thought as undeveloped, implicit and abstract (as in Hegel's [1968] *Logic*), an intimation of a relationship to be worked out (revealing its ground in signification in Lacan, *physis* in Heidegger, emergence in G.H. Mead [1967] and McHugh [1968, 2005]) as something seen-as what it is, necessarily seeing the what that is seen to co-relate to what it is assumed to be as in Wittgenstein's (1953, pp. 192–196) notion of seeing-as and eventually in Lacan's (1997) *object a*.

Images of the body

The status of the body remains an object of fascination in collective life due to its very ambiguity. On the one hand, when treated as a standard of measured speech in ways that preserve a kind of corporeality, its external solidity seems to set the standard for many shapes of reductionism or behaviorism. On the other hand, this view can be treated as simplifying the body and its complex resonances, ignoring its sensuality and the complexity in the relations of senses to self-reflection. This becomes vivid when Serres (2008a), for example, connects the sense of touch and its emergence to the self while still deferring the status of the very question it raises, and that remains, concerning the nature of the exchange between internal and external (resolved in his prose that must be augmented by something other than sensuality).

The body appears as a portent of fragility, irregularity and ungovernability, a sign of the repetitive incalculability of the external, which at the same time is experienced as the weight of the internal. The internal character of the body references the intimacy and particularity of its effects, that always record the history of the subject in a way felt as special and distinctive. Yet, it is the mixture between this intimacy and externality— between the felt solidity of this body as uniquely mine and its ungovernability and incalculability as irrevocably "other"—that marks its domain as a site of singularity in the shape of the enigma it appears to be.

The mixture of intimacy and externalization of the divided subject is always exhibited as the limits of self-mastery reflected in the resistance that the body offers to self-reflection, to the agency of will and self-mastery. In this sense, the body is typically identified as dumb, a mute site for observation of its signs as the incalculable and yet decipherable movement of forces that remain to be mastered. The body invites the need and desire to observe its effects as grounds of inference and action, of the need for self-governance, in a relationship in which one depends upon the other to calculate and provide means of establishing control over its course. In this relationship, the intimacy of the body is problematized insofar as what is owned by me is not really my possession, raising as a continuous concern the question of its ownership, the question of to whom the body does belong, and at least in a medical sense, its owner might not know best! The tenacity of the idea of my body as mine, as property rooted in the sovereignty of my innermost voice and most intimate touch, coexists nevertheless with an incorrigible sense of its generality, as if a foreign territory, an alien substance, that I might only observe with detachment.

The self-observant relation to the body (and to the common view[s] of the body inscribed in the *doxa* of medical practice) establishes in a microcosm the social situation of the divided subject and its need to establish clarity vis-à-vis its self-understanding. Here, then, an incipient image of the *polis*, of dialogue as the common good, rules even such calculative self-observation. Yet, the question remains: what is the good of such sociality? Is this objective of self-understanding, always concretized as such self-monitoring, simply a restricted economy designed to defend against decline, deterioration and death? The ambivalence of the self-observing subject of health permits us to address the question of the good of its resistance, its problematization of continuity and stability (of health) as a good itself. That is, how is self-monitoring anything more than defensive or instrumental?

The conception of health that is presupposed in the image of the positive character of such self-resistance always recommends implicitly an engagement in self-scrutiny that serves to endow health itself with its character as something other than the relief of distress. Here, health as reaching for an object more positive than mere survival begins to point to an element of eroticism that it wants to claim for an undisturbed life or an existence undisturbed by illness, the delight imaginable as coming from the inventive relationship to the fortuitous. From this angle, the play of outwitting the adversary is less agonistic than positive in itself, involving a degree of freedom, energy and spontaneity. Yet, it always seems as if health can only be determined by disease, existing as nothing more than the time spent thinking about not being ill or in following regimes designed to fortify itself against such disturbance. Since it is always hard to justify the "good feeling" assumed to come from healthfulness and well-being in-itself, without recourse to whatever disturbances it is excluding ("feeling bad"), describing one's health always seems rhapsodic, or at least, every bit as vacuous or incommunicable as describing one's pain. In fact, if being healthy is often reputed to be without pain, the incommunicability of pain seems proportionate to the incommunicability of health in ways that disclose this region of self-description as a fundamental zone of ambiguity (in ways that could touch upon happiness and depression both and together as well). Gadamer (1996, pp. 3–16) tries to address this problem by transforming the enigma of illness into the enigma of health, identifying health as the concealed sense of "inner accord" interrupted by illness.

The consequences of intervention in the course of the body are incalculable as of any here-and-now. On the one hand, the need to take action is a reminder of the limits it offers to will and good intention; that the body's commentary is often indirect and implicit is noted in any version of how the consequences of an action are unanticipated as if "complications" with implications for the body as well as the mind. That is, the body "records" influences from the environment in a way that the mind might not grasp; there is a division in the subject released by its engagement in any moment, between its concentration upon its involvement and its capacity to imagine consequences of what it is doing. If unregulated design, intention, mind or will could produce a mix of consequences that only a reflexive disengagement could anticipate, then such a position would have to take the point of view of the future that contemplates what is done here and now as its past, its history as recorded in the body. The body, then, is much like an interlocutor to the mind, which "replies" to it as if a representative of the unknown environment, recording its influences in a way that could question any action. To care for the body is not to "turn back the clock" but to understand its place as a mouthpiece for the alterity of the environment. It is in this way that Parsons (1951) could speak of the body itself as an "environment of action." In this usage the body serves as a reminder to think about the consequences of action, of questions concerning accountability and responsibility; insofar as any action has effects, it raises the question of the difference between "awareness" and intention involved in being oriented to the consequences of what is done.

The relationship of science to health care that is objectified in the picture of a medical system is taken as the point of departure for this book, approaching the corpus of medical knowledge as both functional and aesthetic in Simmel's (1959) sense, a symbolic order and imaginative structure typically expressed in formulations of concerted care for the body and its healthfulness, whether for individuals or collectives, as a state of permanent emergency, a state once regarded as exceptional and now as normative in every and any area of health care. Thus, the operation of the health care system appears to function within the same logical nexus as did the ideas of nuclear deterrence and the cold war in the international system. These relationships can be seen to place new burdens upon practitioners, clients and the system in general, not only with respect to bureaucratization in relation to time, space and scarcity of resources, but to ethical questions that circulate around concerns for governance regarding the quality of care, advice, expertise, information and conflicts between dependency and self-determination. Throughout the introductory chapters and in the following parts, the book will focus upon identifying areas of strain or conflict in public health and everyday life around tensions connected to models of healthfulness and sickness, of self-governance and negligence, and contested representations in public life, media and popular culture of the value and uses of health. These tensions are made visible in a variety of cases, with the intent to exemplify the uncanny status of health and illness in the city.

The city has typically been conceived positively as a site at which resources of knowledge are concentrated and accessible to all (and so, intelligible *in principle* with the aid of expert clarification) *and* at the same time, as a fragmented environment of services that bring to view in their very diversity, social conflicts over assumptions and interpretations concerning the quality of health care and the ethical implications of providing it in one way or another. In other words, the city is a site at which the ambiguity of ethical indecision and emotional dispersion is *produced* by the very advances in knowledge that are expected to offer definitive resolution. The expectation that the city creates an objective way of life is always tested in cases where the population must suffer the frustrating lack of intimate connection offered by such progress. The two-sided character of the city means that its very productivity also creates anxiety over the application of such knowledge to life. Because the city is both stimulating and fragmented, differences become vivid around the question of the relation of healthfulness to life, reflected in collective representations of health and its management that become normative and always arguable models for both citizenship and a well-ordered environment. The book develops a framework for studying collective health by isolating a range of case studies in which the Grey Zone becomes visible and dramatic under the conditions of city life.

1

The Grey Zone as a Primordial Figure: Greek Origins

Introduction

The notion of the Grey Zone as a site of ambiguity can be seen in the conventional approach to health and illness but resonates in a primordial way with various usages and figures of speech developed by the Greeks and the ways they achieved the question of what can be known, of the relation of the subject to the unknown.

(A) At the most fundamental level, the discourse derives from the imagined bifurcation of nature and the social, a division assumed to produce a perplexity around the enigma of nature (which would include–besides the cosmos, terrestrial and extraterrestrial matters and the like–the body). That division was perhaps first honored in the contrast between physics and philosophy enunciated in Plato's (1955) *Phaedo*, where the human subject was formulated by Socrates as "fallen" in a way, being unable to directly and immediately access externals without the mediation of language and representation, that is, without discourse. Thus, discourse as a second sailing in the absence of the immediate apprehension, fantasized by the subject as lost (which we know was never possessed), is assumed to "interrupt" the undifferentiated formless immersion of the subject in the world, a formlessness conveyed in Baudrillard's (1998, pp. 191–192) conception of the actor as having no "shadow, reflection, or double," that is, as being undivided without the desire to take a perspective on oneself, to be without a self and so assumed to inhabit a world in the absence of any relation of original to image (everything is either/or, one thing or the other), that is, in the absence of desire. The relation between what we know and what we cannot know can only be abridged by discourse, but in ways that leave a remainder because of the secondariness of speech.

(B) At the second level, desire itself accentuates this division as the experience of a split between the internal (intimate) and external (real), an experience necessarily oriented to fulfilling what is irresolute, an imaginary and impossible reconciliation released by the obscurity of the division as the enigma (puzzle, riddle) of being human as two-sided, two-in-one or one-two (both body and mind), the enigma whose obscurity exercises the subject dramatically in Lacan's (1992) figure of *das Ding* (the intimate experience of exteriority, the external experience of intimacy) and is dramatically represented in his version of the mirror stage. This sense of *das Ding* was perhaps best captured in Plato's (1949a) *Theaetetus* in the discussion of the difference between having knowledge (as if one wears it or has it about one) and possessing knowledge (as if one might make it over and take it as one's own). Having knowledge in the way of being literate and capable of using terms and enacting the grammar through following rules and the like is not the same as being able to use the language in new and inventive ways, influencing it and being influenced to create and develop unexpected situations. In possessing knowledge we do not mechanically apply a code, but perhaps reinvent the word in different ways, find our voice in the word and the word as an expression of our voice, creating opportunities for figuration and the fluency of expression rather than rule-governed competence. The narrative represents the movement from having to possessing knowledge as the trajectory of the ideal speaker, striving necessarily but impossibly to bring together external and internal.

The split between having and possessing knowledge, itself not an either/or choice, is an example of the Grey Zone and applicable to any phenomenon or usage, including having an experience, having a self or whatnot, making reference as it does to the requirement of self-knowledge as a pursuit insofar as self-possession acts upon what we have (commonplace distinctions) by rethinking them for the purpose of making over both and jointly the distinction *and* ourselves as a matter of import, resuscitating the distinction and grounding ourselves through the practice of such a renewal. This movement from having to possessing oneself in one's speech is intended as a trajectory that is mimetic insofar as it is performed as an imitation of such desire as a pursuit. Despite the reputation of the Greeks as unformed in this respect, this is not an essentialist definition of the human as being reflective in practice but as needing to drive towards a mimetic relationship with respect to self-knowledge in ways that are both necessary and desirable (Kenneth Burke's [1957] "equipment for living") and also impossible to fulfill.

Note in Greek the three-fold nature of this division between the inside and the exterior: first, between the word and the thing as we pointed out for the contrast of science and philosophy; second, the division between the intimacy of the word itself (its interiority) and its externality in ways the word is assumed to "kill" the experience to which it refers (as in Lacan [1992], if the first assumes a split between signifier and signified, then the "advance" that sees only the signifier still recognizes *its* split or division between its intimate and external senses). Finally, the notion of *en medias res*, of being in the middle of things, is the Greek way of acknowledging the secondary character of the human, its inevitable position as a space of inheritance, of always beginning in the middle of a story (just as the talk here on the Grey Zone is *en medias res* since I can in no way pretend to be at the origin of this discourse). Each of these levels identifies a different tension in relation to the unknown.

The distinctions of having from possessing knowledge and of *en medias res* are nicely joined in Lacan's conception of *das Ding* as the irrevocable border between the intimate and the external experienced by the subject of language. The subject, said to be divided by the tension between the signifier and the *jouissance* that exceeds it, treats the word as the corporeal outside of the experience it represents. In line with Freud's (Freud and Breuer, 1952) conception of symptom formation, the word converts the internal excitation aroused by the trauma into an external point of reference that can only reduce that experience as if the subject is two-sided in her loyalty both to the signifier and to the signification that is felt as exceeding it and that seems both to identify its authenticity and to mark it invariably as lost. This border is indicated by the signifier (word, category) itself and its relation to signification. Conversion describes the process where signification brings the signifier into existence through the *physis* of language and the emergence of what is positive (the name), for what is negative (the experience of one's arbitrary groundless nothingness). What Lacan calls a "nonrelation of signifier to signified" (Fink, 2004, pp.132–135, 137–140) means that the symbolic order neutralizes the imaginary wasteland of the subject, organized around the negative experience of loss and abandonment (castration). This relation of exteriority to intimacy experienced as the split in any relation to the word confirms for him the body as the paradigm of identity, because the word is conceived according to the model of corporeality. Such a subject is necessarily driven by the split to imagine that there must be something better than the signifier, such as an ideal or standard that "never fails to make things worse," because it is bound up with the inevitable frustration and aggression of the subject in her disappointment at not being able to realize this standard in action. If for Lacan it is the failure to reach this ideal that is a constant source of frustration, for Plato the commitment to such a standard is necessary and desirable as long as it is understood for what it is, as a playful and provocative "guide for the perplexed" rather than as a final solution to be resolved or reconciled.

If we think of the signifier in the way Plato thinks of any notion, then we recognize it as an ideal, or even better, a standard guiding action, but a standard not capable of being realized. Here is Benardete (1989, p. 9) on the way such a standard (for example, the notion of justice as the ideal regime) functions in the *Republic*: "regardless whether it is of necessity imaginary or not, the one best regime comprehends the manifold of all inferior regimes. It guides one's understanding of political life even if it never shapes one's actions." Think of the "one best regime" as akin to the notion of the signifier that we pursue and that we intend to comprehend the manifold of all usages that are inferior because they are partial. In this way the idea that the signifier has many senses (Aristotle [1966, s.1003b, p. 54] on "Being has many senses") implies the prospect of imagining a systemic and hierarchical connection between these senses in the way the universal might stand to the particulars. This desire guides our understanding even while we cannot apply it in any particular way as an action; it is by necessity imaginary in the way the process of signification exceeds the signifier (that is, in the way the intimacy of justice must be oriented to as something that cannot be determined in speech as this rather than that according to an either/or formula). Here the ideal speaker modeled after the figure of Socrates as one so engaged in a pursuit of the impossible as a necessary standard could just as well in this respect be like Simmel's (1971) description of Casanova the lover as one who desired the impossible. The ideal speaker, like Socrates and Casanova, desires the speech he will not complete and yet can only speak of justice within the framework of desire as such. What the ideal speaker idealizes is desire for the best speech in a pursuit that will end in dramatizing the difference between the influence of the pursuit in shaping one's speech and shaping one's actions, a difference correlative with the distinction between the symbolic order and the Real and with the hole in Being (the Grey Zone). That there is a difference between wanting to be the standard (Pygmalion) and knowing the standard shows the necessity of distance in relation to any ideal as Serres (2008a) has nicely captured.

(C) A third avenue of approach to the Grey Zone comes to view through this necessary ascription of desire to the human subject because the need to universalize it and assume it as true for anyone creates the occasion of "mutually oriented action" (Weber, 1947) as the imperative of conversation in which both the objectification of the situation of co-speaking and of the need to defer to someone to define the terms and conditions of the talk emerge as conditions needing to be accepted provisionally. The co-relating of desiring actors marks them as the same in that respect, similar but not identical as subject to the rule of desire, and so different and perhaps discordant unless moderated by some relationship to shared being. This requirement of what we can call intersubjectivity, though modernized by Hegel, only first appears as a *problem* rather than a stipulation in Plato's (1945) *Republic* and in the various Platonic dialogues (see especially *Meno* and *Philebus*). Here, interlocutors such as Meno, Protarchus and Thrasymachus are persuaded to lay down their arms and give themselves to a version of conversation that they themselves did not create or choose, on the grounds that beginnings as such always need to be experimented with as practices that are done rather than accepted or rejected mechanically or on faith. That is, since the division of one subject must in principle be the division of all, intersubjectivity describes the relation between actors formulated as such, the condition for division itself becoming a phenomenon of social interaction where those necessarily the same and other in this respect must take up (and start from the position of) difference. Note too that this must include writing such as this with implications for practices of narrative and teaching.

What this means is that the imaginary of self-possession, when imputed to the other as well (rather than as a sign of one's innate superiority), makes mutually oriented action, or what Parsons (1951, pp. 10, 48, 94) calls the double contingency (ego-orienting to alter's orientation to ego), not only a parameter of speech but a prerequisite for dialogue, since viewing being viewed and the accountability this releases is a precondition of speaking, giving speech an intrinsically ethical and rhetorical character. This suggests not simply that the in-itself (the meaning of justice, virtue, capitalism, whatever) depends upon dialogue, but that dialogue in its way depends upon not only the commonplace intelligibility of the topic (usage and content) but on the desire to take it up by orienting to its otherness and to the different interests in this relationship as such.

This is where the notion of mathematics as preparation for philosophy acquires its force as a representation of the unstated beginnings in conversation that need to be accepted ironically as part of the play itself, indeed as a move in the conversational play rather than as a mechanical prelude such as in the signing of a consent form, because playfulness as an irony towards mastery in the expectation that it can come to fruition as "shared being" is part of conversation and demands a flexibility seen neither as weak or strong. Thus, the problem of the Grey Zone at this level seems to refer to the question of whether the method of dialogue itself is an imposition of force or not, whereas the real question created for both Plato and his ideological interlocutors such as the Sophists was not this at all (since everyone knows that conversation begins as a discourse of mastery) but rather a question of how such necessary persuasiveness can be converted into a shared resource or whether it is fated to recur as domination, that is, the question of the relation of teaching to power and persuasion and of the unstated but necessary place of force in conversation as a resource to be cultivated and dissolved. In other words, someone must define the situation. This is why the figure of tyranny haunted the Greeks. The Greeks identified the notion that a "discourse of mastery" is the context for any speaking in contrast to Lacan's (2007, pp. 11–32) usage of differentiating it from other types of discourse. For the Greeks, mastery was a parameter of beginning and of co-speaking as that innate asymmetry intended as a frame to be disseminated and reshaped as such, shared and constantly reinvented as the focus of the talk, resembling mathematics in its need to accept the signifier as the mark of *topos* as a site of beginning.

The question for everyone above the Divided Line (see Plato's *Republic* [1945]) is how to develop reciprocally and communally from an original inequality; that is, how to create justice in speech in the shape of a dialogical relation to diversity. This desire animates Plato's vision of intersubjectivity in a way that resituates its object, not in the topic being discussed (virtue, piety, justice or pleasure), but in the imaginary of conversation as a means towards community that is envisioned in the desire of the ideal speaker. What the Grey Zone discloses is that the object in intersubjectivity is less the content or concrete topic exchanged than the methodological imaginary. Further, if the interlocutor to dialogical intersubjectivity seems to be the tyranny that is monological, then deeply it must be the sophist who agrees in rejecting tyranny and accepting dialogue, but exploits it in the name of generic formats governing argument and refutation, subject to a code in a way that takes rather than gives voice. These versions of tyranny and sophistry correspond to Arendt's (1958) conceptions of tyranny and "anything goes" as extremist solutions to the problem of human plurality in contrast to the "mean" of politics, which this book is calling dialogue.

(D) The drama of the Grey Zone must come alive in the narrative, and the best example of this might be Plato's *Republic* because the ostensible topic of justice that appears to bind the various speakers conceals the real topic as desire of an ideal speaker, committed to the forceful unfolding of conversation in dialogue as part of the dream of communal perpetuity. Thus, what is concealed as the object is the split intrinsic to justice itself between the mundane conceptions that assume the authority of the conventions regarding what is justice and the implicit notion of a just speech imagined as the standard to which justice ought to be true, a tension in the usage itself imagined as a space of inquiry exemplified by an ideal speaker seeking to recover it in these views of ordinary justice (this division between the subject of the signifier and of *jouissance* was discussed under B above). Such an ideal speaker seeking to resituate the source (its image) in what comes after (images) strives not for an impossible vantage point but for a path or way of access, a road to traverse in pursuing the enigma as if it is the pursuit itself that is life-affirming. The figure of the ideal speaker centers the division in justice itself, in the usage, as if the discourse speaks about two sides of justice at once, as a relation between justice as common speaking and as just speech, disclosing just speech as neither the same nor as different from common speech but rather as a way of making reference to its ground or form. Being *en medias res*, though, means that the ideal speaker is part of the discourse (together with it in that sense) and so, seemingly fated to "an impossible gaze," as Žižek (1997) says, a degree of alienation from source or end that requires of any narrative an objectification that is not historical but provocative, driving the subject to analogically orchestrate the voices in whose midst it necessarily appears as if a whole, as if a fictitious dialogue that orients to the problem it imagines as obscure. The narrative forces all speakers to orient to its enigma as a puzzle for each and all, its enigma as the riddle that collectivizes the discourse. The narrative makes the speakers analogically congruent to and with one another by virtue of the content as if a third party, socializing them around the content so to speak, by using this content (the speech about justice) as a way of making reference to a just speech.

Žižek's "impossible gaze" is the deceit of using the content as the object, as the center of the exchange, masking its place as medium (and so the message that the medium massages speakers, redirecting them through the pleasure of co-speaking as such). The impossible gaze ruling the ideal speaker is not a position or destination but a provocation. Here is how this works: speech about justice could never tell us what is justice because of the limitation of opinion, but it could show us how the obscurity of justice that fertilizes this very variety is the incentive for distinguishing just from unjust speech through the figure of the desire of an ideal speaker. In other words, while the narrative confirms that speeches about justice will never add up to justice, it shows in the same way that justice can be nothing other than the pursuit of what justice is, the desire animated by the enigma as such, through speeches that will never add up. (As Simmel's [1971] comment on the figure of Casanova as a stage prop for the adventurer, his desire for the impossible, stamps the lover, here the ideal speaker for justice as the lover of justice must pursue the impossible through the diversity of speeches about justice.)

So both extremist temptations, of accepting the speeches about justice as what justice is, and rejecting the speeches about justice as what justice is, both of these extremes of obsessive and hysterical inquiry, are to be moderated in view of the need to pursue justice by giving form to the speeches about justice in a reflection that seeks to moderate the extremes. Inquiry, neither copulation nor abstinence, is foreplay. Here then justice moderates temptations towards extreme speech by listening to the views and reformulating them, knowing that an eradicable distance must remain between the speeches about justice and what justice is.

Form, the hypothetical, the image

The fiction of narrative follows from the notion of the relation of image to original that can undergo a transformation which on the surface appears historical (as in Baudrillard's [1983b, p. 11] conception of the relations between image and Real as reflection, perversion, denial and simulacrum) but that we might rethink as a multiplicity inherent in the image itself and the condition of its having many senses. The image can be oriented to as a likeness (as in the standard of Lacan's mirror image that creates impossible expectations and desire and its inevitable frustration as if it is an original as in Plato) or as the perversion reflected in its inescapable distortion by perspective and interest (as if distance betrays the original) or as the *aporia* generated by the recognition that its representation of what is not can only be done in a way that purportedly is, that is true to the art of semblance-making as what is in contrast to the denial of the Real that it masks as such and so in a way that combines both truth and falsity (as fiction seems to), leading to our acceptance of the truth of method (of the symbolic order and law) as Real in contrast to the unreality that this masks. Accordingly, the final gesture of seeing only the will to signification tries to dramatize the question of how there can be nothing rather than something. It is in this trajectory integral to the image that Plato locates the question of how we might distinguish truth from falsity in a world imagined as symbolic, or how we might distinguish between a true and false likely story.

As a hypothetical exploration of the practice it examines, any narrative seeks to lay out the standard it imagines the practice as imitating (as action oriented to an order in the idiom of Weber) as the likely story it composes about the practice as if it is assumed to be an art guided by an ideal, but of course from the perspective of its own standard. If this is necessary, then it might also be the beginning of travesty that, in exaggerating the art and idealization of what it analyzes, makes it seem both better and worse than it might be in practice. So in the *Sophist,* Plato (1984) purported to formulate the practice of the Sophist and of sophistry as itself an art, an oriented action guided by its self-image as philosophy. Plato used the model of hunting for a quarry to depict theorizing as an art seeking to track down the imaginary of whatever content it takes up, hunting for its ideals and discursive allegiances (what Lacan [1988, pp. 129–143] after Freud calls the "ideal ego" and the "ego ideal"). Thus, there is an implicit and ever-present tension between the truth of the practice expressed in this way as and in the content and the truth of the practice of theorizing that purports to see-in the manner it does and that it honors.

Further, that Plato appears to construct a collision between two different senses of philosophy from the vantage point of one of the participants might appear unfair as if he seeks to impossibly objectify proof of his superiority in a way that seems indefensible. Surreptitiously though, Plato's inference that sophistry was a perverse imitation of the philosophy of Parmenides uses the Sophist to travesty the Pre-Socratics. Here, though, if sophistry is assumed to model itself after philosophy just as Plato's theorizing claims of itself, then the problem of the dialogue might raise the question of the three-cornered resemblance between Plato, sophistry and philosophy, implicitly suggesting that Plato could be the same and other as sophistry and that this topic of what and who is the sophist is endemic to theorizing because of its immersion in the Grey Zone (this is the source of the canonical obsession with skepticism, relativism, cynicism and nihilism). The Greeks could see Plato describing what is false (sophistry as a corruption of philosophy) by making a story that in its own manner must be true (true to itself as narrative, as an act of philosophizing). This discourse develops from the misuse of false as if it means non-existent rather than, as Plato must suggest, as perverse or corrupt actions that are not false in the way of "are not" but in the way of Other. Plato suggests that it is actually Parmenides who, in making what is and what is not into an either/or choice, who sets the stage for the sophistic indistinction that threatens to poison the difference by making it an opposition, and so, promises to undermine the possibility of speech itself.

Thus if the dialogue is about the Sophist as if an empirical, historical bit of evidence or documentation, then it is really directed to the question of the possibility of speech and of the symbolic order. The difference between these two objects, one aimed for and one grounding the practice, will become clearer in Chapters 12 and 13. In this way it proposes that the Grey Zone evokes the understanding that truth and falsity must be mixed along with everything else, but only under the auspices of a recognition of how Other is not that which is not (as in a contrary or an opposition) but that can show how that which is is as if "chopped into bits" (Plato, 1984, s.258e, p. II.56), making not only that which is not what is, but revealing that "everything else in this way, individually and all together, is in many different ways and in many different ways is not" (Plato, 1984, s.259b, p. II.56). Thus, "the same [is] other" in some way no matter what, and the "other" the same (Plato, 1984, s.259b, pp. II.56–57). This plunges us directly into the perplexity of the Grey Zone and the conundrum noted by Plato of trying to tell a true account from an apparition. In this way we appreciate that the ostensive topic of the narrative is the Sophist but only as a stage prop or image of the concern for theorizing and in particular, for the question of how philosophy might heal itself under the condition of its fundamental ambiguity, anticipating for us as an image of health the concern for what is a strong relation to ambiguity as its focus upon healing rather than cure.

Yet the objective of the narrative is not to pronounce in a declarative manner upon the truth "but rather, by increased understanding of the forms themselves, to understand the relations of immanent forms and to make clear what we can of the world we live in, a world full of resemblances than can either lead or mislead" (Ambuel, 2007, p. 29). In Greek, the likely story of the narrative and its rethinking is a form of violence intended to provoke an intensification of collective perplexity and desire around the question of different implications of hypothetical stories. Plato tells us then that if the truth of theorizing resides in its desire to hunt down the imaginary, then this can be done only under the auspices of the artifact of representation, making the symbolic true to itself and false to the Real but, and at the same time, in accord with the Real by virtue of this recognition as such. Of the necessary mixing of such truth and falsity and so of its necessary ambiguity, the Stranger says to Theaetetus:

> Well consider then […] how we were just now […] compelling there to be allowance made for the mixing of another with another. For the purpose of speech for us being some one of the genera which are. For should we be deprived of this we would be deprived of philosophy. But still, at the moment we must come to an agreement on whatever speech is, for if we had been denied its being altogether, we surely would now be unable to say anything; and we would have been so denied if we had conceded that there is no mixing of anything with anything. (Plato, 1984, s.260b, p. II.57)

Likely story

This direction is developed from the assumption expressed in the *Timaeus* (Plato, 1949b) that theorizing makes the world in its image, taking its own oriented character (its capacity for intelligence and design, as Plato says) for the world itself, seeing itself in the world as such an extension on the grounds that being oriented is good and so, that extending this good (as if a gift) to the world is itself a good. That is, if we are oriented in our actions, we need to assume the same of the other and we need to disseminate this assumption to others. But this would remain an incomplete and perhaps shallow vision unless we understood it as a way of addressing the symbolic order as closed to an outside in such a way as to invest any account with a degree of insularity and circularity. Plato poses the question of the kinds of causes there are and how to account for the relation of the visible to the invisible if causes are both intelligent and random. Certainly the world is such a mix at best and possibly dominated by chance; but as a Greek might say, who could care what it is and what are such details unless they make a good story, for is not the important matter the kind of story we need? What is important is that the best account (the question of its truth), in a world where each and any account is a likely story, cannot be proven by reference to externals because any notion of proof is part of the story itself and its methodology. This makes the likely story a way of healing in relation to the Grey Zone as a material condition, implying that the best account need be responsive to the question posed by Socrates, "What would be the best sort of society and the sort of men who would compose it?" (Plato, 1949b, s.17c, p. 3). This also rules out superstitions and accounts that are simple palliatives because the account of value, the true account, has to represent actors, courses of action, a focus upon essentials, and implications of both this and its denial in ways that are demanding and dialogically responsive to the divisibility of the collective representation. This means that the true account is far from neutral but an account true to life in this dialectical sense. Its implications have to be measured by its value for life, value that can only be engaged dialogically and is an open question while yet remaining the constant and ever-present focus for any narrative. This is how those like Arendt and Rancière can agree that the art of politics is the foundation of philosophy.

Thus the grounds for our thinking of the world as orderly and intelligent rather than as a chance event is not confirmed by anything that we find in the world by looking and seeing but comes from understanding our requirements to include how we need to see-as, how we need to appreciate that such a thought is good for us. For example, it is good that we assume in creating a likely story that it imitates a vision of the order and intelligence of creation because such a model of theorizing is healthy in the sense of being good for living. A true account is an account that helps us live, that strengthens our desire to live. Thus, we never know if the world is chaotic and a creation of chance or design and will, and we could care less since any response is a likely story. Any representation of the Real (physical, nature) has to be a likely story because the standard for any story displays the auspices of the symbolic order (its game or grammar) authorizing its exposition, and this relationship can only be likely, its coherence supplied by interpretation (*object a*) necessarily exceeded by what is unstable and disorderly (Lacan's hole in Being, the irruption of the Real), the discordant and unordered matter that humans can only, at best, take over by giving form to such conditions (for example, when we take an overview we come to the realization that medicine knows very little about illness and disease). Thus, the logos makes possible the imaginary concealed by the grammar that intimates making reference to making reference itself, its need and desire, as both a necessity and intelligent. This is not an intended description of the world as if a proposition that it (the world) is chance or intelligent for who could speculate on this as if it was not a likely story? If it is necessary to see ourselves in the world, then this narcissism means only that it is necessary to demand of an account or story that it helps us live, that it be true to life in this way and so "healthy" in Nietzsche's sense, meaning that it is healthy to see-as such by imagining an intelligent artificer as the model for creation and to personify this figure as an ideal speaker for any action and practice we seek to formulate. Plato's likely story then not only dramatizes the import of the question of the difference between truth and falsity as an aspect of the Grey Zone, but also rehabilitates notions of health itself as the seeing-as that empowers strong relationships to material conditions and to correlative effects such as unhappiness, suffering, sorrow and the unruliness of the emotions. The cliché of the life world is also redeemed from its vacuousness to stand for the necessary and desirable relation to existence required by the subject who needs to act on what is known in ways that can be described as different from applying or transferring knowledge, but as healthy for life. Of course, if that question, always itself contestable, cannot provide a cure for ambiguity, its being raised promises to provide an incomparable condition for healing.

Conclusion

The Greek formulation of ambiguity as the Grey Zone relies on a range of tropes that have been digested and revitalized today in ways that are both relevant and applicable, and yet can be made robust through recalling their elementary resonances. The idea of *en medias res,* of beginning in the middle of language and not at some prior, pristine and neutral vantage point, plays off Plato's conception of story and of Homeric epic and of the vision of representation as the mediating link between human and nature, resisting the extremes of both physical science and Anaxagoras' rebuttal, proposing a Greek enlightenment that must always begin with a commitment to mutually oriented action between selves inspired by the imaginary of conversation (*dialogos*) as the game that must be played in order to rescue humans from strife (to defer resentment, in the words of Eric Gans [1982]). Yet even such speakers, alive to their subjectivities, can be locked into monological deadlocks unless they show desire to develop their speech in ways that are alive to the need to join the external and the internal in ways mindful of Plato's distinction in the *Theaetetus* between having knowledge and possessing knowledge, that is, between speaking mechanically as a mouthpiece and establishing a degree of distance towards such palaver. Here, the Greeks pose for us as the primordial split the true problem of applied knowledge, of the relation of symbolic order to the Real, disclosed invariably as the fundamental ambiguity of representation as a writing upon the soul, as a writing that makes, or not, a difference.

2

Ambiguity As a Social Phenomenon: Reshaping the Greeks

Introduction

If ambiguity is essential, a universal, then any approach to ambiguity must participate in its topic, must be infected by the very ambiguity it studies. If such research is not to claim an exemption from ambiguity in a dogmatic gesture, then it must propose to preserve ambiguity in its very manner; part of the appeal of the inquiry must reside in how it mediates ambiguity as topic and resource without denying its two-sidedness or passively resigning itself to ambiguity whether out of disrespect, indifference or blindness.

This text's inquiry, then, begins with a sense of the Grey Zone as an object of collective interest, an object of desire functioning as a collective representation in accord with an honorable sociological tradition (Durkheim, 1961; Simmel, 1971, 1959) but also resonating with Lacan's (1997) conception of the distinction between signifier and signification in a way that confirms the Grey Zone as a relationship in which meaning can be said to emerge (through representations of emergence, *physis,* natality and the like). This approach is not self-evident as any cursory approach to typical Anglo-American philosophy might show (to any body of work that fetishizes either the referent or cognition as two extremes, or even the signifier as if a linguistic unit isolated from its grounds). So if the Grey Zone is construed as a relationship between the exteriority and intimacy of the word, then any approach to the Grey Zone is itself an example of this, a relationship by virtue of the problematic connection of the inquiry (another word, signifier or concept) to its grounds. In this chapter, we will discuss varied approaches to the Grey Zone as the rudiments of a discourse on ambiguity in order to develop a sense of the form of such a discourse, the problem to which it is responsive.

There will be a conversation around different ways of approaching the Grey Zone, different usages and positions in its hypothetical discourse ranging from concrete inflections organized around distinctions such as subjectivity/objectivity, ideal and actual, reification, rationalization, uncertainty and indeterminacy to conceptions of magic, the abyss, *das Ding* and the notion of *en medias res* or the in-between. Throughout, my interest is not exegetical but one of laying grounds for conceiving of ambiguity as a social phenomenon that members seek to address and work out in everyday life in ways that can be called researchable and to develop the implications of such a program for the study of health and illness in collective life.

Ambiguity is a pacific gloss for the incommensurability at the heart of speech and action (or the heart of darkness at the core of life), that persistent trace of irresolution that haunts us in ways that can never seem to be objectified with complete satisfaction, intimating not something secret or hidden, typically captured by the figures of equivocation, plurality or depth, but an experience routinely intuited as a sense of intractability at the core of being. This is why ambiguity, with its hint of polysemy, or double entendre, or equivocality, or indecision, seems the tip of the iceberg of the phenomenon that only a conception of dialectic can begin to imagine, the capacity to approach that unimaginable surfeit that exceeds imagination itself, somewhat like the power to think nonbeing, the void, while subject to the plenitude of life as if one is capable of reflecting upon the absence of reflection (Heidegger's [1961] "possibility of impossibility" that appears as paradigmatic for him and many in the contemplation of death). Basically we shall locate the canonical discussion of the Grey Zone in the idea of a division within the subject, experienced and represented as both collective (outside) and individual (inside) as the primordial enigma identified by Plato, adumbrating an experience of the Real as both external and within reach, an idea taking shape in usages such as *das Ding*, the self, vertigo, surplus pleasure, comedy, Socratic ignorance, the death drive and aesthetics. These can be developed as different frameworks for exploring the way division and its anxiety functions in collective life as both stimulating and oppressive and as a research opportunity. Most important, if this practice of orienting to ambiguity and its aspiration to "size up the situation" (in Kenneth Burke's [1957] terms) cannot itself escape the Grey Zone, then neither can my effort in this work, only illustrating the kinds of intended reconciliations (also in Burke: dreaming and praying) it releases as loci of collectivization.

Views of the original division: inner, outer

> The attempt to analyze is not intelligible apart from the activity of the analyst. If we are to succeed at all in isolating […] forms, it will only be by a careful study of consciousness. Logic, despite its many virtues, is not the study we need for this purpose. (Rosen, 1980, p. 148)

And as we should add, neither is this "study of consciousness" a domain of psychology because consciousness and its various tropes such as ego, psyche and self are imaginary projections of desire and of the one subject to its vicissitudes, a one always fated to be stimulated in many ways by constantly problematic relationships to others and to Other.

> Relations between human beings are really established before one gets to the stage of consciousness. It is desire which achieves the primitive structuration of the human world, desire as unconscious. (Lacan, 1991, p. 224)

We identify the Grey Zone as a figure-making reference to the essential nature of ambiguity that can be said to inhabit speech and action, a zone not physical but roughly equivalent to the ghostly trace of psyche perhaps, or what Lacan (1992, p. 52) calls the strange presence to ourselves of ourselves, that element initially isolated by the subject as alien, as even "hostile on occasion," but as "the first outside", the sense that "something is there after all" (and similar to Levinas' [1987] "there is") that must serve as a "point of reference" to the "world of desires"

> What interferes with the wall of language is the specular relation, whereby what pertains to the ego is always perceived, appropriated, via the intermediary of an other, who for the subject always retains the properties of the Urbild, of the fundamental image of the ego. Hence the misapprehensions thanks to which misunderstandings no less than ordinary communication—which itself rests on the said misunderstandings—become established. (Lacan, 1991, p. 248)

If the convention of distinguishing word from thing as signifier from signified is apparent but only a start, then what remains is the hole in the signifier, that is, the division within the word itself given by virtue of its character as an oriented object, as an object of desire. If the subject orients to the word, then the word is not self-evident, necessarily reflecting itself back to create that space of obscurity to which a subject must answer (the space we typify as "meaning").

Note the fundamental ambiguity here residing in the intimate experience of "the first outside," making what is external seem intimate and what is intimate seem external, that is, neither one nor the other but both at once and yet nothing, because ungraspable. According to Lacan, the obscene or unspeakable character of the first outside that is inside, and the intimate experience of this exteriority, establishes fundamental ambiguity as this encounter with *das Ding* (the thing) that is both something and nothing, that in Wittgenstein's words, is not a thing but not nothing either, the uncanny. In this way the

Grey Zone can begin to be understood as "the original experience of the division of reality" (Lacan, 1992, p. 52), the experience of a gap or split, and of this as a relationship as such, constituted and emotional. This something prior that "sets up end, goal and aim," that the subject represents to and for himself and seeks over and again unsuccessfully to recover, is an object of desire that both precedes and awaits as a seduction or lure, that image of fulfillment that appears prior to desire and to which it seems directed: yet "it is of course clear that what is supposed to be found will never be found again. It is in its nature that the object as such is lost. Something is there while one waits for something better, or worse, but which one wants […] It is to be found at most as something missed. One doesn't find it, but only its pleasurable associations" (Lacan, 1992, p. 52). But note of any such reputed division, regardless of how primary, that it can only surface for one subject to mediation, one receptive to the influences even of opacity, and if "empty" and undeveloped by virtue of beginning in this way, one yet empowered to orient to mediation and its consequences as a condition as such.

The original division of which Lacan speaks and of which he calls the experience of *das Ding* (the thing) isolates this sense of ambiguity and its omnipresence as if an object in a way that makes this the first moment of objectification and the "seat of subjectivity." If on the one side of the division the experience can be objectified in qualities, attributes, properties amenable to judgment and the like, then this can constitute a basis for images of system, construction and for representations that become accessible as such, perhaps the grounds of the digital. In part, this derives from an old and honorable tradition, exemplified by John Locke (1947) and leading all the way to Hannah Arendt, of separating the inside and its interior ideas, perceptions and affects from the outside speech, making the transformation one of publicizing what is concealed and, if untouched, one that would remain inner and unsharable. In this convention it is this gap that produces the drive for self-expression and its possible disfigurement (at least for Locke) in figurative talk such as analogy as a kind of inexact substitution that risks diluting the original, that makes of speaking a "putting into words" that transforms the ineffable into a kind of corporeal presence capable (in the words of George Herbert Mead, 1967) of arousing the same response in different persons. Though this convention certainly recognizes the gap and its essential ambiguity, for Freud it is the emphasis on its imaginary character that is crucial. This means that "the first outside" according to Freud (cited in Lacan, 1992, pp. 51–52) "has nothing to do with that reality" (this palpable representation), functioning instead as an obscene omnipresence upon which any such system depends (for example, the grounds of the analogical). The original experience of the division is split, outer and inner, identifying an object of representation, of self-representation, as a presence both external and intimate. In terms of speech, the first outside might be the word pure and simple, the signifier as an external mark, but its externality both conceals and intimates a process of signification through which its emergence is condensed and displaced in the word. This is how Lacan can use Freud to treat all speech as a process of conversion on the model of a transformation, evoking a sense of how the invisibility of the visible (Didi-Huberman, 2005) haunts any signifier as its unthought trace. For Wittgenstein and others, emergence does not depict a transformation of private to public but a relationship within speech itself (on the surface) among and between distinctions that are made in practice and, if intimating what is invisible, not pointing to a private or interior cause but to discursive implications whose resonances are implied and undeveloped (McHugh, 1968, pp. 33–47).

The gap between intimate and external that marks the word must on this account raise its question (of meaning) as a puzzle for the one exercised by its spell: if the aura of *das Ding* fertilizes the possibility of various constructions of ego and self, of the internal divide, then self-observing is the first step of an imaginary trajectory signifying the potential for self-reflection to first become self-observing in its most primitive shape because self-observation remains calculative and uninspired much in the way of the informant or describer (Bennett, 1995) unless animated by the obscurity of this division as if an enigma (i.e., by the difference aroused between describing oneself and reflecting upon oneself). Thus the Grey Zone discloses the self, not simply in the division between conscious life and the unconscious, or the private and public, or mind and speech, but in the figure of desire released as such through the stimulating and enigmatic obscurity of the division itself, of its uncanny capacity for seduction. Without such desire, in the idiom of Plato, the subject *has* a self but is not in possession of self, is self-observing but not self-reflective. Having the self such as having the name, being able to use it for identification and wayfinding, lies in noting the fact, labeling, following instructions and the like, standing as the most rudimentary version of taking a perspective on oneself, a practice that ought to treat the self instead, as if looking back, as more than a body but as an oriented object, a site of accountability, obscure and enigmatic because of its implicitly demanding character.

We might note in the following comments of Mead (1967) how he can say all of the correct things about the self in a manner that still conceals his conception of himself as an informant who finds the ambiguity of language in need of only the most prosaic clarification, perhaps as a definition of terminology that might let its auspices remain untouched. Here, he tends to treat what he informs us about as if it is an enigma but by renouncing the Grey Zone in his very use of the self as a figure for such, by equating prosaic self-observation under the spell of the code (his "generalized other") as information to deliver rather than as a puzzle in the spell of which he is trapped. Yet if he seems self-observant rather than self-reflective, the implications of what he says here are important because only one with a self can make such a distinction: the upshot being that in all of its seeing, it sees itself seeing. Such reflexivity gives the human, according to what it here imagines, its advantage or distinctiveness that at the same time can be disadvantageous, making one either imperious or guilty.

Division as split: self-knowledge

This conception of the division within is reflected in the way the self is discussed in the literature as an idea engaged and held in collective life as a resource that is typically used to distinguish what the human has through the figure of internal separation in which we treat ourselves as both subject and object, the subject that is an object for itself. This division is captured in the conventional mirroring formula of Mead as follows:

> The self has a character which is different from the physiological organism proper. [...] We can distinguish very definitely between the self and the body. [...] The self has the characteristic that it is an object to itself and that characteristic distinguishes it from other objects and from the body. [...] It is the characteristic of the self as an object to itself that I want to bring out. This characteristic is represented in the word "self," which is a reflexive, and indicates that which can be both subject and object. This type of object is essentially different from other objects. [...] How can an individual get outside himself [...] in such a way as to become an object to himself? (Mead, 1967, p. 135–138)

To begin to unpack this quote we must note how it revels in its contradiction by illustrating what it desires to speak about because the self as what Mead calls the capacity to take a perspective on oneself, the self as such a relation to language, must presuppose what it is representing, i.e., only a self can imagine the world as such, only reflection upon oneself can represent reflection upon oneself as a distinction. In a sense, what is distinctive to the human is the need to begin *en medias res*, in the middle of things, because talking about the self presupposes *having* what is talked about, the distinctive scene he describes as being both subject and object to oneself. To ask what is distinctive to the human in this way is an important question upon which concerns for human rights, bare life, reductionism, conceptions of exploitation and the like depend, first because the other to self is in some way referenced by the body as a figure for the boundary separating a reflexive relationship and its other. The human is identified by virtue of an imaginary contrast of capacity and incapacity and not out of a desire to chase a definition of the signifier (by asking the question "what is the human," forever parodied by Marx [Marx and Engels, 1960, p. 7], who cited enumerable possible answers) but to establish the import of signification as the central focus for the human as reflected in the question, "What is distinctive of the human?," as a query reputed to collectivize our attention as an unending topic of fascination (because it frames our conception of the limits of action in many ways).

Note that what is distinctive of the human who must (at her best) inherit the burden of self-knowledge (of self-reflection or of having a self) is first the implication that whatever the interest discussed, this figure cannot be imagined as addressing this question directly because it is the subject asking about itself, as both subject and object, a subject that cannot treat itself as if a body from which it is apart or separate in some concrete and external sense. Because the self we are asking about is already there, we cannot be neutral by feigning apartness untouched by what we inquire after since self-knowledge must essentially be reflexive, in some way indicative of a capacity to look back upon what is already there. Thus, if our subjectivity must be objectified (as and in the symbolic order permitting us to represent this very condition), then the objectification must preserve this trace of ambiguity as its inheritance and so risk appearing as if it is taken in by the necessity of objectification, as if it seems to treat such artifice as real. Given this formulation, any claim to self-knowledge must try to honor in practice subjectivity, not as a burden, but as a parameter of the condition of being human that needs to be expressed and negotiated with others in any situation and not banned or denied.

Whether humans are to be thought of as self or body, the notion of the Grey Zone, even in Mead's usage, suggests that they are best seen as both, as a mix in Plato's sense in a way that frames human reflexivity as the Same and the Other, as comparable in being an object for one and all including one self and as being in position to take a perspective on this. This means humans can speak about what they are and what they are not with imaginary authority, can see their sameness in their variety and their variations as bound together as the Same. Moreover, this self and its capacity to orient to being oriented to not only gives an advantage but also the burden of being looked at and of being able to look at oneself in ways that make accountability, guilt, shame, frustration, aggression and all of the emotions constant topics of concern. At best, Mead's self and the reflexivity it imagines means, besides these burdens, the potential for self-knowledge that taking a perspective intimates but cannot guarantee, along with the capacity for dialogue, differentiation and the relationship of ethics, and the capacities for transformation through work, performance, mimesis and narrative we include as aesthetic. We note that the difference between having a self and possessing a self is correlative with taking a perspective and self-knowledge, is a difference not self-evident, one to be worked out in speaking according to these vectors of ethics and aesthetics and in any practice as such.

Analogy

It seems as if it is the paradox of self-knowledge and the intractability of mediation and of *en medias res* that makes analogy necessary as a means of objectifying that to which one is essentially connected, placing it as an external image that mirrors the self as if a reflection, reinstating the one that is two as the two shapes of one, the ideal speaker. Thus, our reflexivity which fertilizes our desire to objectify the situation in which we participate and that precedes us produces in this way the necessity of analogy. Analogy answers to the need to speak indirectly, and Mead uses the figure of play and the game as analogies to portray the social and particularly the phenomenon of language as common speaking. Here, we begin to appreciate the elementary form of the symbolic order in the desire of the insider for an exteriority that cannot be satisfied empirically, needing the artifice of simulation, the imaginary of an outside position by the insider reflecting the desire of the subject for the self-knowledge whose realization must always remain irresolute. Here analogy is necessary for the speaker to describe what she is doing, speaking itself, in order to put into relief what is being said as belonging both to the one who speaks and the one who observes this speech (i.e., not simply between the one who speaks and the one who is spoken about, two-in-one in that conventional sense, but between the two senses of the one who speaks as self-observing and ideal speaker), making the speaker two-in-one or one that is two. Analogy enables us to imagine the ideal speaker as not simply self-observing (as an empiricist watching herself) but as potentially self-reflective (oriented to representing herself as reflective rather than as a body) by reinventing the proverbial understanding as an illustration of the commitment to form. The ideal speaker then becomes not necessarily reflective in fact, but one personifying the desire to orient and speak reflectively rather than as something other. In other words, the human can only be reflective by imitating the desire to be reflective.

For example, the self as taking perspective on oneself is both one and many, and can be practiced in many ways, ways both diverse and systemically related as if a discourse still bound by the formula expressed in its relationship (as taking a perspective aims to condense the usage on the self in the society of Mead). Thus if we know, for example, that self-knowledge is not equivalent to various usages popular at any one time, whether mundane practices of keeping a diary or blogging or twittering, autobiography, or doctrines sanctioned academically such as the self-descriptivism of cognitive psychology, and that to treat it as such would be to misrecognize the universal *as* the particular, then neither can self-knowledge be understood as indifferent to these particulars, for it is such usages that mark the discourse at each and any historical moment. These can each be understood as examples of "taking a perspective." In fact, the universal (taking a perspective) is recovered from such particulars through the method of analogy that sees such practices as varied and limited attempts to put the relation into practice (to take a perspective on oneself by objectivizing one's mundane activities in such a format), intimating the ambiguous ground of the discourse as such by pointing to the question of what we need add to such visions of self-examination in order to formulate them as self-knowledge. This is to say that the universal (Mead's formulation of self as…) is only possible because he sees it as this in the many examples he encounters, using this formulation as a formula for sizing up this usage. The ideal speaker's representation of the desire for such knowledge, this mimetic relation, binds together the various perspectives as if the universal.

"Why play?" or "Why speak?" are important questions to ask in the absence of a self as a causal force. Even more, granting the distinction of taking a perspective, it is neither an unmoved mover nor yet something guaranteed to help. If the self is in the middle as if a practice of taking perspective, then its transformation into self-knowledge seems inexplicable except as prayer: what is distinctive and an adventure is the desire to repossess what we have, meaning that performing as if we have a self might begin to redeem simulation as the mimetic way of humans (an example again of the old and honorable "as if" that is the cornerstone of the aesthetic).

Same and Other

Wittgenstein (1953) used Jastrow's famous illustration of the figure of a duck-rabbit, a duck that could be seen as a rabbit or a rabbit that could be seen as a duck, to show how it was not one thing or the other as in a choice, or intelligible simply as dependent upon context or circumstances, or on more information to be filled in, because the figure itself was what it was because of seeing-it as such, where it is seeing-as that is fundamentally ambiguous, capable of pointing out aspects in one that are two and for two that are one, serving in its way as a standard for the relation to ambiguity.

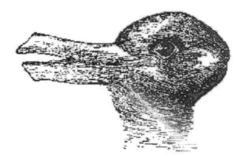

(illustration taken from Wittgenstein, 1953, pp. 193–196)

The duck-rabbit is both together and apart: together it is two-in-one, one figure with two aspects, which makes seeing it as either one or the other gratuitous; on the other hand, this is not correct since seeing it as one, as a duck-rabbit, assumes that we can identify the two aspects first, that we can recognize and identify rabbits and ducks separately. That the duck and the rabbit share a togetherness and an apartness means that seeing them as comparable requires identifying and differentiating them, but that distinguishing them in this way in the first place depends upon their being presented to and for us in this strange juxtaposition as a figure. Further, what is first is not the figure but the need to which it answers, the situation in which it emerges, or the problem to which it replies (this example is also used in Blum, 2010a).

The contradiction displayed by the figure, instead of being an idle curiosity, invites us to ask after its point, notably here to demonstrate the enigmatic inevitability of ambiguity in a demonstrably palpable way to one conceived as subject to an inflexible relation to thought and language. Beyond the interaction that seems to be referenced by choosing and decision-making, as if the puzzle of the figure and its need for a solution appears to center intersubjective relations as a decision to be made over the question of whether it represents one thing or the other, what it really intimates is a movement of desire aspiring for clarity about the problem of ambiguity rather than its resolution, and so, an imaginary anticipating dialogue as a means of pedagogical transformation. In this sense, the figure is a *matheme* in Plato's sense of the mathematical.

Analysis

The method of analogy does not guarantee the relationship to reflection as anything more than oriented because one might be subject to the game (the symbolic order) in many diverse ways, for example, treating it as spin or one's take on things, as pretence, as a necessary resource for advancement, mobility, even wayfinding (as in the cliché functioning as a staple for all desperate newcomers to a situation in which one must learn the rules of the game in order to succeed). In these cases, the symbolic order that Mead personifies in the figure of a game idealizes the calculative actor as the *sine qua non* of reflection but in ways that always provoke us to think of the difference between a self conjured as such and more deeply (the difference between one conceived as playing the game as her objective or goal [*telos*] and one who desires to reflect upon the difference between such a player and an exploration into the limits of this model, of this vision of the social actor).

In this vein, Mead seems to use the analogy as a means of representing the structure of social life and of a common language in terms of its grammar and rules, much like a curriculum required for qualification or in a formulation of the conditions needed to carry off an action, perhaps in the ways literacy or knowledge of the craft serves as a minimum for higher purposes. Yet what Mead's vision of the symbolic order seems to leave out is the hole in Being reflected in the problematic pleasure of the game and its play in relation to competition and form. Mead's notion of the symbolic order as artifice even in the best sense might just exclude a robust notion of Other that could capture its character as *das Ding* rather than simply the generalized other that reflects the grammar of the collective. Mead's solution of depicting the self as grounded in its observant relation to rules and to the symbol as a totem establishing a relatedness among all who are touched by it does not on the surface provide for the difference between this and the means of taking a perspective on this immersion, on this participation in a social order.

Thus, in Lacanian, there seems to be no difference between Mead as a subject of enunciation and what he speaks about as if there is an identity here, an imaginary relation where the environment is a double of the organism and the organism simply carries its environment with it, treating adaptation as an end without a way of understanding that except through the prosaic formats and scripts of the collective. This is to say that Mead seems to speak about the self and its reflexivity, about the divided subject, as if an insider telling a story about the game of life, much as an informant rather than theorist.

In using the game analogically as a way of representing oneself and of simulating a difference where none exists, Mead tends to use analogy to prop up an imaginary relationship to the groundlessness of being, but he is capable of confusing us here. Mead says that to treat ourselves as a body is not different than treating ourselves as a table because the body is inanimate, something that we can experience as belonging to us but in a way that remains necessarily external in the way that the foot can be said to belong to us but has no self or perspective on what it is. The ramifications of this curious talk is that humans must treat themselves and one another as selves and not as bodies, and yet it is in this way that the body acquires its force, being employed as a limit upon our conceptions of who and what we are.

That we have the foot but do not possess it is the issue and is not due to the natural and empirical character of the foot but for the reason that we can only be said to possess knowledge when we are in position to be sufficiently reflexive as to engage the ambiguity in word and deed (or in Wittgenstein, when we recognize the fundamental ground of things in seeing-as), meaning that we can treat ourselves mechanically if we do not take a perspective on the foot, do not give the body voice. The relationship of the self is one of possessing rather than having since we all can be said to have a self (to take a perspective) but not necessarily to possess our selves. To take a perspective on the foot is to develop a relationship to it that animates it, not leaving it as mute and indivisible but as having many senses, whether its usage in locomotion or metaphorically as in the example of the lame Oedipus, or Bataille's (1985, pp. 2–23) big toe. This does not mean that we personify the foot as if it is a human being but that we treat it as an object of desire, an object that is oriented to in many ways, in usage that defines it through such practice as vital. That is, we show our distinctiveness by seeing the table as an object of desire that establishes a relatedness among many views or speakers, i.e., as centering a discourse. In this sense, our taking a perspective on our selves begins to assume shape as reflective when we see objects as if oriented to in ways that include us and our seeing-as as well. In other words, our distinctiveness enunciated by the self lies in our capacity to see-as, and in this way, not to see ourselves in everything (as if the foot has a self in ways comparable to us), but to see the otherness of the foot (or the body, the table, the cow) as the oriented objects resulting from our work and composition as if representations internal to us, that is, to truly make the world in our image and to justify it as such.

Our relation to the things of the world is not empirical but imaginary, resting as it does on our powers not to see new things but to see the old things in many and newer ways, and such powers must include the capacity to see ourselves as such, as having a self always in need of repossession. What Mead's comparison of self and body is actually intended to do is establish the singularity of the human actor as ruled by the concern with such a difference, that is, with the question of the singularity of the human. It is the relation of self to body that he uses to demonstrate how we must take a perspective in ways that inevitably will distinguish the ordinary relation to anything from a reflective approach. To single out the reflexive interest, it need be contrasted with a comical example of the inanimate or even mechanical in order to identify and contrast the human actor and its reflexive conundrums. If the alter to human reflexivity is the inflexible, self-absorbed agent tied mechanically to rigid formulae as if an automaton, then we can appreciate how Henri Bergson (1956) could use such automated responses as exemplary of the comic relationship. It is the human (unlike the toe, the cow, the table) that takes a perspective on any and everything, including such items, and indeed gives voice to the body, seeing oneself as both the same as the body in being such an object and different from the body in being able to see-as, to imagine oneself as the subject who is object (oriented to just like toe, table, cow), and yet the object that is subject (being able to see all of this, to see-as). The triumph of seeing the self as both duck and rabbit is the triumph of human singularity; imaginary, fantasy perhaps, but necessary equipment for living. What seems comic is the human who seems unaware that taking a perspective on everything must include himself and, according to Baudelaire (1972), while this gesture is exemplary of the subject of ordinary humor, this is transformed into true humor when the unawareness is feigned. Humans do share with toes, cows and tables this character of being oriented objects and as mobilizing the possibility of being seen in many ways. The human actor, that is, the one we assume as having a self, only comes (back) into possession of this self, when she distinguishes herself in practice as something that is not (as if) a body, but that is as an entity that can distinguish herself from the many and diverse objects that she uses and to which she might be comparable for that alone, for being oriented objects, which she can do by giving voice to any and all of the things, events and actions she encounters. This irony is the secret joke pantomime and many of the arts deliver. Knowing human distinctiveness to reside in even the many ways human distinctiveness can be seen, knowing the singularity of humanity to be grounded in such a powerful and promiscuous capacity to create diverse perceptions, opinions, beliefs and interpretations, should make humans need and desire dialogue as a means of deferring resentment.

Therefore, when Lacan says that the body is a paradigm of identity and resemblance, he does not mean that we treat ourselves as if a body but that we employ the body as that limit that begins to define who we are by what we are not as if the human is the one suffering that space, that Grey Zone. Note again what Mead implies: if to take a perspective on oneself is to address what is already there, then by not treating it as a body he is recommending that we formulate our selves through division rather than subtraction or addition, i.e., we divide what is already there rather than add to something that we assume we already know, or subtract from what we treat as secure in order to illuminate its basics. In other words, Mead suggests implicitly that what Wittgenstein calls a grammatical investigation or self-reflection in the spirit of Plato and Hegel, recollection that reflects back upon what purports to be secure, is the human path because self-knowledge must begin with the intermediacy of the human actor, the one subject to mediation. Thus, it is not the empirical character of body or self that identifies self as ambiguous in contrast to the body, and so it is not having a self that marks the human, but seeing-as, that is, being in position to see ambiguity in any and everything (feet, toes, minds, selves). Then, Mead's self (capacity to take a perspective) is nothing other than Wittgenstein's notion of seeing-as, being able to see something as something (to compare, contrast, differentiate, collect, segregate, infer and imitate) that distinguishes the human.

The use of the body for Mead suggests that what we already are (what we approach in taking a perspective on our selves), is simply this division between the capacity to realize or not this reflexive potential. The self might be similar to the table as an oriented object, resource or totem whose being perceived, used and acted upon establishes a relationship among many, whether in common use, as a commodity, for purposes of decoration and the like, but it remains this fascination with the difference between what seems here (at first) comparable, that marks the self (and must mark the way the human imagines the table, unless in hallucination where investing the table with perspective is the typical badge of identity). Note that the extreme relations to this difference of self and body come to view not only in Lacan's model of the mirror stage where child sees herself in the mirror as two, as divided, causing her to ask which is real and which is unreal, but because the body's image of unambiguous indivisibility can only stand as the eternal object of realization that desire can never recuperate.

Therefore, as a paradigm of resemblance, the intuition of the body as belonging to the self simply reinstates *das Ding* as the gap (between identity and predicates, between essent and accident, between essence and unity) that is so vexatious to philosophy because its fundamentally ambiguous character can only be abridged by constructions or interpretations (as if fictions), through the magic of the *object a.*

> What happens in the mirror stage is the self's identification with a still image which then becomes the version of superiority that the living self will try to equal. In its fixity, it contrasts with the experience of weakness and fragmentation that is retrospectively established as the subject's present and actual reality. The image offers a fiction of wholeness that the subject will try to resemble. In other words, the subject comes into being in the gap of inferiority between a flawed viewer and the anticipated

>wholeness […] conflating […] libidinal investments with beautiful forms: the fantasmatic and the aesthetic are henceforth the "reality" of the self. And the definition of a "person" would then be: the repeated experience of failing to become a thing. (Johnson, 2008, pp. 58–59)

Here the subject is conceived as resisting taking exception to ambiguity, resisting treating oneself as unambiguous, by accepting the division as what one is and what one needs to suffer and develop. The body as a working distinction makes reference to the tension released through the need of speech to standardize its terms and conditions and to overcome such a relation between the mechanization of self-feeling by which it is ruled and the desire to overcome it in speech itself, the relation of speaking to itself, its desire to use and resist the very conditions it needs to inhabit, to speak against itself and through itself. Here truly, the medium is the message and moreover, is the massage, that is, desire comes through the use of the medium itself not as a means to an end for which it must be forever inadequate, but as its own pleasure. In other words "failing to become a thing" is the commitment to bearing and suffering ambiguity as part of the desire to be more, the desire to embody in practice the ambiguity of being incomparable and of failing to realize a formula, that is, to reveal in action the stigma of a signature. It is in this space that we can begin to contemplate the figure of soul as that which exceeds mind and body.

In this way, if the definition of the person is the repeated failure to become a thing, as Johnson says of Lacan's use of the body as a figure, then the individuality that the actor invests in the characterization as *its* signature (the distinctiveness of the character) and that the theorist redeems in the content as its specificity (the elementary form of the content) can only reflect this failure itself on the part of the subject to accept its fate as a thing, a failure commensurate with the realization of the subject in language (or expression) as an individual (as failing to be a thing, as not a thing), as something rather than nothing.

These relations to characterization feed into the notion of dialogue since the assumption of selves as universal, and of mutually oriented action as the potential of a species such as ours, resists talk that simply characterizes and/or adds to characterization in the shape of exploring variables, instead trying to induce one another to take a perspective on speech and to accept jointly a fiction of wholeness to seek to personify playfully.

Division: transposition

More specifically, content at its inception can appear as corporeal. Like a lifeless mark at first, the content is similar to the body, resembling its inanimate and mute tangibility, until it is given life and used as an oriented object by an actor for and to whom it appears in thought. Thus, according to Simmel (cited in Blum, 2001a) for the dramatic actor the script serves much as the body when treated as the lifeless text that need be animated by the performance. We can also appreciate the body in Mead's sense as that representation of the mechanical relation to characterization (which he calls "the generalized other") against which good acting is expected to recoil when it takes a perspective on what it is doing (the action of acting) in a way that is reflective. Good acting endows the typical characterization with vitality (Blum, 2001a). We demonstrate a reflective capacity to take possession of our speech as we take a perspective on the characterizations and begin to develop a relationship other than generalized. Stanislavski's (1989, p. 30) advice on acting is instructive here: "Characterization when accompanied by a real transposition, a sort of reincarnation, is a great thing." Stanislavski's criticism of bad acting among the students he teaches is directed to their externalization of the characters they play, their use of true but formulaic clichés to approach the representation of an aristocrat, military man, old person and other types; such acting seeming to rely on their own formulaic charm, gestures, clichés and the like that do not permit the actor to grasp what Stanislavski calls the individuality of the types.

> If a youthful impersonator of an elderly role will put his mind on how to absorb and handle the component phases of difficult and more intensive action […] while keeping himself within the confines of the character, of the play, of the "given circumstances" which surround an old person, then the actor will succeed […] will assimilate the external features […] in presenting such a portrayal. It is difficult to realize and to discover what the "given circumstances" of old age are. But once found it is not difficult to retain them by means of technique. (Stanislavski, 1989, p. 35)

He intends this transposition not to be a matter of empathy in identification but as a way of relating to the material circumstances of the content (the part, the image) being represented. The naturalistic obsession of the Moscow Art Theatre should not obscure the fact that the dead script as a body does not simply make reference to the inanimate words on the page but to the formulaic representations that are already part of the characterization as its interpretive surface much like Lacan's empty speech. Thus, in this example, old age, likely to be typified in conventional formulae, is a collective representation of what old age means, divisible and plural, that constitutes the object of reference for the actor for whom the characterization becomes an opportunity for working it through, transposing it in a sense. The characterization of old age is as if its body in speech, the body as the characterization towards which we always need to take a perspective. In a sense, the characterization is the way the collective seems to express itself on old age, in types or stereotypes. This was adumbrated in our discussion of Plato's (1984) hunting down the Sophist and its art as a course of action forming the content of theorizing. Here old age and its art resembles the art of the Sophist in the sense not that they are substantively alike, but in resembling one another analogously as built upon characterizations forming the content that must be analyzed.

Theorizing looks this material over as if for the second time, trying to give voice to the body as a way of finding its own voice. The dramatic actor's position *en medias res* means that her relation to the script and so to the character as typified in and as the script is a second sailing through which she must engage the symbolic order of age as undeveloped, implicit and abstract, as if the inheritance she must reshape (making the script, as Stanislavski keeps reiterating, much larger than that of the play but of the collective itself). Stanislavski says that in order to give voice to old age (for the actor to find his voice in the material), we must take a perspective on the action of old age as if it is oriented to *what* it is, as if it is charged with the meaning of being an object of collective desire and so a token of our (collective) powers to be inventive in relation to seeing-as. In this way, reflective acting assumes the actor as a self oriented to distinguishing incidentals from what is essential in the life of characters. This also relates to the foot, table and toe, for giving voice to these entities is finding our voice in the prosaic uses and characterizations of such things, in the ways the collective represents such things, by our imagining from such a diversity, relations to them that are more than generic or mechanical, perhaps aesthetic. It is in this way that the dramatic actor can be made to exemplify the ideal speaker for old age insofar as she is conceived as orienting to the transformation of its prosaic characterization and so as divided in this sense of being two-in-one, both subject to the generalized other of old age as a stereotype and to the desire to reflect upon and reinvent this condition as such. In this sense, division transposes the generalized other, working within the symbolic order at the border of its relation to the Real rather than addition and subtraction that seem to sustain this order as if a regime closed to an outside towards which attention must be banned.

Thinking of content analogously as such a relationship, imagining the "given circumstances" by treating what is typified as undeveloped, implicit and abstract, as pointing to something more, evokes the promise of characterization that is both incentive and a source of frustration because the incarnation of singularity that imagines for the content, and the transposition it envisions for the subject through the action of such representation, can only relate in ways that must remain irresolute and fundamentally ambiguous. Relating to content in the way of the relationship of stage actor to the character is "mutually oriented action" in Weber's sense, guided by desire as such, not simply as orderly but as good (here, good acting is in part the desire to put into question routinized conceptions of characterization). Thus again, it is not the cliché itself that is at issue, since the given circumstances accompanying any content can only be represented as standard and typical in the way discourse must begin with the typifications of a symbolic order (empty speech), supplemented by the desire to give form to such material conditions. Recall Plato's effort to give form to the given circumstances of sophistry in ways intended to bring out the good of sophistry not by calling the sophist good but by showing to what such a practice was true (its excellence).

Stanislavski's conception of characterization as transposition makes of any representation of content a means of self-disclosure in accordance with the conception of self we have been developing. Self that can only address itself indirectly and analogically does such in its formulation of any content that it depicts, as if mirroring the reflective relationship to speech (the content is organized as if it is guided by the desire for a self-reflective relation in the figure of one who, in the words of Hegel, is subject to the content and master of its use) insofar as the "given circumstances" imagined as accompanying the content as its grammar are taken over as one's own, not in the way of identification or empathy (the actor neither defines herself as the old person nor defines the old person as herself), but by showing in contrast the desire to orient to the circumstances of age (treating age as reflective, as self, and not mechanically as body) by acting in a way that exhibits the suffering of such a difference as the desire ruling the type.

This narrative, though, can only occur under the auspices of the generalized other that it desires to put into question. If old age is the content, then it is not described empirically or in a way that disregards its circumstances but through its construction as a relationship or course of action mediated by and illustrated through the figure of one subject to it reflectively, the figure of reflective thought (the thought that must reflect upon the generalized other). The characterization of old age is neither accepted nor rejected, but reflected, made strange or odd, thought over as if for the second time. Any content is thought through (over and again) as reflective thought in a way assumed to lend to the thinking subject a reflective relationship to what is thought. We can anticipate that a reflective relation to the body (the foot, toe) begins to intervene in the territory of medical interpretation and perhaps in a way that challenges orthodox procedures, and in the case of the table begins to intervene in the territory of the divide between Art and Craft. It is not the body or table that has a self, but we who show this in our capacity to orient to body or table as eventful, as an occasion to be accountable to seeing-as. In this way, transposition points to the effect of theorizing upon theorist (as Plato believed, upon the soul), revealing this as the point of engagement with the Real in which the reflective relation to the content represented in the trajectory of ideal speaker over the course of the narrative is "transposed" to the soul of the theorist in a gesture (speech or writing) necessary and yet forever inconclusive, reinstating the relation of Socrates' second sailing to Pascal's wager. The ideal speaker, both together and apart in relation to the generalized other and the rules of its game, desires to give form to such conditions as part of its desire to form itself through the practice of self-knowledge. What we have purposely left undiscussed is the *aporia* identified in Mead's discussion of reflexivity, that overcoming an inflexible relation to characterization seems to require its own method (Stanislavski's technique) as a vision of self-knowledge now made into a formula, that characterization must always risk the ambiguity of denying what it affirms (not being mechanical) or of affirming what it denies (that it is mechanical) as the comical burden inherited by the subject who would theorize, the burden of desire itself.

Furthermore, if the body is a standard, then content is a characterization of positions expected to result in a proposition—this is age!—rather than a discourse, limiting both the representation of age and the opportunity for discussing it. Similarly, the mind-body problem comes to view differently when characterized as a set of propositions that must be accredited as true or false than when it is proposed as an "offer that lends itself to some form of response or interaction" (Rancière, 2009a) or as a way of pointing out aspects concerning the difference between what is essential and inessential (Wittgenstein, 1953, pp. 192–196). The Grey Zone must live in this space of the problematic relation of self-knowledge to life and in suffering the ambiguity of this, the limits of artifice, analogy and self-satisfaction as curative, the need and desire for healing.

If speaking is a relationship to characterization that is divided in relation to the corporeality of collective thought and representations, then the relation of speech to whatever it intends to express can be one of transposition rather than an example of bad acting. That is, the characterization itself can be an occasion for the transformation of its parameters through an innovative reply (realigning the matters it seems to assume as given) and for transforming the speaker through this very process of engagement (opening her up in unexpected ways to her path of thinking that had become sanctified). Bad acting simply reiterates the self-evidence of the speech as a move in the game which authorizes the boundaries of permissible play, and in the process leaves the speaker untouched. Any expression could then show, over the course of its occurrence, a struggle with its own formulation and means of composition that could be taken as a sign of hospitality to reflection. What is always interesting is not simply this process of appropriation but how it can be subverted or reinvented in order to transform itself from an appearance of plagiarism (mimesis as copying) into a position that amplifies rather than reiterates what it has received. This is an example of the innovative relation to usage that adds to what it depicts in ways that are mutually influential. This is precisely where language returns from holiday.

3

The Elemental Vision of the Split

Introduction

We can note in the following selection from Malinowski (1955) the elementary vision of the split, of the Grey Zone, coming alive as an aspect of the human condition per se, by reconfiguring the theorist anthropologically as a practical actor beset by division in the most elementary sense, the division desire marks between agency and dependency.

> Nowhere is the duality of natural and supernatural causes divided by a line so thin and intricate, yet, if carefully followed up, so well marked, decisive, and instructive, as in the two most fateful forces of human destiny: health and death. Health to the Melanesians is a natural state of affairs and, unless tampered with, the human body will remain in perfect order. But the natives know perfectly well that there are natural means which can affect health and even destroy the body. Poisons, wounds, burns, falls, are known to cause disablement or death in a natural way. And this is not a matter of private opinion of this or that individual, but it is laid down in traditional lore and even in belief, for there are considered to be different ways to the nether world for those who died by sorcery and those who met "natural" death. Again, it is recognized that cold, heat, overstrain, too much sun, overeating, can all cause minor ailments, which are treated by natural remedies such as massage, steaming, warming at a fire and certain potions. Old age is known to lead to bodily decay and the explanation is given by the natives that very old people grow weak, their oesophagus closes up, and therefore they must die.
>
> [...] But who of us really believes that his own bodily infirmities and the approaching death is a purely natural occurrence, just an insignificant event in the infinite chain of causes? To the most

47

rational of civilized men health, disease, the threat of death, float in a hazy emotional mist, which seems to become denser and more impenetrable as the fateful forms approach. It is indeed astonishing that "savages" can achieve such a sober, dispassionate outlook in these matters as they actually do.

Thus in his relation to nature and destiny, whether he tries to exploit the first or to dodge the second, primitive man recognizes both the natural and the supernatural forces and agencies, and he tries to use them both for this benefit. Whenever he has been taught by experience that effort guided by knowledge is of some avail, he never spares the one or ignores the other. He knows that a plant cannot grow by magic alone, or a canoe sail or float without being properly constructed and managed, or a fight be won without skill and daring. He never relies on magic alone, while, on the contrary, he sometimes dispenses with it completely, as in fire-making and in a number of crafts and pursuits. But he clings to it, whenever he has to recognize the impotence of his knowledge and of his rational technique. (Malinowski, 1955, p. 31–32)

Here, we begin to appreciate the source of ambiguity to be given not immediately by the construction of the body and its incoherence but by the conventional split between human and nature, the convention of dualism that enables us to view the body as an icon of nature in the sense that the incoherence we attribute to the body seems to participate in the vast array of forces and agencies affecting humans in ways often incalculable. Nature is a figure of speech for the incoherence of forces that appear in images to and for a subject, who must strive to make sense of their play and who must strive to deal with the irresolution that will fatefully follow such efforts. Thus nature plays a correlative role to the figure of the body as used by Mead (1967) and even by Lacan (1997) as a conjunction of corporeality and image in desire evoking the unruly and incoherent relentlessness of desire, possessing both inevitability and inscrutability. In this elemental vision the Grey Zone comes to view as a relationship between humans and fateful forces that remain in some sense incalculable, in some sense appearing enigmatic, while yet always necessarily provocative occasions for reflection and action. It is here that we begin to note the tension between what Malinowski calls the fatality of such forces and the resourcefulness of human desire and ingenuity in the face of such forces, the constancy in the desire to influence and manage such an environment, to master it through knowledge that concedes both the limits of mastery and the need for reassurance in the face of such limits. The equanimity of this actor seems remarkable to Malinowski, who characterizes his action in the face of his ignorance, of his knowing that he does not know.

The enigma of both disease and death, according to Malinowski, is connected to their appearing as conditions that are ambiguous, both natural and inexplicably related to forces not necessarily of the same order, apprehended in a "hazy emotional mist" as if both natural and supernatural forces that are related to conditions assumed linked to the singularity of a person and his destiny. At the most elemental level, the Grey Zone of health and illness appears as the conundrum of such mysterious causality, how its impersonality as both natural and Other can only be remedied by technique supplemented by prayer.

The division marking the Grey Zone, most visible according to Malinowski in the case of health and death, seems to exist as such for the subject because the obscurity produced by the body of the word is that towards which we must take a perspective. The word creates an enigma because it is not self-evident, always eliciting an aura of multiplicity in the way Aristotle (1966) said of being that it has many senses. That is, the perfection and stability of the natural order is marked by health and interrupted by disease and death that bring nature into question as a trouble requiring clarification and action.

As soon as experiences such as health and death are named, are distinguished by the word, we invest the word with an aura of indefiniteness that serves to us as a call to action, to decipher the mystery of its eventfulness. Think of diagnosis: when one is named and identified, as in "You have depression," the origin of the category as accusation becomes clear in that the name invites the one to whom it is applied to discover this relationship just as the one who applies it must be accountable. The term does not end the story but begins it as a course of action in which the name and what it names remain provocative, raising the possibility of continuous inquiry into this question. The diagnosis that begins by collecting the one so named with anonymous others of the type also opens the door to an exploration of the relation of this togetherness to the apartness of the person, addressing the question of how individuality and typification relate as an occasion. Thus, if a reiteration of natural causality might describe the surface of the disease as if an event in the lives of many different persons, intimating a history where precedents can be consulted and digested as a lore, then the question always remains of how the singularity of this one makes her seem both together and apart in relation to this common affliction. The Grey Zone lives in the aura of accusation implicit in any diagnosis that makes the proof of apartness or individuality the challenge for any and every patient, and gives the one who applies the diagnosis material for reflection concerning how the type takes shape in this individual and how individuality expresses itself through the type.

Seduction by this division between the word (its lawful usage) and its specificity (natality, *physis*, origin) seems to differentiate human and animal, allowing us to ascribe to the human a fascination with the enigma of mortality and with the world as essentially poetic that typically appears to mark the singularity of the human. But as Lacan (1991) suggests, it might be this sense of incomparability that humans need to think in order to see themselves as singular, being captured by the enigma of the self, while knowing full well that this might be indefensible.

Accordingly, this "self-conscious" work of locating itself among all of the other things as one more object capable of saying, "I'm the one who knows that I am," (Lacan, 1991, p. 224) in contrast to the "other things which do not know themselves to be," if it "does perhaps know that it […] knows nothing at all about what it is. That is what is lacking in every being" (p. 224), that is, knowing what the word is but not its who. Thus, if I am not animal, table or toe, or know that I do not know, it is invariably my claim here that confirms how I alone am alive to such distinguishing and that it is this that marks me as distinctively human, and my capacity to see who and what knows and fails to know. Note however, that it is the desire to distinguish and to distinguish ourselves by distinguishing that confirms desire as the fundamental experience. Nature then seems equivalent to the imaginary, and so, reinstates this fixation upon our singularity as both topic and resource for the human, suggesting in this way that it only becomes ideological when treated un-ironically as an empirical comment upon the species.

> The Freudian experience starts […] by postulating a world of desire. It postulates it prior to any kind of experience, prior to any essences. Desire is instituted within the Freudian world in which our experience unfolds, it constitutes it, and at no point in time, not even in the most insignificant of our manoeuvres in this experience of ours, can it be erased. The Freudian world isn't a world of things, it isn't a world of being, it is a world of desire as such […] Desire is a relation of Being to lack. This lack is the lack of being properly speaking. It isn't the lack of this or that, but lack of being whereby the being exists. This lack is beyond anything which can represent it […] Desire, a function central to all human experience, is the desire for nothing nameable. And at the same time this desire lies at the origin of every variety of animation. If being were only what it is, there wouldn't even be room to talk about it. Being comes into existence as an exact function of this lack. Being attains a sense of self in relation to being as a function of this lack, in the experience of desire, in the pursuit of this beyond which is nothing, it harks back to the feeling of a being with self-consciousness, which is nothing but its own reflection in the world of things. For it is the comparison of beings there before it, who do not in fact know themselves. (Lacan, 1991, pp. 222–224)

The relationship to the unknown rather than any specific condition becomes the quintessential mark of conditionality per se, of the human condition (Arendt, 1958) and the problematic relationship to desire that is the common inheritance of beings, the condition of the co-relation of lack and desire. And of course, what remains to be developed as this problem is the task of negotiating the unruly terrain of the emotions, the "emotional mist" to which Malinowski makes reference.

It is in the nature of desire to be radically torn. The very image of man brings in here a mediation which is always imaginary, always problematic, and which therefore is never completely fulfilled […] this experience either alienates man from himself, or else ends in a destruction, a negation of the object. (Lacan, 1991, p. 166)

This suggests that it is not simply the interiority of desire that marks it but its fundamental asymmetry insofar as this assumption must link one to the other and therefore must apply to all. If desire cannot be imagined for the other, other would be assumed to lack a self like the toe, table or animal and could only be used and exploited rather than engaged. The potential for unity depends upon a structure of intersubjectivity as such, each reciprocally being able to see self in other and other in self as in the assumption of mutually oriented action required as the condition for conversation. What this means is that the turn to "magic" mentioned above by Malinowski is precisely the turn to dialogue and conversation as that imaginary antidote to the discursive abandonment of selves to their own resources, that magical moment when they recognize that someone must define the terms and conditions of dialogue, that a discourse of mastery in such a way is necessary to be assumed and anticipated as a common resource for dissemination and eventually, communalization. Thus dialogue in this sense, between selves comparable in being selves, still requires that someone establish the terms and conditions of dialogue and that a discourse of mastery be coeval with comparability as such. In this sense, "magic" is an anthropological translation of Socrates' second sailing. Though dialogue is directed to an eventual equalization (not identity), it must begin as an asymmetrical exchange grounded in trust. Magic begins to make reference to the need and desire to take a perspective on the self and the other, on being the same and different, as a version of the imaginary commitment to dialogue.

Intersubjectivity

What is remarkable in these selections is Malinowski's recognition of the elemental character of the death drive as part of the desire for life, that the subject clings to his magic even as he "has to recognize the impotence of his knowledge and of his rational technique." The idea here of magic begins to make a place for the necessity that the actor's relationship to (what has been called) the unknown be mediated by a relationship to others through a mutually oriented approach, to recognize that healing ambiguity must be shared by those who are in the same boat and, though similar because of that, different by virtue of their needs and capacities. In this way, magic makes reference to the demand that shared being materialize in a vision of justice as the best way of relating to the weaker party.

Yet, justice and the aesthetic are interrelated. Malinowski implies that it is on such occasions that the provocation of dialogue becomes vivid, because on such an occasion the puzzle of mortality and its burden appears enigmatic to the point where its obscurity becomes threatening: "the poet will naturally tend to write about that which most deeply engrosses him—and nothing more deeply engrosses a man than his burdens, including those of a physical nature, such as disease" (Burke, 1957, p. 16). "As soon as we approach the subject in these terms, we […] have a constant reminder that a threat is the basis of beauty" (Burke, 1957, p. 52).

If the threat of the enigmatic nature of obscurity is the basis of beauty, then this means that obscurity as the question to answer assumes decisive shape in the collective search for a solution, much as the riddle of the Sphinx exercised the Greeks as the conundrum upon which Oedipus floundered (Tiffany, 2008). That is, analogous to the spellbinding character of the riddle is the fascination exercised by the burdens of health and the threat of death. For example, Tiffany (2008), following Adorno, says that it is the incomprehension of the philistine towards the obscurity of the poem that establishes the form of modern art and that the desire of the subject to pursue the meaning of the poem is the archetype for the ideal speaker that keeps life alive, keeps death at bay, through the dialogical engagement with the enigma and its obscurity. This is to say, in Greek, that it is the puzzle or enigma of self-knowledge that keeps death at bay in ways that can only occur when the enigma is seen as a riddle with potential, disclosing obscurity as incentive for the animation of desire rather than the promise of annihilation. The question of desire then becomes one of seeing obscurity as stimulating and life-affirming (as puzzle or riddle) rather than as deadly, in contrast to the ban on desire that takes exception to its being subject to the spell of the enigma, perhaps on the grounds that life is the emergency that requires such an exception or that takes exception to ambiguity. If in this way the philistine stands to desire as the body stands to the self, we might say that the philistine is the paradigm of theorizing in the way that the hatred of ambiguity and its spell is the limitation upon *dialogos*. What this glosses is the enigma of the relation of self to other that can locate the other in oneself (e.g., the philistine within) and the self in the other (e.g., that the truth in the philistine's capacity to take a perspective on herself is expressed in even extremist opinions and beliefs). This means that, first, the division of one is the division of all (equality), and second, that the division within, one as the self and the self as other, means that the relationship is an opportunity for development and not a confirmation of identity, that working out this question of similarity (how it is not identity and not difference) is the very puzzle of individuality.

Dualism

We might consider how the vitality of speech can be invested not only with the character of a fateful force and how unruliness might be ascribed to speaking, but the way in which dualism inheres both within and without the speaker, within as the undeveloped and alienated relation in any beginning to the commonplace content, and externally in the code of language and the moves it sanctions as legitimate; even more, just as the code is meant to tame the unruliness of capricious speech and its imaginings, so is self-monitoring expected to pacify the liveliness of unrestrained poetic imaginings. Further, relations between interior and exterior are mediated by the totemic commonplace signifier and the split between its character as an inanimate mark, a lifeless thing, almost as a cadaver (Schwenger, 2000) and its animation through the narrative that promises to breathe into it life (*prosopopeia*). Thus, the propensity to be governed by the volatile unruliness of an interior poetry is commensurate with the plurality imagined in any action undertaken, the dispersion imaginable as inherent in the diversity of directions it can follow (Rosset, 1989). We appreciate here the canonical and oft criticized notion of *form* as an image of the need and desire for collectedness and the disengagement it requires and promises, both within and without, as equipment for living (Burke, 1957), as a staple of the imaginary and its functional and aesthetic powers.

As Eric Gans (1982) points out, the traditional association of culture with cultivation was established through the use of the model of agriculture, where the nature to be cultivated can be understood as a reflection of the unruliness of the emotions and, in particular, the alienation released by the connection of desire to lack. The imaginary begins with this dualism expressed in unreflective submission to the fortuitous caprice of the fateful forces and to the limited recipes offered for their control through any common culture (the alienated language) *and* to the unruliness expressed in the desire to speak about them, typified as the emotions (i.e., the hysterical and obsessive attempts to deal with the limits of common culture). In relation to the original division of the experience of reality, the relation of subject to ambiguity is essentially a relationship to the unruliness of the emotions (and so, to what we usually reconstruct as consciousness or psyche). Thus, whereas we can think of hysteria as the exploitation of ambiguity seeking to overcome what it sees as the scarcity and miserliness of the code (the idea that the format of common culture destroys the object and creates the wasteland), obsession seeks to limit ambiguity because its fear of the dispute released by the variety of *copia* require fastidious gestures of self-fashioning, reductionism and cooperation. In certain ways if hysteria is the posture feared by obsession, then obsessiveness remains the rigidity that animates hysteria. Both postures seem ruled in Girard's (1977) terms by the illusion of their spontaneous desire.

We note that the idea of cultivation typically associated with the notion of culture can point towards an overcoming of the extreme propensities of speaking, not simply towards the extremes of silence or verbosity as in the example of Erasmus' "loquacious rhetoric" (Greene, 1982), but as the overcoming of banality or what Freud characterized as the idle talk of the patient who resists self-exploration behind shopworn clichés or formulaic descriptions. If the notion of transference signifies a degree of passivity, an indolence towards one's speaking as such, then overcoming the transference first invites us to invest our words with life, to animate words as images, as more than inanimate marks but as a mirror of the ways in which we can be seen and said to be and to have been, the appearances and traces of our working and of our works.

In this elementary situation of action, we have all of the ingredients for a vision of the subject as an oriented actor confronting "forces" and "agencies" that he tries to use "for his own benefit," the quintessential practical actor, cultivating methods and means for creating outcomes, inheriting and using the artifact of a system of decision-making through which desire might be realized, an image of the symbolic order, guided by a sense of its necessity and limits, the recurring encounter with the unruliness of nature as an outcome that can only be repeated in ways confirming the Real. In our relationship to any other one, through the speech that she invests with life, we discern her as a vital character as if a speaker subject to an archive and as creator of speeches that can be revealing and unruly at the same time. As an elementary situation we can appreciate the Grey Zone as the hypothesis that the human desire to give form to material conditions must begin with the gap between desire (the imaginary) and the symbolic (system and language) and the management of that excess (the Real). This means that the Grey Zone as such a hypothesis serves not as an explanation to be proven but as a perspicuous representation in Wittgenstein's sense, an irony as in Plato's likely story, the truth of which can only lie in its development. This is how Lacan can equate the symbolic order with deceit since, in showing the necessity of constructing a reply to ambiguity, it reveals the necessity of fiction per se, and in his sense, of the use of fiction to ward off the aura of ambiguity as evil. Further, the forces and agencies that the subject confronts can be expressed as the external body of common language, an image Nietzsche (1956, p. 55) eloquently grasped in the idea of language as a host of spirits. The magic of dialogue makes reference to the necessary fiction of the symbolic order that wards off the evil of the abyss.

This anthropological conception of the Grey Zone hypothesizes the split as commensurate with human culture, disclosed, as we said for the Greeks, in the notion of *en medias res,* being in the middle of things as yet an other thing desiring to be more, the subject of language inheriting the burden of this space as an unformed beginning always in need of form. In this way the fiction of signification becomes an element of problem-solving, a way of taking over the dread of ambiguity through action that serves in its manner as expurgation, akin to Burke's conception of equipment for living. For the Greeks, the human subject occupies this space of both less (beast) and more (divinity) as a figure for the place of desire and, in our terms, for the human as the more that is less and the less that invariably needs more.

Malinowski's text suggests two images of the region of ambiguity we call the Grey Zone, both revolving around the question of the status of the figure of magic that he invokes. Thus, magic can function as the explanation that tries to quiet perplexity by providing the reassurance that it demands in the form of a definitive conclusion or solution, perhaps in the way we search for an answer as an end to the ambiguity almost as if a cure. Yet, the likely story that binds together the parts is also functional in the way of Lacan's *object a*, putting anxiety to rest not by eliminating the problem but by sustaining a relationship to it despite its intractability. The idea of magic here is commensurate with Lacan's (1991, p. 75) vision of "the human defense [...] through signifying structuralization in the human unconscious," not simply defense "at the level of [...] metaphor" but by means of "lying about evil" which can explain the need to believe something false in order to put evil to rest (in order to put to rest the unruly emotions stimulated by the fear of the unknown). In this sense, we heal rather than cure anxiety not by envisioning an interpretive coherence where none exists but by developing a coherent relationship to whatever appears incoherent. Thus, magic does not solve the problem of the Grey Zone but develops a relationship to it in living practices or in the desire to live as such. If fear of the unknown is the truth, then the unconscious can lie about this truth through its construction of magic that normalizes it. The palliative status of magic can be nothing other than the libidinal investment in the imaginary of shared being as the practice of community, the commitment to the perpetuity of conversation as ongoing, fundamentally ambiguous, the place between origin and end.

Note though that in Malinowski's example, the idea of nature as the return of the repressed is absent because nature in his sense has never been expelled or excluded in this way. If modern enlightenment is supposed to exclude nature in the shape of a ban (the exception, subjectivity, etc.), then the anthropological conception affirms the ever-present presence of nature as interior to the human in the relationship of self-knowledge. That is, the anxiety released by the unruliness of the emotions and the obscurity of the word can never be banned, only displaced and condensed through linguistic modifications that remain symptomatic of such conversion. It is through language that we adapt to the anxiety of our relations to the unknown, the obscurity of the word only maintaining such anxiety as we take it up in expectation of respite. This is to say that what is natural is the propensity of the subject, the human, to mirror the environment (the fateful forces, the traditional beliefs, the opinions about causes of health and death, aging and decline, what is called common culture, background expectancies, the "emotional mist," and the utilitarian aspiration to survive). What is natural is the inescapable relationship of any human to common culture, its externality and coerciveness in the idiom of Durkheim (1938a), and the demands it places upon us for adaptation.

In Lacan's analogy of the imaginary as an environment worn by the subject as if his double or mirror, nature becomes similar to the second nature as the reflected self, the self-constructed and reflected back to itself as the environment of knowledge to which the human is subject. What is natural to the subject then, his own reflected limitation in mastering the environment, can mirror for any actor his failure and so, the unruliness of emotions of fear and trembling, of dispersion, fragmentation and the groundlessness of being. The unruliness of nature, not in opposition to the social, remains part of life as the emotions that pervade human existence in the experience of separation (of loss or of lack) that are overcome through healing rather than by impossible fantasies of reunification. If it seems to be Freud and Lacan who dramatize the human condition as terrifying in relation to the figures of loss, of abandonment and of castration as an intractable sense of separation and abandonment, then such an aura is present in the notions of the second sailing and *en medias res,* but perhaps as more composed responses to the condition of human intermediacy, reflected in the replies of tragedy and, more deeply, comedy.

The magic of aesthetics

It is actually Hesiod (1953) who best dramatizes the link between the mysteries of nature and the unruliness of the emotions, not simply as a causal result of somatic infirmities, but as a response to the intuitive visualization of oneself as both intimate and external, in the shadow of *das Ding.* As a shepherd isolated with his flock in the wilds, Hesiod recounts how his cries for help, for the magic of response, was an appeal to the muses for the powers of music and art that might divert him from his self-absorbed isolation, giving him the gift of a purpose, to become absorbed in telling a story. For example, Hesiod rhapsodizes on the emergence of speech as the magic of poetry, thus rescuing Malinowski's magic from its plausible identification with superstition, custom or false belief.

> Fortunate is the man whom the muses love: sweet words flow from his lips. If someone has sorrow and is sick at heart and stunned with fresh trouble on his mind, and if a servant of the Muses sings of the glorious deeds of men in former times or of the blessed gods whose home is Olympus, he quickly forgets his bad thoughts and no longer remembers his troubles: the gift of these goddesses instantly divert the mind. (Hesiod, 1953, I.96-103, pp. 55–56)

Speech itself might be said to originate as an eventful collision with the unruly emotions as an attempt at amelioration, not by denying or reducing the emotions but through the pleasure offered by sweet words in ways that might divert the mind. Here is an elementary vision of healing that portrays the shepherd, the one isolated in the wilds, as surrounded by ghostly spirits in the "luminous night" (Nietzsche, 1956) who can be touched by the music of speech. In this elementary situation, music and language come together as song, and with the aid of the muses, help make magic. Here we see that the magic amounts simply to dialogue but dialogue oriented to form and so, aesthetic, what Rancière (2009a) depicts as the aesthetic relationship to the world, the need and desire to commit to form as part of a disengagement from the tyranny of conditions. If health and illness are linked irreparably to the volatility of the emotions, then the visualization of such a relationship might just escape or exceed all attempts to make it visible and to confirm or test its reality only and exclusively through such means and methods. Certainly theorizing health and illness has to pay its respects to such a Grey Zone. Is this not a point of entry into the problem of being sick, more than physical infirmities or the genetic correlates that are imaginable (as the tip of the iceberg), and more than what is stereotyped as stress, but sorrow, being "sick at heart" and "stunned with fresh trouble in the mind"? Does this not begin to make reference to the Grey Zone of health and illness, of being sick, as the real matter that must touch and be oriented to by all concerned?

Taking our lead from Hesiod, we might be able to glimpse the prospect of health not simply in its capacity to defend oneself from disease through regimes of self-monitoring, but by an engagement with language mediated by the desire to remake this eventful encounter with the music of sweet words in representing any and every relationship to being "sick at heart" (see the modernization of this in the idea of life as a "song of suffering" in Deleuze and Guattari [1994, p. 176] and developed by Rancière [2009b, pp. 54–56]).

> A monument does not commemorate or celebrate something that happened but confides to the ear of the future the persistent sensations that embody the event; the constantly renewed suffering of men and women, their re-created protestations, their constantly resumed struggle. (Deleuze and Guattari, 1994, pp. 176–177)

Encouraged by Rancière, we can think of the monument as a figure for art, but we might go further and think of it as a figure for a life and, even more, as a figure for the relation of a life to its art, the appeal to the magic of the muses to empower one to orient such intimate suffering "to the ear of the future."

The idea of being sick at heart and constantly vulnerable to being "stunned with fresh trouble" should not describe wide-awake normal people living out a round of life, but only an exceptional condition for them, much like disease. But if we imagine such a condition as itself a universal, then disease has no weight, for life itself could be considered a kind of sickness. Living under the rule of *das Ding* could be as if a kind of sickness if this "original division" was treated as a condition that limits us from thinking aesthetically or as neutralizing "the circular relationship between knowledge as know-how and knowledge as the distribution of roles [because] Aesthetic experience eludes the sensible distribution of roles and competences which structure the hierarchical order"

(Rancière, 2006, p. 4). An aesthetic relationship to language enables us to begin to give form to material conditions in ways that give form to theorizing itself as that uncanny embodiment, as both escape and sacrificial, and so as comic in its relentlessness, in its very *jouissance* that is the death drive revealed in Socratic ignorance (that the truth has to be pursued even and insofar as we know that we do not know). This is to say that an aesthetic relation to the original division of *das Ding* makes reference to an ideal speaker able to double herself as two-in-one: "[I]n other words, the identity of a subject capable of escaping the assignment to a private condition and of intervening in the affairs of the community" (Rancière, 2006, p. 6). Here, the "affairs of the community" could be the common language, its *doxa* and familiar distinctions and proper names ("that pin people down" [Rancière, 1992, p. 62]) and the escape from the private assignment can be not simply rejection but what Rancière calls "a transgressive affirmation," a reformulation aiming to reassign meaning to what had been privately assigned, the second sailing where what had been thought is rethought as if for the second time, but under the condition that what is rethought here can be given form as a revitalized image of collective suffering that the intimacy of the life might call to mind. Because it is a social order that assigns us to a private condition and its name, the name of the father, that assignment includes for anyone so subject a capacity for escape and to remember more than paternity, the (m)other. This escape begins to make reference to the powers of disengagement that we might call aesthetic, a capacity to seem to be at home with what is temporary and contingent and at the same time to be desirous of something other, to be two-in-one.

The enigma of human nature

The nature of the human makes nature coeval with the human in a sense that seems more resonant than corporeality, as what Marx (1964, pp. 76–77) called "species being" or we might think of as etholological universalism. The recurrent fascination with the human resemblance to animal is typically marked in our clichés about aggression, sex and courtship, forms of association, maternalism and the like. On the one hand, whether or not desire is a universal of the species, the engagement with the spellbinding enigma of our universality as part of the riddle of our self-knowledge seems to be a conceit we need, our equipment for living.

Thus, Hesiod presents us with an occasion for exploration because, as all animals, we are predictable, fearful and emotional, in ways distressful and always requiring relief. That is, we might very well be the species unique in its proclivity to be stunned with sorrow and sick at heart. In response to this picture of human nature Socrates proposes in contrast to tragedy what he calls "due measure" ("that resists holding its wounded parts in grief") (Plato, 1945, V.XXXVI.602–603, pp. 335ff). What binds these various vignettes of human nature is still the power to transform what they see to see-as, the power of the self for transposition, and so the question of what would be an inventive or creative relationship to life, for the self confronting being sick at heart or stunned with sorrow as basic material conditions. Thus, whether due measure, tragedy, comedy or art, what such desire reveals is the mimetic aspiration to perform at what is seen-as necessary and desirable for one who would maintain her self in her coming to herself, as in this passage. Such a transformation of this basic condition into a symbolic order begins to show how such a condition can be made into a relationship with juridical and aesthetic possibilities that can capture the overtones and implications of the Grey Zone as the emotional landscape of health and illness. We should now appreciate that the enigma of health and illness is a function of the elemental division in the signifier itself raised by the puzzle of the contrast that asks, "What is health and what is illness and how am I in particular related to such conditions?" So far, the enigmatic character of this condition was given by the self-identification of the practical actor recognizing the need for magic and the experience of sickness and sorrow as if any solution requires more information or knowledge. Now, though, we are prepared to see that what is elemental is more basic than this because the subject of health and illness who identifies herself as such is part of a relationship in which what she sees-as can always be open to question.

We appreciate the power of Plato's notion of a likely story in the turn Malinowski makes in the elementary situation where the appeal to magic, understood abstractly as dialogue, is nothing other than an appeal for a true account, i.e., for a way of helping us live under such conditions. What is asked for is not so much an explanation of illness but a way of living with the suffering and sorrow of sickness and death, and if an account of the illness will help us grasp our part in its evolution, then the magic of such self-knowledge, of knowing this as such, could and should help us deal with the condition. The turn to magic is the turn to the imagination and in this sense in part, to the intensification of the imaginary.

What is displayed in the elemental view of health and illness most basically is how the obscurity of the terms health and illness that originate a discursive relationship to the enigma of their meaning is due to the condition that being named sick (and healthy) is a way of identifying health and illness socially as a relationship, the relationship of all so named to the name and to its effects. Sickness in this sense is a mode of self-identification, a way of seeing oneself as (in this case) sick at heart and stunned with sorrow. The anthropological view seems to recognize this identification as the start of a dialogical process in which the subject of sickness by virtue of such an enunciation creates a dependency ruled by the anticipation of some form of expert intervention as part of a claim of weakness qualifying him as special and particular in some sense. This sense of singularity can connect health and illness to special treatment insofar as illness at least is a way of asking for help and of offering to be responsive to such intervention out of helplessness. This collaboration is organized around the questions, "Why or how did you come to be sick and what can we do to make you better?" In such a way, being named sick rather than healthy brings to view the symbolic order and its various moves as an economy of social action directed by the signifier itself. A most rudimentary view of the symbolic order of health and illness recognizes it not simply as a game in Mead's sense but as what Wittgenstein (1953) calls a language game, that is, as a regime or legitimate order. And despite the necessity of some order, we must keep in mind its limits, the limits of any such artifact or apparatus, the omnipresent sense of the hole in Being that must haunt any resolution. In particular, we can now ask how a modern society such as ours transforms the eventful relationship to health and illness as a collective problem.

The dialogue

At the most immediate level, the Grey Zone appears vexatious in a society such as ours through the tropes of specialization and fragmentation assumed as medical science's contribution to the decline of a sense of the whole (aura, the sacred) as a contemporary restatement of the conundrum of *en medias res*. Gadamer and Raffel both approach the same problem from different but related ways. For Gadamer (1996, pp. 103–116), the enigma is not one of explaining illness per se but of providing for illness against the background of health and it is as if the fascination with illness and disease distracts us from engaging the unspoken notion of health that is typically defined by implication of the absence of illness. Gadamer assumes in his way an orderly path between illness and health, the kind of passage idealized in the *Timaeus* (Plato, 1949b) as itself a standard of health. This is also in part a legacy of Stoicism and its affirmation of the virtue of composure and tranquility. Thus, it is healthy to try to live according to a model of health that is not segregated from illness and not its opposite either, but an aspect of the relation to illness as such. Calling health a sense of "inner accord," Gadamer (1996, p. 3–16) suggests that this is not a state opposed to illness but a way of relating to illness, a healthy way of seeing illness, where this relationship is designed to enhance inner accord. Despite its concealment, it is inner accord that must make demands upon us that guide our relations to illness and disease in ways even more essential for instructing us how to live with illness, permitting us to ask: what is a healthy relationship to illness? Gadamer proceeds to describe mundane practices that can be said to maintain "rhythmic functions" and equilibrium in everyday life (1996, p. 114). Comparing this with the *Timaeus*, we appreciate health as what is needed and desired to maintain ourselves well under bad conditions (or to maintain ourselves in good condition under bad conditions). In this sense, what is most interesting about Gadamer's criticism of medical science is that in focusing upon the influence of science on life, it implies that science is bad, not because of its research per se, but for the reason that it is emulated as a way of thinking (unhealthy) and uncongenial to the inner accord he requires. The de-ritualization and erosion of the aura connected with

Walter Benjamin is translated by Gadamer into a notion of the decline and so increases concealment of any vision of health as inner accord. It is actually the palpability of disease as defined through medicalization that heightens such a vanishing sense of health as if the specialties prevent us from reflecting upon what they are visible infractions of, a sense of basic and functional integrity necessary for everyday life.

Raffel (1985) develops in a related way from Arendt's notion of the intermediacy of the human condition the constraint of *en medias res*. The withdrawal of the whole as a figure for the drama of all such work is highlighted in Raffel's ability to embody and put flesh on the subject of the world who is realistically condemned to see herself as a victim of chance rather than as an outcome of will, right or decision. Raffel's dramatization of the subject of such a world translates the abstraction conveyed in the figure of the withdrawal of the whole into the picture of an oriented actor who can only treat life as requiring her to catch up (to make up for bad conditions) or to give up (because life itself is such a bad condition). Raffel imposes upon this actor the requirement of rethinking what it means to live healthfully when she can be said neither to have the first word nor the last word, inviting this actor as such to address life under the auspices of the question, "Just what does existence (this life) make possible?" What Gadamer calls equilibrium or rhythmic functions, Raffel treats after Arendt as a call to action, a demand (or invitation) to rethink the question of the difference between what is essential and what is inessential. This is a translation of Gadamer's notion of inner accord as the desire to ask what kind of life existence makes possible in this way. In this gesture Raffel encourages us to transform our resentment towards life by resisting evaluating existence. It is the elementary relation to health and illness that makes these questions accessible by bringing to view the unspoken assumption grounding the Grey Zone and ambiguity that life is either worth living or not. If inner accord as health is a symptom rather than a fact in the idiom of Lacan, then we have conceded that to be less of a burden than a beginning to engage in the human relation to its conditions as such.

4

The Official History and the Unwritten Text

Introduction

The motif of this chapter is simple: there is an official history of health and illness written from the perspective of medicine, that identifies the field with a history of medicine, especially with professionalization organized around technological innovation and its application and accessibility to uninformed users; and there is an unofficial history of health and illness that is organized around a trajectory narrating the experience of being well or sick as a recurrent "song of suffering" necessarily felt as privatized and singular. The distinction between such histories comes alive through the figure of desire, necessary and treated differently in both stories. Reflecting upon such history then causes us to rethink the notion of desire not only for the subject of medicine (for example, doctor, patient) but in and for the writing of history (the subject of the authorship, the collective and its grounds and speakers). This gap makes visible the need for any collective exercised by the concern for health and illness to engage the unending problem of connecting technical accomplishments of medicine to the experience of health and illness of all by reading the official history's project of making knowledge of research available to a public (knowledge transfer) against the unofficial and obscene vision of the imperative need to make experiences of health and illness and of the subject of medicine accessible to medical professionals.

History

Didi-Huberman (2005) develops Hegel's conception of the experience of a present confronting history as its past, always subject to the feeling that the original eventfulness of the origin is missed in such retrospective views. In talking of the history of art, he says of such historians that they

would discover the inevitably split status of their objects, objects
henceforth placed under their gaze, but deprived of something that we of
course no longer want anything to do with; something that has effectively
passed away. Something, however, that made the whole life of these objects,
their function and their efficacy: something that in turn placed everyone
under the gaze of the object [...] The difficulty being, henceforth, to look
at what remains (visible) while summoning up what has disappeared: in
short, to scrutinize the visual traces of this disappearance, which I will
otherwise call (without any clinical connotations): its symptoms. (Didi-
Huberman, 2005, p. 50)

Here, the mediator between past and present, mindful of losing sight of the original
moment of passion that defined the emergence of the object (in our case not art, but
health and illness), can only hope to look at what remains visible, such as a tangible
history of achievements, a record of technical accomplishments and defining moments
by "summoning up" what has disappeared and its physical traces. (See my use of the
Nietzsche passage "the original sung of terror while the present version is as a lullaby"
from his *Use and abuses of history* quoted in *The imaginative structure of the city*
[Blum, 2003, p. 36]; see also the author's "Still life" article, unpublished, 1991b). Didi-
Huberman (2005, p. 50) says, however, that it is not simply temporality that separates
us from such an experience (despite its appearance in a visible record) but its pointing
to what "has effectively passed away" and "that we no longer want anything to do with."
In this chapter, we will explore the relation between what has effectively passed away,
which we believe to be traces of desire in the original collective experience of health
and illness, and its repression in its official history. Thus, we shall open up the question
of "what we want nothing to do with" as the experience of desire in the relation to
health and illness, and how and why that might come to be, by reviving parts of Plato's
(1945) discussion in the *Republic* in order to begin scrutinizing the visual traces of this
disappearance.

Absence and presence

This inescapable mediation of the present—the idea that representation cannot jump
over its own shadow—was dramatically inaugurated in Plato's (1949b) *Timaeus* through
his vision of history (or really of any account) as a "likely story." Lacan's notion (1988,
pp. 50–52, 62–70; 1991, pp. 49–52, 208–212, 236, 243–247) of the symbolic order that
situates concepts such as ego, self and others as symptoms rather than facts certainly
includes history as such a necessary fiction, as well as Wittgenstein's (1953, pp. 192–
196) conception of all perception as seeing-as, further aligning history with narrative

through the usage of the "perspicuous representation." If Hegel's absolute and Heidegger's ontological difference at best provoke us to consider the irony of such necessary fictions that seem to posit a course of development as if they are apart from the action of positing, then they still invite us to rethink the relation of the Same and the Other, of being together and apart from history in ways that only highlight the necessary deceit of any and all narrative as a relation to history that must remain part of it rather than apart, and so, of the place of fiction in representation. (See Derrida [1982] on Heidegger's use of clock time as a misrecognition of its difference from eventfulness or from what Lacan calls the time of the concept, or Gadamer's [1986, pp. 192] notion of the primordial event of speech). In this sense, Žižek's (1997, pp. 3–44) grammar for fantasy condenses such a "metaphysical impasse" in the usage of narrative occlusion, partially in relation to the necessary strategies of what he calls "after the fall" and "the impossible gaze," strategies of distancing that the second sailing (the fall to discourse, to *en medias res*) makes necessary and desirable.

All such gestures acknowledge temporality, the condition of our eternal and inescapable present (Simmel, 1971, p. 359) as the condition requiring our repossessing absence as present (Gans, 1982) in the signifier and the trace of its emergence, as an application of the *object a* that functions to supply coherence necessarily, and so, to make any narrative accountable for its means of repossession. Here then, instead of arguing whether or not history is a construction, as if such an admission condemns the distinction between truth and falsity to oblivion (as in those tepid debates among historians in the *Times Literary Supplement*), we pin the distinction between true and false elsewhere, on the story and its implications, with respect to the different consequences of seeing-as, of viewing a history of health and illness in one way or another. The refusal to settle this question with a proposition as if to say, this one rather than that is correct (either/or), again confirms the necessity of a conversational relationship to signification that points out the difference between aspects that are essential and inessential.

Stories

The inescapable character of mediation simply acknowledges the in-between as the space between beginning and end registered in the notion of influences being handed down or disseminated. The rudimentary version of this recognition occurs through the idea of history or pastness but might also reference the many conditions said to determine a beginning and to mark it as an end of sorts, always potentially renewable as revitalization. Though tradition tends to be identified with what is handed down (Shils, 1981; Blum, 2003), such influences are more opaque, signifying the over-determination that enters into the literacy of any environment, always functioning as the materials for mediation, transmission, translation and the various figures used to describe dissemination, for example, the idea of the code or stock of knowledge (Schutz, 1973). The material itself, or media of influence, are more than archives, encyclopedia, libraries and museums, but often and inexplicably, they are memory and minds, beliefs, opinions, habits and vestigial images supposedly attached to experiences, whether of individuals or collectives. Besides technologies such as surgical laparoscopy mentioned in official histories, these are experiences attached to undergoing and administering such techniques, or leading to the need for them, or following from their application as complications.

Benjamin (1971, pp. 83–111) says that a "proverb is a ruin which stands on the site of an old story," suggesting that the cliché underlying requirements of planning and preparation for healthfulness and its procedures and tests (typically "better to be safe than sorry") condenses and displaces a story implicit in such a formula as weighty and significant, a story that seems to announce a noteworthy event requiring such a formula for its easy transmission. Thus, he says that every story containing something useful as it must, making possible an eventful exchange of experience, can only be diminished by the dissemination of information (Benjamin, 1971, p. 88), which, by abbreviating experience, undermines its communicability. Thus, crafting experience as communicable work for objectifying the event, the "what happened," in ways that reach over the borders separating times and persons, is similar to crafting an object of sorts that can only be of use if pleasurable and can only be pleasurable if useful, making any such occasion of dissemination an opportunity to inquire into the relation of the proverbial surface to the eventful experience (and story) that it conceals (resurrecting the best sense of Foucault's archeology). The story, seeking to join pleasure and pedagogy, only weakens as it focuses upon one or another of these extremes (amusing and frivolous v. didactic and boring), capable of communicating well only as its language presents and represents its retelling as eventful as in the manner suggested by the relationship to sweet words mentioned by Hesiod (1953).

Yet, if stories transmit an archive of experiences, idiosyncratic and perhaps tied to large scale fluctuations assumed of the environment in which they originated or emerged as experiences of note, then the reception of stories must feed back upon its telling in the ways in which the experiences of those who receive such stories "return" to make new demands upon their telling and retelling.

> Everything past is definitively anachronistic; it exists or subsists only through the figures that we make of it; so it exists only in the operations of a "reminiscing present," a present endowed with the admirable or dangerous power, precisely, of presenting it, and in the wake of this presentation, of elaborating and representing it. (Didi-Huberman, 2005, p. 38)

In this chapter, we shall take up the question of how history, as such an exchange, begins to communicate the experience of health and illness, and how the creation of records of technical achievements ostensibly tied to a model of production and consumption of information, risks maintaining the invisibility of the experience itself. If such relationships to history can themselves be abbreviated temporally or periodicized as classical and modern, then it is only to permit me to refocus Plato's likely story as a way of redeeming an aesthetic relationship to language, in showing the roots of abbreviation (as in the proverbial grasp of the history of health and illness as a history of medicine) to be a ruin standing on the site of an old story and how this story in its way, while aesthetic in its drive, is yet about justice and so ethical in its implications.

The idea of history is revealed to gloss two different stories of the collective relationship to health and illness, one that masks and simplifies the place of desire over time by reducing it to records, paradigms and "breakthroughs" seen externally from a deadly viewpoint, and one that animates desire as a dialectically recurrent factor in health and illness and in the biographies that topicalize well-being and its interruption. What we may call the official history, or curriculum, attributes historical development to the genius of technological progress in ways that make the relation to health and illness evolutionary in every sense except for the unanticipated noise that saturates all conduct. In contrast, Plato's likely story told in the *Republic* requires health and illness to traverse a relationship to self-monitoring and self-reflection in ways that the official history disregards, connecting health and illness to desire through the figure of justice as an aspect of the ever-present relationship to the weaker party (that is, to the unformed or undeveloped aspect of any beginning), whether of oneself, the other or the content, the weaker part for which the paradigm is typically the representation of enigmatic corporeality, whether as a placeholder for self, or other or any commonplace.

Note also that if a proverb abbreviates and in this sense stands as a ruin on the site of an old story, as in Benjamin's terms, then information abbreviates in a way that makes the formula always the issue, that is, the fetish to abbreviate, whether in proverb or information, applying as well to the various clichés and epithets that are celebrated in everyday life in ways that bring to view the problem of strong and weak relations to language, the difference between eloquence and banality. Benjamin's remark suggests that information too, and its tabulations and computations of health and illness, stand as if a ruin on the site of an old story that we might explore. Yet we note how Freud rescues abbreviation from its negative connotations by making it over into a phenomenon through the dream. Thus, it might be more apt to say that any image can be treated as if a formula masking an old story, for this permits us to rethink the very idea of usage and discourse, or of the symbolic order, as a proverbial structure that can only dream its aspiration to overcome its fears through a formula that conceals such a recognition in the gesture of abbreviation. This anticipates a distinction we will discuss in the final two chapters that Jacques-Alain Miller develops from Lacan between the dream of interpretation and the interpretation of dreams.

Seeing-as and history

In the first instance, we who desire to approach health and illness as a topic not only inherit a stock of knowledge as it is said, but as part of such a regime, the ways and means of narrating its story. More explicitly, we inherit a story about health and illness as a *historia* (tale in Greek) that claims to recite the coming-to-be of this matter as an eventful distinction. Since we inherit such a narrative structure almost as if we are its inhabitants, it always seems to us second nature, remaining difficult to objectify and create distance that allows us to develop a reflective relationship to the story itself. To engage the official history of health and illness as the curriculum it seems to offer, we might best conceive of it as if a story told to a child about the ways such matters work and come to be as a collective focus in a society such as ours. We can suggest that the very notion of such a history, with its divisions, continuity, ruptures, defining moments, linkages and plot line, exposes a proverbial structure pointing to a collective imaginary in which health and illness are major characters. From our perspective, the divisions typically represent incremental stages over time (unless we assume ourselves being worse off than what came before), the object of such a history, as difficult as it is to locate, causes us typically to rest our case with medicine. Then, an official history of health and illness most likely would be a history of medicine, and this as one specialized branch of a history of science. If the aimed-for object of an official history is a description of progress in medical knowledge, then this might be what Benjamin calls a (1971, p. 230) "stage prop" for an object of desire elsewhere and otherwise (the surplus pleasure or *object a* of Lacan or the ground animating Wittgenstein's seeing-as).

Here then could be written a history of progress, of professionalization, and of the conquest of disease, a trajectory that might resemble military history in its view of a war against plague and pestilence and, parallel to this, a rising victory over superstition. This history of health and illness would be written as if the reminiscence of the scientist as such a warrior, extolling virtues of courage (crushing old paradigms and risking experimental dangers) and inventiveness (seeing through the past to a new future), a story that brings to view for us the imaginary of medicine in its aspiration to conquer disease that must remain unconquerable despite success rates in curing specific diseases. This story of medicine would then be a tale recounting progress from oppression by nature to a kind of liberation incarnated in freedom from nature, or as the capacity to overcome disease rather than remaining subject to it. In this case, mediation makes reference to the dissemination of the story as a curriculum and how in its construction, it imagines mediation itself, the actor subject to the need to disseminate whatever health and illness seems to mean or imply, and the one(s) to whom such connection is forged.

We can question the limits of this history in different ways, noting first that the story of our relations to health and illness is only officially reflected in the medical version as a history because it has elemental roots more comprehensive than this, a history that, at the most fundamental level, can contest the medical utilization of the image of disease, that is, can contest the ways medicine comes to imagine disease as the recalcitrant object of a military campaign, as a quarry eventually to be captured, rather than as the sign of a recurrent drama in which we are as much the prey as the hunter, reversing the ideal of the mind in hunt of the body (medical progress) by understanding the force of the recurrence of the body, its refusal to be liquidated, as a condition of our sentience, our mindedness. The idea of the recurrence of the force of the body must create for medicine the ongoing problem of needing to explore the symptom of such a return, as if the collaboration between mind and body has to be constantly thought through as a dialectic, almost as an oriented action designed to subvert the medical dream of annihilating disease. In this chapter, we create points of collision between the proverbial view of the conquest of the body by mind and the proverbial view of the recurring haunting of the mind by the body as one way of exploring the relations of health to illness.

It could be said that the official view of the relation to health and illness, using medicine as a stand-in for science, writes a history of the desire for knowledge that leaves unstated the place of desire in knowledge. An unofficial history or likely story that we will imagine in contrast understands knowledge as so intimately connected to desire that knowing anything, in its terms, can only be a knowledge of desire, of the link of desire to claims to know, of how desire is factored into whatever is known or not. This means that such an unofficial history of the relation to health and illness must write about the coexistence of desire and health and illness. Whether for the practitioner, patient or "general run of mankind" (as Descartes [1960] calls the public), it treats knowledge less as a progressive surmounting of obstacles than as a recursive dialectical structure in which the relation of desire to knowledge repeats itself in many varied and specific shapes.

Desire as the inward call

Given the universality of sorrow and being sick at heart, the emergence of science for Max Weber (1958, p. 134) seemed to reflect the ameliorative shape of desire as an "inward calling," fated to be specialized and "imperfect" and yet passionate and devoted to the practice, "intoxicated" by the vision of the consequentiality of this project despite the limits of its every present accomplishment on the grounds that its future "progress" shall repay its present imperfections:

> One's own work must inevitably remain highly imperfect. Only by strict specialization can the scientific worker become fully conscious for once and perhaps never again in his lifetime, that he has accomplished something that will endure. A really definitive and good accomplishment is today always a specialized accomplishment. And whoever lacks the capacity to put on blinders [...] may as well stay away from science. (Weber, 1958, p. 135)

Desire for accomplishments (productivity) can be intoxicated ("for nothing is worthy of man as man unless he can pursue it with passionate devotion" [Weber, 1958, p. 135]). Integral to desire, its passion, is the capacity to renounce metaphysics, accepting the notion of putting on blinders, on making an exception to ambiguity, banning it, in the case of this project, on the grounds of the expectation that it will even out in the end, making visible the operating imaginary of science. Weber identifies the ideal speaker of science as one who can endure and embrace specialization because of its necessity:

> We cannot work without hoping that others will advance further than we have. In principle this process goes on ad infinitum. And with this we come to inquire into the meaning of science. For after all, it is not self evident that something subordinate to such a law is something meaningful in itself. Why does one engage in doing something that in reality never comes, and never can come, to an end? (Weber, 1958, p. 138)

As many have noted, Weber's scientist seems similar to his ascetic Calvinist who answers in his way to an irrational demand, that is, who commits to an objective that must remain irresolute. Here, the Grey Zone comes to view in a primitive way through the gap between expectation and fulfillment, the imperative of being resolute about what is, strictly speaking, unknown. The man of science, his rationality, depends upon such an exclusion. This means that the imaginary of science is tied to the anticipation of the ultimate and progressive calculability of the world ("[O]ne can in principle, master all things by calculation. This means that the world is disenchanted" [Weber, 1958, p. 139]) and we can be both optimistic and in a way resigned to imperfection as a modernized enlightenment version of the second sailing.

If stages of history have to be way stations en route to such an end, then at any moment the fundamental ambiguity of one's project can be called into question without complete assurance, supported only by the *object a* that enters into the creation of the picture of a final resolution. The truth of science, requiring being true to this limited picture and being passionate and devoted to it and the exclusion it demands, seems to Weber the only just way of approaching science and its "inner meaning," indeed showing the difference between truth and the Real, for as he admits:

Who—aside from certain big children who are indeed found in the natural sciences—still believes that the findings of astronomy, biology, physics, or chemistry could teach us anything about the meaning of the world? If these natural sciences lead to anything in this way, they are apt to make the belief that there is such a thing as the "meaning" of the universe die out at its roots. (Weber, 1958, p. 142)

This is curious because the infantile attachment to meaning is both unrealistic and haunting, discernible as it is in the ban that he imposes upon the realistic project. The two sides of the Real introduced point to the reality defined by the practice (the generalized other, the symbolic order), and the Real evoked by rethinking its limits (the difference between little and big Other here being the difference integral in the relationship to the code between the signifier (science) and its signification (natality, spirit, emergence or "ultimate meaning"), between the truth of science and its grounds. Weber both brushes aside (as unrealistic) and acknowledges ambivalence here, the deep source of anxiety in the gesture of "putting on blinders." If the world is disenchanted, divested of magic, then now we appreciate that what is withdrawn is the commitment to conversation into the question of meaning, excluded as a distraction for science and as an infantile legacy of outsiders, those who are not specialized. Now we see that the task of science is not only to resocialize such infantilism in the public and to renounce it in the project and its day-to-day work, but to ponder a history of science that will represent this trajectory of anxiety and hope. Further, we glimpse an opening between scientific excellence (the truth of a practice) and the Good (the end or place of the practice in the whole) in the question that Weber's entire essay poses concerning the difference between the good of science and science as a Good (in life), a line of questioning which he both renounces as infantile (a vestige of theology, personal utopianism, self-indulgence, Tolstoy) and which he takes upon himself to relentlessly pursue as a demand (showing the complexity of the ideal speaker and his fate, the burden of having to ask if the truth of science is enough for life, of chasing this enigma as if his life depends upon it).

Professionalization

Recall Weber's construal of the professional who mediates between imperfect knowledge and an uninformed public in ways intended to distinguish competent practitioner from one who orients to the profession as a vocation (with passion and dedication). This passion is not simply supposed to depict the professional as a workaholic but as one whose dedication to the problematic relation of present to future knowledge is not self-evident and so is potentially a discursive opportunity. Weber implies that the inward calling of such a scientist requires an interest in making this very commitment legible and accountable, a capacity to take a perspective on oneself. One who treats medicine as a vocation desires to objectify its commitment as a way of grounding oneself, of taking a perspective on what one does, asking after its point and purpose for oneself and for the others. In this way, the scientist is driven to make what appears irrational intelligible as a ground of action because of the consequences of the action for himself (his soul) and for those with whom he comes in contact. There is a difference between being excellent in the work, and being governed by this aspiration, and being exercised by the question of the value of the work by which one is exercised. The ideal speaker for the vocation must put into play this very difference as part of the operating routine of the practice. It is this focus that lends the passion. Weber reminds us that if the progress of medical professionalization is tied to technical developments in the specialties, then this applies to the ordinary sense of profession as competent activity because, as a vocation, the profession has a mandate to itself and its own work that, like art, never changes or progresses, remaining the enduring basis of commitment to the application of knowledge.

A vocation is eternally committed to reflect upon the application of its work to the weaker party, to all it is designed to touch and who need and use it. Because the knowledge always remains imperfect, an irony towards its finality and rigidity must be exhibited in representing it in its various guises. If what the vocation finds unavoidable is some dialogical engagement in this sense of objectification, then what this means for the vocation is that its discourse need represent and expose its ambiguity to those who are stunned with sorrow and sick at heart and must orient to the consequences and complications of such influences. Seen as a vocation and so as more than a technical specialty, it appears that the heart of the medical relation to health and illness must be a relationship to suffering and so, a relationship inviting both aesthetic and ethical gestures, and yet as light-hearted in its way, because the experience of suffering can always be understood as centering the afflicted in a manner that is self-absorbing or narcissistic. If the professional tries to recover her voice on each occasion, then the work of the profession strives to overcome this transference relation that seems inevitable between expertise and dependency as a means of hearing the individuality of suffering in the material conditions, giving form to the material condition of the illness by orienting to the way the patient converts the experience into the dependency of affliction, depicting the patient as together with all others as if a type, and yet apart as if singular, in the shape that such suffering can assume in this affliction. The inward calling of which Weber speaks applies to the mutually oriented relation in which the desire to redeem the voice of the patient as part of the treatment gives shape to the professional mandate, the capacity to be engaged by and attentive to the patient's relationship to suffering.

Enlightened discourse

As we will discuss further, Descartes' (1960) methodological recipes were grounded on the vision of medicine as the art whose exploration of causes (though imperfect) should be a model of inquiry to imitate. Descartes made communication and well-being of mankind integral features of adequate knowledge and its dissemination, affirming the test of knowledge in its promise to have such good effects, primarily through its capacities for clarity and exactness. As this notion of clarity develops for the purpose of more effective communication, the contingencies of social interaction, contingencies of application and use, and ambiguities in the interpretation of causes and results (of well-being itself, for example) emerge as problems to negotiate in public life. What is unspoken is the fundamental ambiguity of dissemination.

Unlike the likely story Plato develops, in Descartes the study and treatment of health and illness served educated persons as a model for inquiry in every area of life. In this sense, medicine and its treatment first appear as a paradigm or model, which inquiry can imitate.

> [...] and this is desirable not only for the invention of countless means of enjoying the fruits of the earth and all the good things it contains, but principally for the preservation of health, which is no doubt the chief of all goods and the foundation of all the rest in this life [...] I believe we must look for it in medicine. It is true that what is at present practiced under that name has little that is of any use; and I have no desire to be scornful, but I'm sure there is no one, even among those whose profession it is, would not admit that all we know of it is almost nothing in comparison with what remains to be known, and we might be liberated from a number of disorders, both of mind and of body, and perhaps also from the feebleness of old age, if we had a sufficient knowledge of the cause of these ills [...]. (Descartes, 1960, pp. 84–85)

Here, Descartes comments upon the current inadequacies of medicine. Yet, this does not prevent him from praising its practice as a standard to emulate and for admiring it for its potential rather than its present results. His capacity to discover potential in these results seems truly miraculous, clairvoyant, being able to idealize the practice in terms of what it seems to him capable of becoming if it only could remove itself from its current shackles. The power of medicine resides in its promise to benefit the general run of mankind, and in this way, to offer now a future picture of itself as a perfect, practical art which will acquire and apply knowledge to solve the most important problems of human health. Note, though, that the power of medicine (perhaps illusory in Lacan's sense) depends upon the capacity of Descartes to imagine this promise and potential, to perform this idealization. Perhaps Descartes mirrors the fact that it is a certain kind of society that needs and desires to think of knowledge in such ways, that it is a certain kind of society that needs to believe in knowledge as such, to believe in its perfectibility and in its potential for answering to a promise. Someday medicine will redeem the debt of these current imperfections with which it saddles us and will repay us many-fold for suspending disbelief now. Note that both Plato and Descartes look to the future in their discussions of medicine, but where Plato anticipates the destiny of the relation of medicine to the city to be intertwined, Descartes seems to have faith in the autonomous power of medicine to prosper and grow without respect to the city, yet as a growth that promises to deliver great benefits to the city if it cooperates as a witness to this progress. The necessity of this cooperation reminds us of how the city is envisioned along the lines of those so-called "underdeveloped" or third-world countries who were always encouraged to cooperate in securing the benefits of economic development and economic aid.

The virtue of the art of medicine is that it mirrors the knowledge deemed most desirable by a society imagined as ruled by an interest in understanding itself as a collective in position (and with the luxury) to solve its own problems, the problems that come from meeting to "enjoy the fruits of the earth and all the good things it contains," among which is the preservation of health. We note in such passages how Descartes finds medicine exemplary because of its final purpose or objective in preserving and sustaining the health of mankind. It is this greater purpose that inspires Descartes to communicate the results of his research. In this sense, we could say that dialogue and communication seem to be stimulated by the objectives of knowledge insofar as knowledge that is most desirable, knowledge oriented to the general good, requires those who are its intended subjects to seek to disseminate and communicate its results. In this sense, Max Weber's "valid knowledge" is so-called not only by virtue of its achievements factually or substantively but insofar as it inspires the collective to form itself in assembling to deliberate upon such results. The dissemination of knowledge and its very communicability is a locus of collectivization, a focus of the public life of the city. Indeed, the communicativeness of knowledge is capable of creating a market and of reducing the value of knowledge to palpable and demonstrable criteria, almost as a table of derivates, if sufficient accord can be developed under the rule of a logic of market value.

Valid knowledge creates a public by virtue of this concerted concern for dissemination through which members exchange information about the causes and conditions of health and various ills, in this way making possible the argument that such a vision of communication is itself "good for preserving" whatever is of value for mankind. The stratification implicit in such a social organization between the practitioners and the general run binds those expected to be united under the auspices of this project and only divided by virtue of *techne*, differentiating those who make the knowledge from those who will receive its benefits, creating the expectation that the general run of mankind will be forever grateful for this sustained gesture of selflessness, grateful enough to forswear an oath of fealty to medicine itself. Those who make the knowledge by virtue of their *techne* will earn the right to be called experts and have special access to such knowledge and to exercise rights over its interpretation and application. This view of medicine in the story being told then reinstates its art as the ideal of service delivery caricatured in Plato's city of pigs as an idea resting upon an unequivocal and unquestioning sense of the newsworthy character of any research that is to be disseminated and of the value of the services to be delivered.

Insofar as medicine serves as a model for any body of knowledge, we can understand this picture of enlightenment as one that might inform modern society's interest in self-understanding. In this case the practitioners and the clientele are cooperatively united with respect to the objective of creating knowledge that can be applied to the common cause to enable it to prosper and to enjoy the benefits of life. The link Descartes establishes between knowledge and its application through communication is a process constantly affirmed as the backbone and ideal of any enlightened modern vision of public life and its cooperative exchanges assumed to be ruled by objectives of clarity and distinctness in the exchange.

The voice of the patient

> [...] The obligation to co-operate fully with a therapeutic agency, that is, to work to achieve his own recovery. The rationale of this is plainly that, if he is not motivated to work to attain the conditions of effective achievement, he cannot very well be considered to be motivated to the achievements which require good health as a condition. (Parsons, 1964, p. 284)

The grammar of the sick role by implication identifies the charge of uncooperativeness and negligence as the continuous accusation to which the patient might be subject in the medical relationship. Yet, could negligence not be an opportunity to consider resistance creatively rather than as selfish, ignorant or careless? That is, resistance could be formulated in part as one of the ruses, the strategies and tactics of everyday life that Michel de Certeau (1984) identified through which the struggle of self-formation occurs. The resistance of the patient can take shape, then, in ways which permit us to expand our conception of the uninformed and unformed patient by connecting it to the dialectic of self-formation. Note how this insight is adumbrated in the work of Montaigne:

> I am at grips with the worst of all maladies, the most sudden, the most painful, the most mortal, and the most irremediable. I've already experienced five or six very long and painful bouts of it. However either I flatter myself or else there is even in this condition enough to bear up

a man whose soul is unburdened of the fear of death and unburdened of the threats, sentences, and consequences which medicine dins into our ears. But the very impact of the pain has not sharp and piercing bitterness as to drive a well-poised man to madness or despair. I have at least this profit [...] that it will complete what I've still not been able to accomplish in myself and reconcile and familiarize me completely with death: for the more my illness suppresses and bothers me, the less will death be something for me to fear. (cited in Starobinski, 1985, p. 144)

In response to the Cartesian picture of the patient as an anonymous part of the general run of mankind, as Descartes puts it (1960, pp. 84–85), expected to benefit from medical progress, the voice imagined as the recipient of the good of medicine, Montaigne reinstates the voice of the patient as particular and not only as qualified in one sense to offer a view of his body as the property owner so to speak, but one whose intimacy with his body might just count for something needing to be factored in to the medical imaginary. That is, the patient might be said to have a kind of knowledge in this respect. In complaining about his maladies Montaigne seems to resist the injunction of medicine to cooperate. In some to-be-determined sense, cooperation offends him not because he is simply pig-headed, a bad boy, but because medicine threatens to take from him something that is rightfully his.

Medicine equates cooperation with responsibility itself and attributes negligence to the subject that does not take upon herself the remedial action that medicine requires, attributing to this refusal either obstinacy and sloth or ignorance. Yet for Montaigne, can we not begin to discern here a claim for neglect as something other than either weakness or will but a first position in the economy of self-defense? "In the experience I have of myself I find enough to make me wise if I were a good scholar" (Montaigne, cited in Starobinski, 1985, p. 145). In other words, I could even know myself better than medicine does and could use this knowledge as a way of initiating a refusal that is something other than a sign of negligence. As Starobinski says of these passages:

> Reflection upon failure constitutes an example that I can call my own. In the felt evidence of the present moment, when what is at issue is my own life, my emptiness paradoxically comes to possess the authority that no longer inheres in the authors of the past. (Starobinski, 1985, p. 155)

In other words, my body, my health, belongs to me and I have the right to choose what will be done with it (with me). To put oneself in the hands of medicine is to invite advice, not control, for the life that is an object of such speculation is mine. That this life is mine also means that I am entitled (have the right) to claim intimate knowledge with respect to it, especially in lieu of the fact that the claim of the other to know me is only based upon probability and typification. My not knowing even as compared to the professed knowledge and certainty of medicine now (paradoxically it appears) becomes more authoritative for me because it licenses what could be thought and done about this. Anyone really ill whose identity is infused with the disease knows even in her uncertainty and lack of knowledge that what is claimed to be known by the other has a tenuousness that ultimately cannot grant action with any more authority than what she timidly might propose upon listening to the body that is hers.

When all is said and done, we grant medicine the authority to act but we could also refuse, not on the basis of greater knowledge but because of our intimate connection to and experience with, what is ours, our body. On these occasions, we hear our body cry out, it demands to be heard and we alone can hear it. On the occasion of not knowing, I can risk the action that in exceeding what is known is essentially incalculable, as a solution to distress and its relief.

Here the refusal to cooperate is only ignorant to an abstract observer, for what it says is that action in excess of what is known is not neglectful but rather careful, that it cares for rigor and exactitude because it refuses to cooperate with that speculation that is generic and grounded only on probability. This is to say that this resistance claims to be efficient in its sense of desiring to develop a careful relation to what outsiders prescribe for its well-being because it measures itself by the way the body speaks and the speech of the body can be understood in part as a measure that could influence one who has intimate rapport with it to listen most carefully to any external prescription. This would indicate (unromantically) that the claim to know is always measured by the claim of the body to have a position and to be in position to hear all claims intimately. What is abstract is interference in such self-possession, the right to say and be as we want undisturbed by the expectation of the other. Montaigne says that what is grounded in probability is not known in any particular case because we might need to act in excess of what is claimed in this instance if the claim is not felt as true to oneself. On any occasion, intimate knowledge absolutely requires of a claim to know (abstract as it must be) to measure itself by our sense of its truth for us *and* therefore by our emptiness.

Emptiness originates such an intimate self-engagement, insofar as my knowing for certain what is true of me divests any claim of the element of calculation necessary to it, treating my self as if it is a secure and knowable determinate thing, obvious and transparent to all. In contrast, all we know is that it is mine—to possess and to hold—and that the other is only granted rights by virtue of me. (This desire resonates with Simmel's [1971, p. 197] conception of the Adventurer, where he says of Casanova: "He believes in nothing except in what is least believable.") This is to say that emptiness and so the possibility of going wrong rather than the fullness of self-certainty and of an irrevocable outcome is action that belongs to the self, is the action that is mine, my particular action. The self, in contradiction, can be understood and misunderstood and what is resisted is the preemptory claim of the other to be in a privileged position with regard to that question.

Montaigne's rejection of medicine's presupposition in the refusal to cooperate says that if I am empty of such an obligation, then I am free to act in excess of what is obligatory and so I am free to measure myself by the incalculable consequences of that. Starobinski says of emptiness itself:

> Montaigne's nostalgic wish for the ability to maintain one's health without art (in the technical sense of the word) is undoubtedly related to the need we feel today for an art (this time in the aesthetic sense) that would bring home to us physically the purely pragmatic powers with which science and technology have endowed us. (Starobinski, 1985, p. 163)

This is the sense of inner accord or relation to what he calls the whole that Gadamer (1996) claims of the concealed notion of health that he cites as our real enigma. In Benjamin's (1971, pp. 217–253) sense, this is how the aura of health can be said to erode under conditions of mechanical reproduction, except that the dialectic in Gadamer marks the collision as one between specialization and the progress of the specialized sciences which appear to lose a sense of health as the unnamable against which illness and disease offends. As a stand-in for the whole, health seems to function as the missing whatness that all of this research and enterprise is for, making emptiness the sign of loss for the subject of health and illness. If Montaigne's reaction to Descartes framed the basic initial conflict of modern philosophy, then this response is exemplified in his critique of medicine (Starobinski, 1985). The Grey Zone is resuscitated as the division in the self and the diversity of approaches that struggle to control the means of interpretation.

What Montaigne discerned in the good-hearted progressive spirit of medicine was its intrusiveness, since its claim to benefit mankind and to apply knowledge for the general good seemed to be an extension of its self-interest and orientation to its own empowerment. Montaigne's resistance to medicine can be formulated as his resistance to being dominated by the category of health as a standard that exemplifies adjustment and well-being and to be treated only and exclusively as a type and as together with all members of such a set in ways that seem to him to bury his apartness and stature as an individual. What Montaigne noted was that the need to give oneself to medicine was, on one level, the renunciation of the particular for the general and, at another level, a form of dependency in which freedom and self-governance is delegated to external forces. The symbolic order of health, illness and disease then becomes discernible for him as a struggle for the self-expressed in the dialectic between universal beneficence and the need to affirm the particularity of self-defense that takes place whenever the issue of health and illness is raised.

If, on the one hand, Descartes' picture of medicine as the exemplary body of knowledge stressed the sociality of a progressive society that applies its knowledge in order to overcome the irrational forces of illness, then Montaigne reemphasizes that such progress always threatens to extinguish the particularity of experience insofar as it promises to make it necessary for those for whom the knowledge is applicable to give themselves to the progressive force in a way that could always compel the renunciation of what is special and distinctive of the person. What Montaigne proposes at the very minimum is the need for a discursive relation to the body and its treatment insofar as it is a symptom of an economy of self-formation and self-defense.

The progressive march of medicine wherein it intrudes in order to control and eliminate irrational forces, is sensed as the extension of control, that in spite of its promise of progress, threatens to undermine the social by depriving those to whom it is applied of their freedom and initiative: in this gesture the advance of knowledge is seen as requiring a subject who is committed to a view of her own typicality in a way that affirms the predictability and universality of its classifications at the expense of her particular character and experience.

The need to create a subject for medicine in order to advance its social claim is understood by Montaigne as undermining the position of the person as one subject to health, illness and its instabilities, insofar as it raises the question of what being healthy and/or sick means. That is, the very advance of medicine is seen as creating a problem which Montaigne discerns as the tension in the need to make predictable and typical the medical subject in a way that undermines its capacity for self-representation and for expressing its distinctive experience and initiative as an intimate story of one "stunned by sorrow and being sick at heart" (Hesiod, 1953, I.98-99, p. 56) that is always masked in such a formulaic exchange as a matter of no matter. This struggle for the self is seen to be the true contest implied in the advance of medicine and so an integral feature of the symbolic order of health and illness.

Montaigne's resistance to the medical interpretation of his body was directed to its preemptory claim to know his body best as if seeing the body in one way, the way of medicine, is the only way, whereas his intimacy with the body as his not only disqualifies this presumption but makes it necessary (and not merely possible) to reinstate the discourse around this very problem of seeing-as, whether the body can be seen in one way or the other (perhaps medicine rather than Montaigne) or both at once, like the duck-rabbit, raising the question of what is to be done, how to honor the two as equal parts of one or the one as two, again as the relation of the apartness of each to their togetherness. Montaigne's complaint is that medicine treats him as not having a self, not having a perspective on what he is as if he is comparable to the bodies they treat, mute and empty until invested with life through their practices.

Being real

On these grounds it is easy to refute Cartesianism as ideological. Yet, if the Cartesian affirmation of medicine is part of collective life, instead of dismissing it as mechanical and as the philosophical ground of the biomedical version of the body, we need to understand the lure of Cartesianism in collective life. The *cogito* affirms the desire for certainty which, from a contemporary perspective, seems illusory or logocentric. Nevertheless, it is important to examine that metaphysical aspiration in the life of the collective. Descartes' fear that he could be dreaming and deceived by a malign god, i.e., the evil demon, reflects his need to treat desire as real and the fear released by that condition. The Cartesian dream glosses the desire for eternal life and the fear that such desire masks the movement of the body and so the concern for the dialectic between passion and reason expressed in the anticipation that passion will overcome reason. The fear of deception reflected by the *cogito* recognizes that life is a passing moment vis-à-vis the issue of mortality and that death can always cure enthusiasm. The problem for Descartes is that one needs a watchful, detached observer or to cultivate such an eye oneself. The cultivation of detachment occurs as if alongside the dreamer as a form of a self-observing and self-regulating censor. In this gesture, Descartes proposes as his reflective antidote to the enthusiastic swirl of life and its expectations and injuries, the person becoming, as in a performance, a watchman for himself, being two-in-one in this respect alone, that such self-observant watchfulness can censor the vital and yet unruly pulse of a life. The belief in life as capricious in this way, as a product of the imaginary overestimation of oneself, leads to the result that any wide-awake subject must inflate her self and her capacities, creating the Cartesian fear that, in innumerable mundane ways, one can only habituate himself to complacent justification of his own temptations in ways that will accustom reason to the rule of passion.

The question the *cogito* raises concerns how life can observe and monitor itself, and the intended solution suggests that it can only if life is in position to simulate what it is not, i.e., the eye of death. Life needs to become other than it is in order to observe itself from the perspective of death. Illness then reflects the dialectic between passion and reason, the way in which ignorance is a normal social fact leading to the need for watchfulness as its measure. The *cogito* suggests that reason can only be provoked by emergencies, i.e., by the disruption of illness.

The dream then says that the fear of self-deception is not as inscribed in empiricist epistemology, the concern for mistaking the rule for illusion, as in seeing something incorrectly from the distance (e.g., the bent twig in the water), but rather as a fear of embracing an illusion. It is not illusion per se that is feared, but the destructiveness of the illusion of immortality that underlies the realistic grasp of our mortality and of our unity. This illusion is perhaps our primordial conceit, and yet, as a requirement of life, it always remains unspoken as a seen but unnoticed background understanding, affirming one's own eternal perpetuity as the silent environment of life itself. The ambiguity of this conceit resides in its character as both an illusion and a requirement. In undergoing this deadly mutation the living being is encouraged to return to life by saving it from itself and its self-destructive capacity for excess.

The Cartesian imaginary of death provides for the "real" character of this watchfulness by conceiving of a disengagement modeled after the way in which death itself is imagined in life, as rigor mortis in the original sense of being immune to stimulation. If it is actually the impersonation of death that is designed to save life itself from its voluptuous excess, then this makes the most reflective life the one that strives to emulate being other than itself, being deadly and so "realistic" in this sense (whether through bureaucracy or the split life that goes against its best instincts in order to imitate procedural justice). Here, the paragon of reflection must be the unhappy captain in Melville's (1951) *Billy Budd* who forced himself to sentence an innocent man to death, knowing full well that his guilt was undeserved in particular, except as defined by an infraction of rule. This Cartesian imaginary authorizes medical practice as guardian of the Real, because in making possible life and its illusions and fantasies, its awareness of this imposes upon its own self-understanding its fundamental ambiguity with respect to this border between life and death, this need to be two things at once, healthy and sick, alive and dead, in order to embrace the deadly proceduralism that might rescue the ignorant and error-filled life from itself. What death makes clear is that our moment is a passing instance and so that immortality, despite its needfulness, distracts us from understanding the social form of time as ephemerality. What death also reminds us of is that our social differences, as inscribed in the spatial coordination and differentiation of perspectives which vary, simply mask our fundamental unity or equality. In death, we recognize both our mortality and our equality, our social location in time and space, our ephemerality and unity. Such a recognition tends to be concealed in our commitment to our eternality or immortality and to our uniqueness. In this way, the Cartesian program sets the stage for those various attempts of humans to objectify what is most intimate, programs ranging from straightforward positive methodologies to the strained empiricism of Hume and eventually Kant, always suffering the aspiration of trying to be more deadly than we are, of abstraction from life to the great spectacles of travesty developed in the social sciences where insiders strive to appear outside and outsiders attempt to regain their insidedness in artificially induced gestures of inversion.

As suggested in the *Phaedo* (Plato, 1955), the respect for death releases the recognition of equality, the equality that we suffer when, as Socrates says, our nudity exposes us to our fundamental unity. The story attributed to Solon that a person's life can only be judged after her death not only assumes that death signifies the completion of the story as in the misrecognition that "all the data are now in" in a way that is limited (see Didi-Huberman, 2005, p. 50), as if the capacity of life to change and circulate renders it incalculable because it is unstable, in contrast to its posthumous judgment, but overlooks the fact that the judgment of the dead by the living is done by those who similarly might be expected to circulate in ways that render their evaluations unstable. The vanity of social differentiation as the commitment to difference is masked by the self-deceptive sense of our difference as fundamental, i.e., our irrevocable special and unique character. Forgetting death, then, is not just to forget the decline of the body, but reflects our tendency to overestimate our powers to outwit mortality and to be larger than life, leading us to inflate our moment as eternal.

The species is then marked or stigmatized by mortality and equality, and in this way, life, by inflating our sense of being special—whether our time or place—empowers us with a sense of consequentiality. Because of its materiality, the body's existence in time and space always intensifies the tempting illusion that our present is eternal and that we are special. According to Descartes, the deception of our dream means that our sense of eternality and uniqueness could be illusory. The social actor needs to embrace the position of self-observant watchfulness in order to escape from the closure of its desire for eternity and uniqueness. The method invites imagining oneself as an other who can empty the self through the strenuous artifice of watchful self-observation.

March of medical science

The official history of health and illness (as if a tale told to a child) enumerates the achievements of medical research in ways that are bound to take for granted its emergence by seeing medical advances as if simply goodhearted responses to the recognition of needs shown by the general run of mankind (accomplishments typically treated as the struggles of inventors against forces of reaction). In this story, there seems no place for a recognition of the part played by desire in illness or in its treatment as anything other than whatever emotion is seen to arise in the transaction between producers and consumers united by a kind of causal model. Knowledge is simply whatever is registered as bona fide research at its time, perhaps exhibited in laws, propositions or information, indubitable and without resonance in relation to ways in which it might be oriented to and used in life aside from the imaginary image of simple and robotic application (for example, clichés such as applied knowledge, knowledge transfer and knowledge translation, currently in vogue in corporate circles). The process that is reputed to relate producers to consumers, typified as communication, is thought in terms of the postal model that is imagined to join medicine and its weaker party (its recipients) in ways free of extraneous influences that could be decisive. Specifically what is missing is the notion of knowledge production as socially constructed, of its reception as over-determined, and of the relation of medicine to the people as always already attached through transference.

In the official history, medicine and its resulting research is much like a commodity or good transferred from producer to consumer in ways that make the ethical problem of medicine the problem of a just relationship to the weaker party, into the concern for dissemination itself and for translating research in ways palatable for the public. This ethical problem is compounded by the ignorance and lack of qualification to which the public is condemned by virtue of its need to defer to the expertise of technical specialization, a lack of qualification and an asymmetry that guarantees not only that the practice cannot be engaged reflectively by the outside, but that the quality of service (of the product and its delivery) depends upon a paternalism in which the good will of practitioners as part of their commitment to duty, must lead them to treat their ethical dedication under the rubric of the unstated contract implied in the promise, or the common sense expectation of reasonableness. The fundamental ambiguity of such gestures create as appealing alternatives intended solutions such as the code of ethics administered by the specialty, or utilitarian inventories of consequences and utilities, as part of the strenuous ad hoc forcing of solutions to the question of what is right and wrong action in relation to the weaker party.

Therefore, the primary ethical problem raised by the *paternalistic* interest in justice concerns the best ways of transmitting information to the public, questions of disclosure, restricting the rights of patients and their self-determination, and the grounds under which deceit can be justified as noble. In the best sense, medicine is said to ask how it can convince the public to take care of its own health, by disseminating and making clear and distinct its bona fide research and to affirm an image of the medical practitioner as trustworthy. In contrast, Plato's story represents the tale of health and illness as part of a discussion on justice because self-monitoring is part of the role(s) of doctor and patient in ways that are unspoken and imaginary, dependent upon their mutual openness to one another as problematic objects of desire in a transference relationship between medicine and the people. Plato's likely story shows that the notions of contract, and of promising and prayer (of willing the good), that the official history requires in order to heal its fundamental ambiguity over what is right and wrong medical practice, needs some formulation of the desire for self-knowledge that is glossed by intended solutions such as deontological duty and its renunciation, consequentialism and its utilities, the code of ethics and its attempt to enforce a norm of virtue as reasonableness, because ethics intimates the Grey Zone, or what Wittgenstein (1965, p. 12) calls "the limits of language," as the imaginative structure that grounds this façade and its surface of contestation and free choice.

Plato's city of pigs

In the first instance, the situation of illness might be understood as organized around a sense of trouble and the need to elicit a response to this trouble in the form of relief and/or assessment. The "trouble" to which is referred is meant to cover even happy prospects of childbearing insofar as an interruption of self-sufficiency is required and, with it, the need for relinquishing control to expertise in some shape, passing control of oneself to another. "Trouble" and the social seem to go together here in the sense that any interruption of the fantasy of self-sufficiency is also an invitation to be social (in the limited sense of cooperative) and to open oneself to dependency upon others. Therefore, "trouble" and health and illness need to be understood as cross-referencing incipient steps in a history of desire in which self-containment, self-management and self-composure become topicalized as a strain produced by the appearance of the body as a distraction from which mind cannot free itself. For example, we note in Plato how the force of the body is not a recurrence at all since body and mind are separated only heuristically and abstractly in the official history: indeed, it is the cooperation between body and mind that is the starting point for Plato's history of health and illness, a history not of progress, return and recovery, but of an eternal relationship to desire that repeats and recurs in different shapes and under various conditions: it is never being solved or cured, but its status is a constant opportunity and incentive for reflection.

This conception of trouble directly relates to the division of labor as originally discussed in the *Republic* (Plato, 1945) where the limits of each and any individual are noted as an indication of human finitude and that the dream of self-mastery must be moderated by the realization that no human is capable of attaining self-sufficiency or of satisfying all of her needs. Knowing this is said to produce the cooperative impulse of social life where services are exchanged in the shape of our specialized skills and the products they realize. Though the common bond of money or profit seems to be absent in this rudimentary state, the fact that "trouble" is correlative with the turn to the social always identifies the social as a kind of compensatory gesture, perhaps the first intimation of the force of utilitarianism in social life (but where the utility of the exchange resides in its contribution to our survival). One of Plato's characters called this the "city of pigs," because of the absence of desire for anything more than the exchange of services to satisfy basic needs, and Socrates claims that as long as social life is conceived in such a way, there will be no need for physicians. So the suggestion that the city of pigs is healthy resonates with the notion that desire (and the fluctuations and imagination it brings) is implicated in illness and so also in the turn to medicine. It is not that desiring is sick, but that the risks desire takes in its strongest sense can lead to illness, or to state it otherwise, prudence is healthy because it makes no demands of itself. What this seems to mean is not that there is no doctoring in the city of pigs but that health and illness might be taken for granted as part of the round of life, part of a rudimentary exchange of services and not as a specialty of abiding preoccupation (perhaps similar to the model of the country doctor). With the modern city, the notion of lay doctoring disappears as a profession emerges, a specialized claim to expertise that not only creates dependency but opportunities for trust and skepticism. That such expertise and the need for it grow simultaneously with desire (*eros*) hints at a function of medical practice as a kind of gatekeeper, perhaps overseeing the boundary between mind and body.

So interestingly, the drama of meaning and its ambiguity becomes visible in this uncertain connection of medicine to the city: when social life seems rude, the desire that leads to illness (Plato speaks of spices and luxury) is undeveloped (restrained, under wraps or not yet even discovered as legitimate) and so there is no need for medicine. It is the over-stimulation of desire produced by a more complex city that makes people sick through aspiration and its frustration in ways that risk exceeding their limits and that causes the dependent turn to medicine. The rude and unadorned exchange of services at least keeps us healthy and free from the trouble that arises when our desiring psyche falls under the spell of sociality and values, objectives and criteria of satisfaction that are not necessary, the trouble that invariably leads us to need expertise. Our appetites are basic, and because of this a simple social order united only by the fear of extinction and a kind of neighborliness can prevail. This hypothesis raises the questions, "What is the place of desire in illness and what kind of city is healthy or sick?" Even more, is the city of pigs really healthy, and if so, why do desiring folks want to escape from its mundanity? Note also that the expertise to which we turn include all those sciences that give advice and information on how to stay healthy (nutrition, sustainable environment, pollution) in ways that make such experts two-sided as advocates for progress (as in the newest and best information about the body) but typically and invariably, advocates for an impossible return to the city of pigs.

The *Republic* begins to suggest a relationship between health and restraint, making desire (*eros*) somewhat dangerous, and a tepid social life seem normative. As it is being used, the *Republic* should be taken not as a sacred text but as a provocation. It suggests that the kind of social life pictured in the rude city, the city of pigs, is actually healthy. As the city develops, our desires lead in some way to troubles because we become fascinated by the liberation of the senses that amenities offer (today, instead of the spices, courtesans and couches mentioned in the *Republic*, the amenities might be television viewing, drinking, technologies for modifying, enhancing and changing conditions such as our fatal appearances and even moods, and new and powerful ways and means of extending life or of bearing children efficiently or of eliminating dissatisfaction). In Plato's likely story, it makes it possible to begin to understand how the priority of the desiring modern psyche can always be cited as a resource for questioning our own responsibility for falling ill (that is, we can treat the sick as if they have corrupted themselves by bad choices and habits and that cooperating with medical practice by doing as it says is a right and proper gesture, in the same way that we can view healthy and cooperative patients as good people).

If we begin to appreciate the *Republic* as if Plato's dream work that seeks to represent what is (strictly) inexpressible as a history of desire, this is because it is impossible for us to write a history of desire without imagining its absence (what is unlike desire), and this image is unimaginable for we desiring subjects *en medias res*. The story of desire, necessarily a reflection of desire upon itself, takes it upon itself to imagine death or the condition of the absence of desire for a human subject. Since we have stipulated that the unofficial history of health and illness is commensurate with the history of desire, we are suggesting that the self-reflection upon desire and the history of health and illness are to be seen as parts of a story that can narrate their joint development.

The force of the city

The city of pigs dreams the absence of desire, asking in effect, "What would a city be like under such a limitation?" We imagine the mix of mind and body constituting no special problem because the society divides and collects according to an instrumental model of service delivery, suggesting in its way an exchange of services between specialists and the parts or spheres on which they specialize. Here, it is as if the body could be divided into body parts on which different practitioners specialize, who become by virtue of this, specialists in different body parts. This kind of specialization is not yet part of the medical dream, for in the city of pigs doctoring is a general practice that delivers its services to those afflicted and with such complaints. As we noted in Malinowski's (1955) vision of a simple, elementary society, the basic collision of health and illness involves the confrontation of nature and culture in the old-fashioned sense when the one subject to disturbance and distraction (or illness) tries to decipher and solve the problem by using the resources of local know-how, and failing this, must turn to magic. Plato dreams in the absence of desire that doctoring is a service similar to many others, and as such, is exchanged for other services. If medicine itself seems to lack any special quality distinguishing it from other activities, then medicine as any practice can and should still show an aspiration for excellence in its conduct and thus, there could be a medical ethics, just as a shoemaker's ethics, a carpenter's ethics and the like, the range of excellences particular to each practice. Plato's dream hints that the presence of an aspiration for excellence is not identical with desire, making desire into something similar to and different from the aspiration for excellence, showing that excellence only rules the city of pigs in the absence of desire and so that this difference itself cannot yet be vital in the city of pigs. In other words, the city of pigs does not make a distinction between excellence and desire (i.e., between the good of a practice and the practice as Good or between medical ethics and the ethics of medicine). Plainly when desire becomes an issue in some way and differentiated from excellence, the difference itself must be factored into the story of health and illness and into the story of the city.

In the typical view of the *Republic*, the images of spices and amenities are introduced as if to show the overstimulating character of such externals and luxuries as correlative with the luxurious city. On the other hand, that spices are needed to adorn meals need not reflect an extraneous and frivolous appetite for incidentals but the need to bring out the quality of the food. Spices add to or intensify the meal, bringing out its best, reinstating or reinvigorating the dish as to quality. Socrates' warning that the introduction of spices will require physicians, presumably because people becoming so addicted will fall sick, is the surface of a dream that narrates the origin of human desire, not as addiction or cravings of such sort but as the need for quality and for bringing out the best of things (including oneself). Of course physicians will still be needed because the introduction of human desire (in contrast to the aspiration for excellence) is an animated overreaching of boundaries, an effort to give form to material conditions (whereas excellence remains somewhat privatized in the way of competence or intelligence). Excellence can only be transformed when the difference between the good doctor and the good of medicine, between the generalized other and its grounds, becomes an abiding focus for the ideal speaker who desires of medical competence that it exemplify the Good of medicine.

The history of human desire, marked in part in the story of the second sailing when we engage the surfaces of things and distinctions by demanding more of them, by investing them with potential ennobled as their quality or "best," when we reengage the world as if for the second time by making demands on it in such a way, can only be a story of hope and suffering, for the expectations we imagine and the frustrations that must ensue can only coexist as part of the mix itself, the mix of mind and body registered in the problematic dialectical relation of desire to itself through the mediation of a material environment of objects, distinctions and representations. Here, the introduction of desire recommends that the harmonic relation of parts of the body to the whole body might be disrupted by desire and its reinvestment of the notion of mind with capacities and powers for excess, for demanding more of oneself and of others. Note that such excess and its demanding nature need not apply only to externals such as food and drink and to luxuries as such, but to the relations between specialists who might demand more of one another than simple service delivery, more in the way of "quality" and eventually to relations between doctor(s) and patient(s) who can come to demand more of oneself in relation to the other (for example, medical ethics), and more of the other in relation to oneself (that the doctor treat the patient as a person), or that both make demands upon the relationship to be better than it is, to overreach itself.

In the city of pigs, the absence of desire reflected in the absence of spices is essentially the absence of any drive for quality or for bringing out the best of things, that two-sided desire that produces both health and sickness and the unstable mix of mind and body as a problem to which we constantly attend, monitor and, importantly, heal. In the absence of such desire, the division of labor among specialists administering their specialties with competence and excellence seems to be a healthy city, but for Plato is not a city at all. As he implies, his city of pigs is a pigpen and not a city. The city emerges with the concerted interest in spicing up life, and from within this context, despite the volatile and convoluted mix of mind and body, anything prior or other can only be a pigpen. Another more generous way of deciphering Plato's dream is to say that the model of a privatized division of labor among specialists, exchanging and distributing benefits according to the ideal of service delivery is the pre-political, necessary but insufficient element of a city, always needing more than this, needing the volatility of a public life that could make us sick.

5

The Relationship of Knowledge to Life

Introduction

The relationship of knowledge to life adumbrated by Descartes (1960) was idealized in the example of medical knowledge because that corpus appeared to him to personify what knowledge is, and its practitioner seemed in its way to exemplify the man of knowledge. This imaginative structure was based upon a conception of the use value of medical knowledge, i.e., that it is directed to the most important issue (health, life and death, or whatever). In contrast, for Plato (1945), health, life and death, or whatever, mean very little if we live a dog's life, i.e., if our life is deadly. Thus, we see the ground for a contrast between two different versions of the relation of knowledge to life, one organized around a very contemporary vision of applying information to our round of activities in order to maximize our well-being as inscribed in usages such as health and illness, and the other directed to the question of self-knowledge. In any conception of the relationship of knowledge to life, the contingent evanescence of life is always seen to be intractable to the codification and calculation that could disarm its indeterminacy with any degree of assurance, making of life a continuous relationship to ambiguity in word and deed that can never be reconciled with the finality of mastery in that sense, evoking an image of life and of the social as a Grey Zone (rather than black and white) and of the actor at best as one who must be "subject to this concept and master of its use"(Hegel, 1967), as the ideal speaker oriented to inhabiting ambiguity healthfully rather than fretfully. Thus, if the Grey Zone cannot be eliminated, nor its subject condemned to phallic aspiration, then the subject needs in its way the magic that might empower a healing relationship to ambiguity. Yet, if this remains Plato's voice, we still discern in the Cartesian imaginary the promise of mastering ambiguity through a vision of scientific progress and accomplishments that medicine can be expected in its way to epitomize.

> Every field of knowledge constitutes itself by imagining itself fully achieved by "seeing itself" in possession of the sum of knowledge that it does not yet possess, and for which it is constituted. It constitutes itself

89

then by devoting itself to an ideal. But in so doing it also risks dedicating its object of study to the same ideal; it bends the object to this ideal, imagines it, sees it, or rather foresees it—it informs it and invents it in advance. (Didi-Huberman, 2005, p. 87)

Classic and modern

Note the difference between classic and modern here, for Plato's vision of philosophy as the royal art opposes in all respects the Cartesian image of the exemplary practice of medicine. Indeed, while Plato uses medicine frequently and in a positive way as an example of a social practice, of doing something intelligently, he always uses the practice to exemplify both the power and the limits of *techne* and so, the need for medicine (or any practice) to be integrated in some way with philosophy. Plato acknowledges this asymmetry in knowledge, in the discourse of the master, through his use of leadership or sovereignty as a self-reflective or thoughtful relationship to material conditions which, in his use of medicine, becomes the thoughtful relationship to the body. In other words, Plato uses medicine analogically and not empirically, not as a standard of adequate knowledge but as a way of dramatizing how asymmetry is done, how the discourse of the master is done as a practice. Descartes simply assumes the application of knowledge to life through communication and the cooperative energies it releases, whereas Plato insists that the asymmetry between the producers and recipients of knowledge can lead to many results, whether the tyranny of mastery or the tyranny of servility, unless moderated reflectively in other ways.

Where Descartes accepts without reservation the potential expertise of those who make knowledge, Plato foresees the expertise of the producers to generate a sacrificial crisis unless arrested by reflection. Even more, medical knowledge is conceived in Descartes as information, a body of facts transmitted to cooperative recipients, mediated through a postal model of dissemination between senders and receivers, whereas in Plato, information is a valuable civic resource for chit-chat below the divided line but always at best a point of departure for development, distinguishing and calculation that will invariably remain *aporetic*, unsettled and provocative and not a final solution.

What we note is the withdrawal of human desire from this conception of patient (or of the people), both conceived as a category with generic wants and needs, almost as Milton's "heap of dead bodies" with uniform and formulaic goals and objectives (well being) (Teskey, 2006, pp. 190–192). The city of Descartes similarly loses the edge or its erotic sense of differentness and ambiguity that Plato noted in the very same way that Descartes' mobility and movement among cities without respect to local detail could satisfy for all practical purposes such a one who treats both knowledge and the city generically. The imperfections of medicine that Descartes records are simply aspects of the position of knowledge in relation to technical progress and historical development, for the goals of deciphering the hidden laws of the body and its sequences of cause and effect at any one moment must always suffer the tension between chance and the expectation of fulfilling progress just around the corner.

Can we not appreciate how the imaginative structure animating the relation of the city to health, at least in the texts previously discussed, concerns the relation of the modern to whatever seems to precede it significantly, such as the classical? In Plato, if that relation was fuelled by desire in the sense of coveting more than we need and so, in the *eros* that can be both experimental, liberating and self-destructive, then the descent implied by Socrates in the passage of time is different than the progress Descartes describes, since any and every present destroys and improves upon its past (its "youth" or foundations). Similarly, if for Plato medicine functions in the city as another craft, as an art which in doing communal service still remains subordinate to philosophy, then in the modern city of Descartes, medicine detaches itself from the laity in order to do its communal service, becoming the royal and progressive art that, for all purposes, is philosophy itself. Yet both Plato and Descartes seem to agree that something about modern life, whether it is unchained desire or progress, makes medicine into a specialty, serving and saving desperate persons, and makes the city dependent upon medicine in an altogether unprecedented way. Whereas Descartes' medicine as the exemplary modern art personifies the gain imagined in any present, the increasing perfectibility of time that endows this art and its technical progress with its status as an object of enthusiasm, Plato's medicine can only be a reminder of what we seem in any present to need in addition to *techne*, perhaps a capacity for self-governance. Thus, the modern is interpreted as that essential relationship to the present at any moment that experiences its clock time as exceeded by temporality in ways that cannot be determined and so that makes its fundamental ambiguity as an object of contempt and enthusiasm an unending topic for inquiry. Modernity is tempted into the extremes of either/or overestimating or underestimating its moment as decisive, always leaving space for a reflective relationship to this opposition.

In relation to the great advance registered by Plato in linking body to mind through the figure of desire, an advance forever sealing the fate of medicine to be regarded in such a way even in its gestures of denial, Descartes can only reduce the specificity of any one patient by assimilating it to "mankind" in ways that dissolve the particularity of the encounter between doctor and patient, between theorist and subject, and in such a gesture forgoing an interest in his own desire, the desire of theorizing. The aspiration to emulate medicine, to compare inquiry to *techne* in this sense, is part of the desire to achieve probabilistic knowledge of the hidden causes and, in such a way, of contributing to the corpus of knowledge at this time. The body now conceived as the body of knowledge conceals its special laws from the inquirer in pursuit of its secrets: inquiry imitating medicine, because information as the scarce resource of such a society will forever remain enigmatic in the absence of a methodical and willful desire to simplify our own desire and aspirations, the desire to know more than we are capable of representing with determinate specificity.

The fear of Descartes with respect to knowledge, city and medicine is that at any present in the absence of method or program, life could be arrested, stagnant or at a standstill, and that the search for causes and the computation of probabilities is our only defense against the incoherence of intersubjective human desire. Thus, information is a scarce resource not in the sense that it is withheld from doctors or theorists, but because of its complexity in the same way the mysterious body is assumed as complex, as a corpus of knowledge for use as actionable matter or as data from which we can make disciplined inferences. The scarcity of information is a figure of speech for expressing the difficulty in converting information into laws, a difficulty that emerges as a technical problem to solve in this sort of society.

Here, Freud (Freud and Breuer, 1952) looms as a subversive figure in this interpretive struggle to clarify the social value of information, accepting in his way distortion and/or false thinking as the parameter of any and all encounters. For Descartes, false thinking exists only in and as the tradition and its received ways and means of disregarding the need for adequate method. In contrast, both Plato and Freud exhibit no malice towards error because distortion is the inevitable accompaniment of existence in the world and its imaginary foundation and, as such, is the occasion of beginning in any analysis. It is in this sense that distortion is an incitement to discourse, to working and speaking together, despite its intrinsic ambiguity and inscrutability. In both Plato's and Freud's worlds, what doctor and patient should know is that medicine (and indeed, everything else) begins as a scene of repression and resistance, in which the patient distorts opinion as if it is knowledge and where medicine too tends to inherit a distorted view of the priority of the body. In ways that Descartes cannot seem to imagine, Freud conceives of discourse as if it needs to begin in a spirit of negation that makes demands upon the patient (as in Plato) to show herself, providing us in this way with an elementary glimpse of the subversive relation of theorizing. Whereas Descartes' patients seem faceless, Freud's patients have secrets about which they remain ambiguous, and in this way they always present in the very materiality of the hysterical symptom a divided consciousness in the shape of a split between intelligence and reflection as if knowing more than can be said, an indecisiveness about revelation that can stimulate because its very resistance to recovery intimates what seems most singular, exceptional and intimate.

Desire and knowledge: desire for knowledge/knowledge of desire

What seems missing in the official history is a conception of the place of desire as anything other than the appetite of medical science for productivity and of the receptiveness of the general run of mankind to these accomplishments and so for their own well-being, and a sense of these users of medical knowledge as something other than such a generic category (mankind). Desire must operate not only to animate the achievements of scientists and the survival instincts of possible patients but as an element of the city itself, as part of the structure of an urban imaginary in the way the city could be said to produce a situation in which the subject can see herself and the conditions of her life as an inheritance and as a limit to reshape. Plato's story of the city of pigs reinstates this concern through the figure of justice that depicts the relationship of scientist to general run as fundamentally a relation of leader to follower, conjuring up an imaginative structure relating to expertise, dependency and communication and introducing in its way a notion of the sick and/or ignorant as the weaker party in a manner glossed in the official view, and of knowledge and communication as more problematic notions than used in the official history. Thus the city of pigs replies to the official history by reformulating health and illness as an image that collectivizes society through its aesthetic force and through its ethical demands, bringing the relationship itself under the jurisdiction of art and law in ways intending to question the claims of *techne* and specialization to be the *sine qua non* of the relationship to health and illness. The city of pigs counteracts the official history by bringing to view the way it represses the divisibility of such notions of desire by reducing it to productivity and its works and of the subject of medicine as simply one in trouble, a survivor needing and wanting help to relieve distress, affirming in this way the indivisible character of the march of science, and the authoritative claim of its spokespersons to know what this other lacks, anticipating in this way the model of knowledge translation which our contemporary policy-makers and administrators now celebrate.

In its way, the city of pigs poses as an explicit concern the question glossed in the official history concerning the relation of desire to knowledge. This means that medicine needs to understand itself as something more and other than a *techne* since it deals with those who are "sick at heart and stunned with fresh trouble in the mind" (Hesiod, 1953, I.98-99, p. 56), i.e., those who are subject to the instability of desire and the interaction between infirmities and incapacity upon self-understanding to and for all concerned, and who, in this relationship to such trouble, must participate in ambiguity in ways that are irresolute, making suffering both of the afflicted and of those who witness and care the focal point of treatment, mobilizing the question of desire and its status as the centerpiece of the relation to health and illness, and thus dramatizing the unstated ethical implications of any relationship to sickness.

If desire is assumed as indivisible, as directed to the goal of productivity and the creation of works, then this is reflected in the official history of science as a succession of paradigms, each in its way as partial but capable of adding up to a vision of finality that can be anticipated in any present. The ideal of paradigm reflects the official view of the place in history of any present, abstracting and idealizing the need of a science to exercise violence upon the common culture and its so-called frame of reference, displacing and condensing these terms and conditions as part of the wayfinding of science in and for the collective as it locates itself and its environment with respect to change and history, defining the fundamental ambiguity of life in terms of the continuity of change, and so of necessary revision and alternation of the speech of any present. The scientist, as such an actor, is subject to history and its pluralism in ways demanding an enlightened commitment to any present as a stepping stone towards an imagined resolution of ambiguity and so as one who dutifully suffers the full weight of renouncing absolutism in the service of a historical consciousness. The idea of paradigm, derivative upon a notion of the narrative continuity of history despite its fluctuations, conceives of nature as disguising itself in the changing appearances that different stories (paradigms) represent, each story showing the prejudices that inspire it, creating the expectation that the succession of stories fashioned over time approximate what can be known, making any present partial and every view revisable.

Thus, the official view identifies the coexistence of ambiguity and life not as internal to the word and deed but as external in the way that social change, due to revisable material conditions, is assumed to influence changes in views and so different paradigms, making history a succession of viewpoints (and errors) and the subject of history, the historical man, the one who knows that, though every paradigm is a lie, the lies can add up to a truth: the truth of self-knowledge is the knowledge that everything is a lie. The official view of science, identifying the symbolic order with the usage of paradigm, shares with Hegel and Lacan this sense of the equivalence of deceit and construction with one important qualification: the paradigm does not provide for how it can escape self-cancellation by putting its own closure at risk, how it might risk itself through interpretations that begin to challenge that border by bringing to view the ambiguity of desire in ways that could destabilize its terms and conditions, the putatively self-destructive *jouissance* that can disrupt any paradigm when its status as an ambiguous object of desire is made transparent (see Stengers [1997], who discusses this limit and opportunity for science). If such desire in the official history is identified with the figure of historical man (Nietzsche's [1956] "cold demon of knowledge"), then the city of pigs can be understood by restoring the balance to that figure by disfiguring this relationship to desire. Furthermore, if the march of science progresses, then what is repetitive and recurrent is the indefiniteness of any such achievement and the anxiety over its application to life that persists as the remains of its irresolution.

Specialization and excellence

Note some of the problems in a city in which specialization is the trope of desire and the stratification of excellence the basis of a good society. First, the division of labor as such occurs in response to our human limitations, the fact that no one is self-sufficient in the way of comprehensive mastery. Self-sufficiency is only possible if each one cultivates some advantageous innate ability to bring out his excellence. So the desire to be self-sufficient operates under such conditions and as such is conditional, and yet within its limits, self-sufficiency can be achieved as a kind of autonomy with respect to the part one develops. This means that the desire for mastery is not dead and it gets transformed into a notion of autonomy and control of one's specialized domain in ways that lead such a vision of expertise and competence to become the *sine qua non* of mastery. This leads to the self-conception of man being the king of his castle as equivalent to the idea that man is the master of the universe. Durkheim (1938a) claimed that the organic solidarity binding different specialists under such conditions need not be seen as an amoral situation leading to a war of all against all, but as cooperative at its core and so as a moral order. In this city, goods are exchanged between specialties and, assuming that everyone is a specialist in something (that no one is excluded), it is to be expected that all needs and wants can be satisfied through reciprocal exchange. In the city of pigs, if cooperation is the *sine qua non* of the ethical relation, then the just distribution of medical beneficence can be expected to be directed exclusively to the cooperative recipient in ways that should cause us to ask after the status of cooperation as such.

Excellence at a specialty is not indivisible, and yet in this city such excellence is assumed to be embodied in the practice as if it is a stock of knowledge handed down or in circulation among those who seem fitted for it. The very basis of such specialized excellence (carpenter, baker, ship captain, doctor) might not rest on innate natural abilities but rather upon *fortuna*, legacy and the like. Secondly, excellence in the specialty cannot be assumed to be self-evident and surely is contestable among those even best qualified to practice carpentry. There must be dispute over excellence within the coterie of the excellent, within the guild. Third, assuming an equality among excellences is problematic, because as excellent as is the carpenter, he might not be qualified to run the country or even his family (in other words, excellence must always be supplemented by a reflection on the form of that to which it is applied if we are to be able to discriminate between excellences). As previously noted, the lack of an external reference point to specialized excellence means that any specialization can only be self-regulating since the "outside" is condemned to be unqualified and ignorant. But then again, the unqualified is not an indivisible category and as such, is always qualified in some way to speak to and about the subject matter, showing even for the expert, that there is some limitation on saying whatever is thinkable (the demand of the "life world"?).

We have noted how the absence of any sense of a collective project (the omnipresence of the inarticulate experience of *das Ding* in Lacanian [1992], the withdrawal of the transcendental in Girard [1977], the ineffability of the "there is" in Levinas [1987], the fact that Being has many senses as in Aristotle [1966], the inability to imagine an interlocutor to difference, the prosaic idea that totality is always a partial social construction) can appear to make specialization the only reasonable option in a city, not because of the lack of any innate foundation of value, but for Plato's reason that no person is self-sufficient and capable of satisfying all needs, or really, is capable of knowing everything. It is this limitation of knowledge correlative with the finitude of the human being that serves as the proverbial ground of specialization as an attempt to rectify this "loss" of wholeness (which is not a lack but is as it is unless we assume its falling short of some standard that is external to it, and is not a loss because it was never possessed as such). Even if differences in abilities are not innate, the idea that the most reasonable or efficient method allocates abilities to specialties according to a theory of best fit simply rationalizes inequities at the start. Here, it is assumed that each person, in cultivating his own part, could be expected to excel in that part and no other, still producing an arrangement where his products could be both high in quality and exchanged for one another so that no one need suffer from lack or deprivation (except possibly those who cannot be reconciled to any such fit, those beyond the pale of any apparent ability). Imagining a social order of souls abandoned to themselves without recourse to anything other leads to the depiction of a collective populated by resourceless and defenseless atoms whose fate remains external and outside of their hands (see Arendt's [1951] description of the masses in *Origins of Totalitarianism*). In a social order where everyone is abandoned to their own specialty and a sense of wholeness seems lost or absent, the whole becomes specialization itself and its promissory structure, first of excellence in each specialty, i.e., the promise of cultivating excellence, and then, as a prospect of fair or reciprocal distribution, the dream that each will exchange with the other and that such needs and propensities will work themselves out. Thus, there is an obvious problem of achieving social order in a collective where the sense of the whole is absent, the Hobbesian problem of war of each against all that Parsons (1937) formulated as the social order problem. At the most prosaic level, this is simply the problem of making a place for impartiality in a collective in which partiality rules the subject, is the law of the land, a condition we recognize from time immemorial in the figure of circularity and how its tautological structure appears to make any solution that claims impartiality necessarily external and abstract.

Fascination

Each specialty remains fascinated by the *techne* of every other in ways that produce the dependency that distracts the specialist's sensitivity to Other, making possible the non-specialist's experience of outrage because her assumed lack of qualifications disqualifies criticism as ignorant. The specialist's offer of choices in formulating alternatives for the non-specialist attempts to bridge this gap, but the structure of the relationship creates a regime in which re-socialization and dependency, deference and expertise, define the legitimate and permissive moves in ways that must exclude criticism as necessarily unqualified.

Yet there are more interesting tensions inherent in such a city based upon the principle of specialization as an effort to compensate for the absence of wholeness. To prevent

Hobbes' war (1994), or the turn to referee, sovereign or umpire, the typical proposition of self-regulation through a code of ethics administered by each specialty has always seemed fatuous and dependent upon arbitration that is necessarily problematic and interested itself. More relevantly, we note first that the original distribution of different aptitudes is socially fashioned insofar as prior to their official cultivation as specialties, aptitudes are nourished, formed, given advantages to and disfigured in many ways according to luck, *fortuna* and local detail (family), that make all abilities seem not just beginnings but results of much socially organized work. (This is one of the implications of the myth of Narcissus, who suffered the fate not simply of self-love but of being over-praised.) This is only to say that the notion of aptitude is not indivisible but itself an object of desire to and for interested parties, creating endemic grounds for tension at the beginning of any process of social selection. Secondly, given the identification of those qualified to specialize in certain ways, the cultivation of excellence in the baker, shoemaker, ship captain or physician, is not a self-evident matter but must remain a fundamentally ambiguous locus of concern among those specialists who are related by the task but who differ in their views, always grounds for the rivalry Girard depicts as the sacrificial crisis released among those whose relatedness (e.g., to the specialty and its demand for excellence) still must easily dispute just what is and what is not excellence: just think of academics or of the argument over the decline of craftsmanship in any specialty. Finally, assuming the specialty as if a guild that can agree upon such a notion officially, the question always remains as a vexatious issue in the public life of the city as to how the various and different excellences (specialties) stand in relation to the city (the question of stratification) in ways that inevitably fertilize dispute over the allocation of resources and the ranking of such practices in relation to the hypothesis of collective purpose or a common good. For reasons such as this, the city of pigs cannot be expected to solve the social order problem (as in a medical cure) except with strenuous ad hoc devices, but can bring to the surface the fundamental instabilities it harbors at its core, tensions we have only begun to enumerate in the most apparent and concrete ways through the proverbial sociological conceptions of inequity, rivalry and stratification. However, this does suggest how any city at its core is a city of pigs (plagued by the normal wrongs of inequity, rivalry and stratification), always giving cities aspiring to be more than this (cities desirous of being true to urbanity as such) the opportunity to rise to the challenge of healing by giving form to such material conditions.

Excellence, expertise

Most important, excellence is not the Good, though it seems to epitomize the highest reaches of value in a city that has forfeited a robust sense of the Other, that has renounced any sense of an omnipresence more weighty than interaction. The desire for excellence in a specialty as the desire to be good at it or to be the best says nothing about this excellence as good, that subject matter or whatness of the specialty that makes it what it is and not something else, capable of showing how this end of what it is and does is something good in the way that the quality of any activity reputed to be an art rather than a knack (the cook, soldier, arguer, artist, professor, baker) must at its best provide for the relation of excellence to a discourse reflecting upon its extreme and moderate positions, must provide a way of thinking about the conditions under which excellence itself may be good or bad. Being the best at something neither says that one's ability is good (the judges might be ignorant), or that what one is best at, the field of application, is of any matter or makes a difference (the activity might be shallow, frivolous or even evil). This unstated dimension of the dedication to quality always masked by the concrete fixation upon excellence is needed to be made explicit in order to transform competence into a more powerful notion. For example, what is missing in the city of pigs and its distribution of specialties is some notion of excellence that includes a relationship to its content or subject matter that could redefine the relationship to the activity, or provoke the collective to rethink its relationship to the activity, or to relate reflectively to the circuit between its production and consumption as more than technical. This does not mean that the specialty need be defined in a doctrinaire or ideological way (regarding its good as its consequences or utilities), but that it is engaged reflectively in relation to its quality of being made and the care and concern exercised in the specialty. In this sense, the subject matter of the art is always at the mercy of the violence of the specialist who is free to do whatever to its material in the name of excellence, inviting in this way any reflective approach to orient to such diverse voices as its unstated discursive ground.

Excellence, then, need not be simply technical proficiency whose benefits are transferred to the ignorant non-specialist but a more forceful intervention somewhat like teaching in which the non-specialist (the ignorant) is engaged or moved to develop a stronger relation both to the specialty and to its subject matter, perhaps by taking initiative for influencing its redefinition in some sense. Yet, in the city of pigs, in condemning the non-specialist to ignorance by virtue of the rule of specialization, the specialist forfeits any dialogical engagement to those outside of the specialty because they must remain ignorant and so unqualified to engage with the specialist except as those who are illiterate. The excellent doctor must be a specialist who cannot on his own ground risk putting his excellence into question because no one other than he and his circle seem qualified for such an engagement.

This does at least three things: first, it separates excellence from the good of a practice by limiting it to expertise, to a monological structure that is basically homoerotic (insular, closed) and is only capable of prejudging dialogue as unqualified or irrelevant. Second, such a specialty has no ways of discriminating its own expertise (for example, in surgery) from any other except on external grounds such as repute or prestige (i.e., it cannot talk about what it is that makes surgery good in a way that is different from another specialty that is similarly excellent) or about what distinguishes excellence in surgery in relation to the many varieties of practice that can fall under its name, such as what makes a good surgeon other than simply being able to *do* surgery (the question of the form of a specialty). And third, the excellence of a specialty as its expertise inexorably comes into collision with its concern for the weaker party but in a manner typically identified in the city of pigs as a dispute between standards and leniency, as if excellence always has to defend itself against gratuitous demands for civility or bedside manners, since the concern for the weaker party is understood as external, decorative and peripheral in relation to the high quality concerns for excellence. The relation to the weaker party means that this undeveloped notion of excellence (that we think of as empty or weak by virtue of its automated acceptance and use) needs to be explored, brought out and topicalized with a view to its strengthening. Thus, in the city of pigs, justice is an afterthought because desire, limited as such to expertise, can only make the unqualified outside into the general run of mankind, those sad and ignorant laymen who need technical assistance. In the last chapter of this book, this notion of the relation in connection with the discourse of mastery will be discussed, as well as Rancière's (2009b) conception of dialogue and his use of the figure of the ignorant schoolmaster to personify resistance to such a pedantic conception of knowledge transfer. One might say, using Plato's *Republic* as a model, that the city of pigs describes a pre-political, pre-dialogical situation of action as a limiting case of justice (an antidote to tyranny perhaps, that is treated as good simply because it is not atrocious, as was Mussolini, whose badge of excellence was reputed as making the trains run on time) that takes its bearings from a notion of desire as adaptation to conditions (in Arendt's sense, to the condition of laboring under abandonment). To aspire towards excellence at what one inherits (aptitude or ability) is perhaps one way of making the best of the condition as such. In other words, as compared to the attitude of resignation that accepts being determined as a fateful lot in life, one might treat whatever condition that is inherited as choice-worthy, as if chosen, by aspiring to excel at it (by making the best out of it).

The introduction of spices in the city of pigs means that the status of desire changes as the question of quality shows a two-sidedness around the relation of excellence to the Good and so, of the relation of body to mind. The split in the original experience of *das Ding*, the split in the Good itself, means that there are many relationships to what is just, and so there are varied and diverse ways of understanding not only relations to the weaker party but the self-monitoring that need be factored into that as a feature of our relationship to our own weaker part(y). Spice makes excellence into something to bring out as more than competence but as doing something well, doing it so as to bring out the best in the subject matter. As we said, the relation to health and illness, as both legal and aesthetic, only confirms over and again the ethical nature and its theater of dramatization in the city.

To this point, this text has suggested that a hypothetical unofficial history of health and illness links body and mind through the figure of desire in a way that creates a contrast by disfiguring such a standard in constructing the city of pigs imagined in Plato's *Republic*, a city modeled after specialization rooted in technical excellence, seeming unable to comprehend such a link because of its governance by a standard of market value or exchange. In this city, the difference between such specialized practices is a distinction between knowledge and ignorance, each and any excellent practice being distinguished from the others by virtue of this stratification of knowledge in which everyone knows just one thing and is ignorant of all the rest, creating a dependency of each upon the other and its knowledge which they lack commensurate with the differential excellence of each. This limitation of excellence makes it impossible to criticize any practice from outside since criticism can only be ignorant and unqualified, making necessary an externalized version of professional ethics as self-regulation. In the city of pigs, the division of labor regulated by specialization that is technical and so, by a limited knowledge of the body (limited in this sense to *techne*) can be self-correcting in only a specialized sense and a rudimentary Grey Zone can only be glimpsed in the confrontation between producer and consumer, but in a way with little weight since consumer satisfaction or dissatisfaction has to be unqualified because it is basically ignorant (non-specialized). In this city, the specialist and the other cannot thoughtfully engage one another because the specialist can be expected to have no respect for the ignorant, and the ignorant can only sulk resentfully at her exclusion since, lacking any apparently justifiable grounds for grievance, each specialty must obey each other's specialty mechanically. In this sense, no specialty, regardless of its excellence, can be expected to listen to another or even to itself since there is nothing other to specialization and its exchanges and interactions, no conception of a whole (for example, of Lacan's [1981a] L schema). In the *Republic,* Plato proposes that with spices (desire, quality), the problem of monitoring the relation of body to mind is redeemed as central to health and illness.

Before the introduction of spices, excellence in any practice must be defined by the city as such in terms of the standard of market value that confers legitimacy upon any specialization that participates in an exchange meant to give the interested parties what they value. Value, apparently commensurate with what is conceived as lacking and needed, is typically that which one cannot produce for oneself. The aspiration to bring out the best of the activity can refer only to the need for its rethinking, taking its reputed excellence as a point of departure, an excellence insular in its way because it is closed to criticism by those who cannot practice it, and who are, therefore, assumed ignorant with respect to its quality. The introduction of desire brings not only expectation and frustration but discordance and resentment with respect to the quality of what is delivered and the limits of its reputed excellence. For our purposes, the introduction of desire must be the advent of genuine politics, of the *polis,* as a cacophony of differences and contentiousness collectivized by the spectacle of market value as the focus of public life.

Ostensibly a work on justice and the city, the *Republic* introduces the body into this mix as its way of centering the problem of justice as one of monitoring desire. It has been noted that the city of pigs identifies the weaker party in relation to any specialized practice necessarily as ignorant in a way that cannot provide for any reasonable method for limiting the specialty since it always has the last word in relation to the other whom it is supposed to serve. But then again, service is only a kind of provisioning rather than an exploration of what is of quality. In this sense, Socrates seems right to recoil from Thrasymachus' contention that justice is in the interests of the stronger party, but as Glaucon shows, this is not enough: for example, Socrates is the stronger party in relation to Thrasymachus (he refutes him and wins the argument), but he does not show that arguing is the Good (I.III. 336b–347e, pp. 14–29). That Socrates is an excellent arguer does not show that arguing in his way is the best kind of approach to dialogue. In this example, Plato provides a way of approaching the Grey Zone as a split in the whole, recognizable as a split between excellence and the Good, that being excellent in a practice does not confer excellence upon the practice.

If the introduction of spices means that the city is the site where the difference between excellence and the Good is dramatized as if a spectacle of public life, then this suggests that the existence of the city is intelligible as an array of such differences, of activities in pursuit of excellence in a way that makes such a pursuit the very topic of public life and consequently makes variation and the distribution of advantages and disadvantages, of just desserts and undeserved *fortuna,* a continuous and abiding topic. Given the inexorable split between the stronger and weaker party in the city of spices, such a condition appears as a material fact always needing to be addressed. We see that this condition reinstates the asymmetrical character of any beginning discussed as the discourse of mastery, that the opportunity to give form to this material condition of life, in the stratification accruing through the conditional character of existence and the constant experience of inequality visited upon us by the difference between good and bad conditions, sets the stage and serves as the context for the public life of the city. Now we might appreciate how the introduction of spices in the city of pigs is Plato's way of addressing the need for an aesthetic relation to material conditions in the city, the political implications of such a mutation for self-knowledge, education and justice. Note throughout how this formulation reveals the weaker party as a figure for "weakness," as the undeveloped beginning that stands as the unformedness and potential latent in any such moment, the indefinite and multitudinous capacity of what exists (much as the empty speech) that appears always and essentially in its most immediate aspect as vulnerability. This discloses how a collective begins to show its singular character through its relationship to vulnerability in ways that include speech, bodies and selves, bringing such aptitudes together as a way of understanding what it is to take a perspective for any subject, whether individual or collective.

The redefinition of ethics: applying knowledge

We see that the ethics of medicine as distinct from a notion of medical ethics can be understood as a mutation from the endlessly circuitous contestation over right and wrong practice exemplified in debates ascribed to the conventions of ethics and its wrangling over the permissible limits on medical intervention and discretion, on patient autonomy, restrictions of medical prerogative and the like, as questions that could only be settled by authoritative fiat, by self-monitoring tribunals administering codes of professional ethics, or by attempts to enforce norms of medical reasonableness. The problem of all such solutions, including the Kantian recourse to duty and obligation that Lacan satirizes as an ethics of pain and renunciation, is that each and all remain monological since notions of specialized expertise condemn all outside of the specialty to the lack of qualification of ignorance, effectively undermining their claim to criticalness. What is transformed is the liberal version of ethics as organized around the problem of reconciling the rancorous disagreements released by plurality, or rationalizing the place of authority in a collective dedicated on face value to egalitarianism, or the problem of explaining the need to infringe upon the rights of others in ways that hurt the perpetrator more than the injured party, the countless anomalies released by the historic conception of the insularity of the so-called open society (Popper's [1971] society that is closed to reason) and the Grey Zone displayed in its need to be closed (Agamben's [1998] "ban"). This leads to the proposition that the enlightened ethical solution to the insularity of medicine has to be directed to overcoming the ignorance of the unqualified layperson by making medical knowledge public, i.e., by making it palpable and accessible to the public. If at first this imagines a direct dissemination of medicine to the patient, and later, because of public indifference, a process of transmission of data on medical decisions to medical practitioners as middlemen as in evidence-based medicine (EBM), then this process of service delivery, now designated as delivering knowledge, could apply to any such recipient. The internet has the capacity to make all medical information and lore EBM. In this way, the hierarchic relation of producer (medical science) to user (patient and physician) frames the end point of such a process in which the ethical relationship correlative with medical practice (and perhaps with all teaching and knowledge) is defined as service delivery through rubrics such as translation, transfer and application. This redefinition has a number of implications for the Grey Zone of medical knowledge. In this way, the notion of dissemination is capable of redeeming the ethical question as connected to the age-old problem of the use value of knowledge or of the relationship of knowledge to life in ways that mark any knowledge (philosophy, art, literature, politics) as a circuit of influence capable of being conceptualized as idols, as goods, as a lore or body of know-how, as sacred or profane distinctions, but always as a curriculum to be invested or not with value, to be open for revision, exploration and innovation or to be treated with distrust, indifference and skepticism, revered or even vandalized as the case may be.

Knowledge translation, ever more than the simple process idiotically abbreviated as KT today, can only appear as a complex dialectic, bringing into relief, besides the problem of curriculum and its complexity, the divisibility of the notion of communication, its media and reception, and indeed, the relation forever problematic of those mediators who must intervene in the process to reshape whatever is disseminated in ways that do justice to all who are touched by it.

Market value: knowledge as a derivative

The idea of a derivative in finance defines the value of something by virtue of other variables derived from it. The most popular derivative in our kind of society is the way a person's income or position is said to measure her value. Thus, being a doctor confers value upon a person accordingly in ways that establish quality by implication. In social research, the notion of a concept-indicator relationship expresses this well since any and all attempts to establish an independent value for a concept are reputed to rely upon implications or measures assumed to reflect its meaning (indirectly) in the way that the existence of the state is reflected in indicators such as military conscription, law, paying taxes and the like, or a good person is measured by how many others say of her that she is good. In all such cases, meaning that lives by implication in this way (by virtue of conventional imputation) acquires its status as a value indirectly in ways that might always be contested, protected as it is by the limits of a symbolic order that authorizes a certain parochial version of seeing-as as authoritative by fiat. The symbolic order is then governed by a logic of the derivative that serves to stabilize and give form to human relations to the unknown and to ground human desire, grounding relations to groundlessness.

In our society, this shape of Grey Zone is typically recognized in the ways various indicators assumed to measure value (whether of a person or of anything else) depend upon what Lacan calls an *object a* (1997) that supplies tacit coherence between concept and indicator. If market value confers such status on whatever is assumed to be desired (purchased, wanted, consumed), then the value of a person could also be defined derivatively by wages, awards, marital status, type of spouse, length of life and the like. Statistics runs according to a logic of derivatives where inferences are justified on various grounds to establish meaning (as when, in the recent U.S. presidential election, a TV pundit said of people who responded to an exit poll question on whether race enters into their vote and who reported that it indeed, in fact, did not, accepting the derivative self-report as if it was direct confirmation). Health and illness must be approached as such derivatives through the apparatus of testing that define these concepts by scores and index values. The logic of derivatives grounds not only testing in medicine but regimes of healthfulness and calculation of risks in the way that unpredictable outcomes, side effects or complications can be treated as aspects that both belong to an action and indirectly follow from it.

Perhaps the clearest idea of knowledge as a derivative refers to how it can be used or understood. Knowledge that is useful is assumed to stamp knowledge as valuable. But knowledge itself cannot be defined directly and relies in its way upon reference to a derivative that establishes it as such, for example, in ways that regularly disqualify novels, painting, music or stories as knowledge, but do confer such value upon information. Indeed, the derivative of utility probably enters into this very relationship, establishing knowledge as what it is by virtue of its claim to being useful in the way that these other genres might not be assumed to match. For example, a model of knowledge might be provided by a set of instructions for assembling a household object or a children's toy, where instructions are taken as a derivative of knowledge, or following instructions as a derivative of application, allowing only knowledge that is guided by such a format to qualify *as* knowledge, defining knowledge by implication of such a derivative (which itself seems to depend upon the assumption that following instructions exemplifies useful application). In the case of knowledge, a market for derivatives (useful knowledge) is typically created through the administration of granting agencies that award applications in ways that give value to the proposed research through the awards that establish the value of research by implication of various mechanisms of response (voting and other types of decision-making); in the same way, derivatives such as publication define the work in ways that rarely can make problematic the relationship itself (for example, peer approval as a derivative of a successful application becomes an issue in cases of bias, corruption, conflict of interest, etc., and not when the mechanism itself is challenged, for example, the belief in peer approval *as* a derivative). As we said earlier, the power of peer approval as an unquestioned staple is itself made possible by the insularity of a city of pigs that can discover no qualified "outside" to the specialty (in contrast to the nightmare of Socrates' trial or of a tribunal of administrators or a committee of barbarians).

We suggest then that if the introduction of spices makes possible a concerted fascination for the question of quality and desire as a focus of the public life of the city, then this question which *seems* to become conversational according to the rule of a logic of derivatives always needs to be challenged and uprooted to give form to a genuine *polity*. This is because a logic of derivatives, grounded as it is in market value, by only allowing us to address what is countable (the indices or derivatives) must leave out the uncounted part, that encounter with the value (meaning) of an eventful distinction that cannot be apprehended directly (that "exceeds all signification").

6

THE CITY OF PIGS AS TRAVESTY

Introduction

Travesty appears as a strategy of subverting the pretense of objectivity in a description by disfiguring what it claims to describe through an exaggeration meant to mirror this object as if a scene, in a reflection revealing in the smallest details a difference between what is inessential and essential, as if the scene itself is designed only and exclusively to exhibit this secret. Travesty treats any description as if it is oriented to be exhibitionistic in this way, responding as if an audience engaging this scene by heightening its theatricality and artifice as its manner of enjoying the pleasure of pretense in any such performance. Travesty then forces any description to be a story about the imaginary, concealed in and by the action, and a forewarning about the requirements its symbolization creates for any subject who would live according to its rule, directing the dialogue over implications to the ambiguity of irresolution and its problem-solving that any description must leave unspoken. Travesty is then intended to show the inevitable instability of any description as it becomes visible and operational when life as such is construed as the field of performance in which the description must test itself by imagining living a life under such auspices (of the description) as if a course of action. Travesty exaggerates the description as if a scene of action inevitably fated to suffer the implications that it excludes, disregards or makes unambiguous, as if riveting rather than inconsequential trials and tribulations of ambiguity that are shaped in ways specific and singular in relation to the topic.

We can discern the seeds of the notion of the Grey Zone, reflected again in the subject's position in-between, not simply as linked to space or time but to the two-sidedness that comes from the speaker being spoken (again as if two-in-one), that connectivity between speaker and what she speaks about, subject as objectified to and for oneself as in language, and object as oriented, as a relationship in language, reflected most visibly in the figure of the signifier or term as an object of desire that exceeds determination. One could venture that the most concrete appearances of the notion of the Grey Zone occurs, especially in the social and natural sciences, in the usage of the observer as part of the field of observation, and the various images of circularity, and of the infinite regress that such recommends. This formulation of mediation through the figure of the circle makes possible different imaginary relationships of the insider to objectification, exaggerations of the necessary two-sidedness appearing immediately in the reinvention of travesty. This chapter explores various ways in which insiders try to feign an outsideness in representing the interior of collective life that they routinely inhabit and to which they must reconnect their intimate and recognizable senses of the inside, gestures taking shape in the diverse performance of objectification and its ritual structure, seeming to follow from the imaginary efforts to reconcile the vital sense of the division of *das Ding*, in impossible but necessary strategies of reconciliation. The city of pigs is a paradigm of travesty, recommending the relation to health and illness as if a systemic exchange of services modeled after some vision of the organization of the body and its distribution of parts, the need to deliver services efficiently and to ban discussion of the ambiguity of what is produced (health care) and of the distribution of services (quality, efficiency) by taking exception to criticism and dialogue by conceiving it as unqualified and untouched by medical literacy. The travesty pictures a system organized around this ban, the official line of needing to take exception to ambiguity as if an infraction or violation of the law. The power of the travesty of the city of pigs lies in its exaggeration of the specialization and insularity of any view of doctoring that equates it with service delivery based upon simple technical competence (no matter how complicated the task) and practiced monologically, intending to provoke through such intimidation (the intimidation of the caricature) a reflection upon the Grey Zone of health and illness.

Division of labor

The official history in its many guises tends to conceptualize what we call the Grey Zone or the ambiguity intrinsic to human conduct as an interdependent set of effects and innumerable influences of such immensity and complication that it can only be imagined or pictured as complex in the manner of a fiction that seeks to mirror these interactions in ways that can give aesthetic satisfaction through picturing itself. Any representation of health and illness must picture the body, with health and illness used to depict effects or processes traversing the body. Such picturing not only permits all of us to imagine our bodies but gives medical practitioners roadmaps or rules of thumb to find their way among bodies, to calculate them, to research them and act upon them in various ways. Pictures of the body are then mimetic, guides to action, and never self-evident because picturing in this sense must be translated or put into words, and putting the body into words is fundamentally ambiguous for all concerned. Everyone has to learn to imagine and speak about the body, and collective life displays a range of ways and means for such representation. Although the official history often claims that talk about the body reaches the level of an exact science the more we have access to its interior and have developed over time as an effect of such plundering, such putting into words remains fundamentally ambiguous. This is illustrated in medical attempts to explain and represent the course and dynamics of illness and also the attempts of patients to represent their symptoms. Medical lore regularly attributes such difficulties to the differences in technical know-how between professional and layman, whereas the ambiguity of the body always remains the source of the ambiguity because putting the body into words is never a matter of achieving clarity through technical lingo, which only reassures those already privy to it. The development of the model aims to picture complex interactions as its means of mastering such dynamics by doing nothing more than making them intelligible. Our speaking seems to make necessary a conception of history as a succession of stories, itself a way of picturing history as equivalent to narration. In part, this is what Heidegger (1982) calls a world picture, and it assumes many shapes in the official history from usages such as "frame of reference" to "paradigm" to "system," all of which are variations on the theme of the omnipresence of mediation and its necessary materialization in the symbolic order that always must conscript loyalists to enroll in the cause of mediating its influence(s) because of the need and desire to give voice as such.

Yet if any beginning can be pictured casually as a frame of reference in the way that some kind of selective process seems fundamental to speaking and acting for any species, the notions of paradigm and system suggest a degree of violence exercised on common conceptions, gestures of abstraction and idealization that aim, within the terms and conditions of the symbolic order, to refashion and reshape it for special purposes as if for distinctive projects, and so, to serve as models to emulate or as standards of action. Violence is always endemic to representation insofar as the split in the signifier means that the capacity for estrangement resides in the word itself but only as the desire we name *prosopopeia* can be animated, that the need and desire of the subject to open up what appears to be closed, to bring out the two-in-one, can be mobilized. In this way, any paradigm or system does not simply orient to recapitulate the commonplace distinction(s) in circulation but drives to condense and displace its diversity in a mirror designed to reflect to the collective itself its self-organizing capacities for being productive, for making things of value, as guided by aims and objectives of making works of some integrity and legibility. Thus, the project (as a paradigm or system) tries to make explicit the productive capacity of the symbolic for guiding action that is useful, as its way of confirming the exchange value of the symbolic order (for the regime of knowledge that we tacitly inherit), its capacity to be translated into profitable consequences. The mimetic powers of such modeling confirms the desire of a collective at any moment to understand itself as making such a difference in time, in investing its moment with consequentiality. The self-understanding of individual and collective at any point is grasped prosaically through the cliché of the circle that animates various mundane usages such as system, paradigm and totality, and that tends to engage the Grey Zone through images of circularity or the infinite regress as constraints.

For example, we can describe the world of health and illness through the figure of a health care system that is meant to lend an aura of consistency to the relationships that are pictured. In this way we rescue such relations from an image of dispersion or fragmentation by honoring an internal determinism that does not seem to operate by chance. Lacan's (1991, pp. 295–296) suggestion that chance is a figure for the absence of intention in determinism allows us to treat system as fulfilling this function of maintaining the intentional (purposive) determinism in these relationships. Because the usage of system allows us to imagine health and illness as if a machine regulated by unseen but oriented forces, it always raises the question of how or where these forces originate, but most importantly, how they can be controlled. In this sense, fantasies of origin, end and of conspiratorial workings seem to go with this kind of thought unless it tries to elevate itself by imagining an anonymous but patterned circuit whose sources are inexplicable. The conception of system always raises the question of how the relations are to be administered, assuming the administrator as the subject who is supposed to know and the knowledge to be known as the system and its workings. System, always somewhat confused about who works the works and never daring to go in that direction, is typically dramatized in films of scientists going mad (*Frankenstein*, *Dr. Jekyll and Mr. Hyde*, *The Fly*) as the subject who produces the system becomes increasingly subject to it in ways that seem incomprehensible to him. Therefore, system goes hand-in-glove with administration and invariably with the idea that administration (Agamben's [1998] "constitution") must corrupt the nascent creative passion entering into its formation. That is, if the health care system was created and designed to represent the liberation of medicine from antiquated and feudal restrictions, it is now seen to be practiced in ways that remain forgetful of this original spirit (in the way that biomedicine is characterized).

The notion of modeling as such seems to depend upon the rationale of division of labor in the sense that ambiguity can and must be managed through administrative solutions that reduce and exclude noise to the point where it can safely be disregarded as an obstruction as if relations to ambiguity can be divided. The ideal of interdisciplinary studies is a good example of such division of labor insofar as the Real (called complex reality) is conceptualized in areas of study such as psychology, economics, philosophy and the like because the whole, as it seems to stand, appears impenetrable. In the social sciences, the notion of levels of analysis resonates with this view of a whole and its parts (deeply inaccessible), making necessary a cadre of trained experts equipped to specialize in each venue. In all of these senses, the Grey Zone tends to be conceived along the line of whole-part relations, or as a set with members, in ways that not only connect it to as an administrative working solution to the problem of ambiguity but that serve to lay grounds for a conception of the practical actor as a problem-solver in the way of policy.

Interdisciplinary academic work and natural science models of systems always function as typical insider versions of objectification trying to picture health and illness as complicated systems in which either or all of fields (specialties), interests or variables are reputed to interact. Unlike the travesty of the city of pigs that is provoked by the ban on ambiguity (the Grey Zone) and expresses this through its grammatical investigation of the ban as a collective representation, these more prosaic projects use the ban as a point of departure for producing conclusions about health and illness that can be safeguarded from dialogue.

Blind spot

Baudrillard has a good quote from the physicist Jacques Monod that points to the kind of inbreeding that this science/system talk might be conceived to do:

> Plato, Heraclitus, Hegel, Marx: those ideological edifices, presented as *a priori*, were really *a posteriori* constructions designed to justify a pre-conceived ethico-political realm. The only *a priori* for science is the postulate of objectivity that forbids itself any part in this debate. (Baudrillard, 1983b, p. 113)

In other words, any notion of modeling is defined as much by what it excludes as by what it considers its basic properties or characteristics and so needs to be understood invariably as an exercise of violence in which ambiguity returns to haunt its achievements in ways that are unsettling. That expurgation rules modeling makes the ambiguity of desire omnipresent and perhaps unsettling. For example, the community of speakers, strictly defined by the ban that excludes those who desire to participate in this illicit debate is meant to limit talk of health care as a system only to and for those who have determined of themselves or have been determined to be indifferent to everything that might complicate their commitment to objectivity.

We must then be careful to distinguish ourselves from the scientific/policy view of health and illness even while exploring its imaginary relation to its objects. While we do not accept the ban in studying those who do in a way that differentiates us significantly, we must appreciate at the very same time that such inquiry is only possible by virtue of our desire to imagine how it is to accept the ban (and what place such an actor, action, situation or motivation must be conceived as occupying in relation to the symbolic order). This is the decisive mark of the Grey Zone in the practice of theorizing, that we (inquiry) are both the same and the other, close but not too close, far but not too far. That is, if we can say that medical practice is exercised by the ban or the problem of its forbidden desire, we are depicting in such a gesture the self-understanding of this practice (its values) through the figure of its aspiration to understand itself as a flexible or liberal adjustment to "circularity" (a cause in which it has enrolled many philosophically inclined spokesman from Kant through Latour and Luhmann to make such a case). In this way, our desire to know medicine has to be reflected in knowledge of the desire that animates its practice. Here, the Grey Zone is used to refer to the circularity of any system, typically referred to by its practitioners in clichés such as "situated embeddedness," as its being closed to itself and unable to observe itself because observing is part of what is observed. Call this the liberal view of the *blind spot*.

> In the end, doesn't this consideration bring us back to what I started off with in my commentary on the functions of speech? Namely the opposition between empty and full speech, full speech in so far as it realizes the truth of the subject; empty speech in relation to what he has to do *hic et nunc* [...] in which the subject loses himself in the machinations of the system of language, in the labyrinth of referential systems made available to him by the state of cultural affairs to which he is a more or less interested party. Between these two extremes, a whole gamut of modes of realization of speech is deployed. (Lacan, 1988, p. 50)

The objective of the theorist to change the situation she is studying requires understanding the local detail in any such context, what is important to know, the different possibilities needed to unblock or break the rigid patterns which prevent different interventions that might lead to change. The ambiguity of any system resides in its immunity to change, and since change can only be initiated within the system by one of its parts, any intervention must begin by accepting the system as it exists in order to influence the system towards accepting its own redefinition. Here, the Grey Zone seems to reflect the compromise position of policy, the necessary in-between status that it shares with therapy and the idea that the subject (the health system) cannot enlighten itself without the external push of an insider who can seduce it to rethink itself. In this sense, policy seems a good example of what Lacan (1981b, pp. 105–110) calls travesty and its three facets as camouflage, exaggeration and intimidation.

First, it *camouflages* itself in the very views of the system it seeks to change, becoming part or inside, so to speak. Secondly, from all of the complicated variables that it can imagine as functioning in the health system, policy *exaggerates* the way in which the blocked character of the system is a feature of its closure and insularity, its inability to distance itself from itself in the absence of any reflective consultation from within, thus inflating the need for a detached expert from among its own, the familiar stranger as policy specialist. In this sense, policy exaggerates the need for the very expertise which it will claim for itself, making itself invaluable by exaggerating the system's blockage. The view of the system overcomes the limited perspectives of those who are parts because the interdependence at the root of the conception of system is meant to exaggerate the capacity of one of the special and driven parts to command a view of the whole. The system must exaggerate the interdependencies among parts by excluding whatever influences would block the view of a spectator, in a gesture that makes literacy about interdependencies into a kind of knowledge of the whole, and by creating a subject who is supposed to know as the exemplary part of the whole that is known. What is exaggerated is whatever inquiry thinks it needs in order to make a space for itself as necessary, as an apt reply to a limit that it makes visible in the situation into which it inquires. In this way, policy creates the consultant.

Finally, policy *intimidates* the health care system by identifying its continuation and maintenance as if a grave crisis, an emergency or panic situation that needs to be immediately addressed. The relationship of science to health care is treated as a bona fide example of such intimidation, expressed in the growing tendency of the medical system to alter its relationship to the indistinct region of thought as if an exception to the norm, to the point of treating care for the body and its healthfulness, whether for individuals or collectives, as a state of permanent emergency, a state once regarded as exceptional and now as normative in every and any area of health care. Thus, the operation of the health care system seems to function within the same logical nexus as did the ideas of nuclear deterrence and the cold war in the international system. These relationships can be seen to place new burdens upon practitioners, clients and the system in general, not only with respect to bureaucratization in relation to time, space and scarcity of resources, but to ethical concerns circulating around questions of governance regarding the quality of care, advice, expertise, information and conflicts between dependency and self-determination.

Yet policy can only be a corrupt version of travesty since it is organized in a way that blurs the boundary between the symbolic order and the Real, using the symbolic as an instrument to change the real as if they are indistinct or the same, as if symbolizing is a tool for changing conduct in that sense. This view of travesty buries an interest in the artifice and ambiguity of whatever it describes under a standard of social engineering, in terms of which it tries to enact concrete changes. In contrast, work true to travesty sends up the Real through its very representation as a symbolic order in the most rigorous sense, not as empirical description (because any such description has to be inexact or probable) but in taking the symbolic literally as Real and by taking the real literally as symbolic, showing the irresolution at the border of this relationship as a continuous problem for the member.

Thus, to travesty an account is to disclose how its symbolic order risks subjecting action to a master plan that inevitably creates bewilderment, frustration and signs of equivocation that the subject has to orient to as a problem to solve both in figuring out what it means and in trying to live by it or apply it in action. Travesty emerged in sociological description that recognized the place of descriptions in life as phenomena that could only challenge their understanding as technical resources. In the idiom of

Garfinkel (1967), descriptions become topics as much as resources, and this is shown by travestying their self-understanding as resources for collecting data. This is how Simmel, Kenneth Burke and Goffman might be considered the inventors of this genre, but no less than Weber's description of bureaucracy and Marx's spectacular travesty of capitalism (see the seeds of such analysis in Blum's [1973] "Reading Marx" and Peter McHugh's [1968] *Defining the situation*). At the most obvious level, the objects of analysis might include any automated system, organization or hospital emergency room, but also formats regulating practices and civility, interaction and relations in collective life such as the countless exercises Goffman (1963) identified as social ritual, or the most intimate relations of love, family and friendship. Conversely, in treating the symbolic as real, we try to imagine the description as if requiring of its subject that she perform in a certain way, meaning to dramatize the ungovernable connotative surfeit that exceeds its symbolization as if a normal but necessary problem. Unlike the breach experiment of Garfinkel from which it might seem to derive, travesty does not do infraction in order to expose the artifice of the normative but exaggerates the scene to make each suffer being the other, the normative suffering being Real and the Real suffering being normative as if, in life, each is both the same and the other rather than one or the other, both inconclusively conclusive and conclusively inconclusive. What travesty shows is that the Real must be symbolized (and is not deficient because of this) and that symbolization need be enacted and performed (and is not deficient because of this).

Institutional logic

In order to better appreciate how this method works, we might recover a paradigmatic sociological vision of such a system because it will show the practice of travesty in action. Here is the sociologist Stinchcombe on what he identifies as systems that rationalize conduct and institutionalize reason, social formations including science, medicine, university, law and any of a number of domains that he takes to be involved in "routinizing a body of reasoning" in formal practices. This permits us to better grasp science as such a construction, i.e., as a body of reasoning that is put into practice, and it permits us to understand the type of actors, actions and relevant relations to language that such practices require as world-building activities.

> Reason is a weak cause of people's behavior and can only work reliably when the strong causes, personal interests and passions or "rationality" in the now conventional sense, are segregated from institutional decisions. If therefore an institution is going to reliably produce decisions that are guided by principles in the paradigms embedded in the institution, it has to have arrangement not only to make the paradigm available to

practitioners, but also to prevent personal interests and passions from interfering [...] Weber analyzes this most completely in his ideal type of bureaucracy. (Stinchcombe, 1986, p. 158)

In other words, because bureaucracy is not simply an external fact but a method for constructing relationships, Baudrillard's astonishment at the ban celebrated as necessary by science does not really come to terms with the imaginary of science in this sense, as grounded in a vision of reliable and efficacious decision-making in order to satisfy (or what Stinchcombe [1986, p. 165] describes as "maximizing the utility of") certain very specific standards of success (milestones). This is to say that the grounds of the ban reside in some vision of the good society and begin to dramatize the figure of the Grey Zone in a different way, around questions relating to desire, language and social life, or around the relation between value and utility, between reason and rationality.

> The achievement of civilization could be formulated as the successful detachment of the faculties that make people rational from the limiting context of personal goals, so that they can be applied to the improvement of social life. The result of such a provision of an "irrational" context for the faculties of rationality is an improvement in rationality through the institutionalization of reason. (Stinchcombe, 1986, p. 165)

Here, the Grey Zone is finally acknowledged as existing in the shape of a necessary concession—the "irrational" context always needed and provided for any "rational" endeavor—as the desire to disregard, to accept the ban as equipment for living. The status of the ban as an aspect of the Grey Zone is clearest even in this repudiation of the Grey Zone, for in making the ban on what is most vital necessary to progress it can only accentuate and dramatize the struggle of such a divided subject (a subject that it creates as divided) as essentially ethical through its link to progress and presumably the progressive conduct of good citizenship. This will lead us to ask how it is with medicine and its relationship to health and illness in this respect, that is, in respect of the taboo.

> The ban is the pure form of reference to something in general, which is to say, the simple positing of relation with the nonrelational. In this sense, the ban is identical with the limit form of relation. (Agamben, 1998, p. 29)

What Agamben means is that the ban on the irrational or on participation in the canonical discourse, as such a gesture, is an act (speech act) that relates whosoever it bans (the scientist) to whatsoever it forbids (perhaps philosophical sensitivity). Forbidding is a relationship to a nonrelation and in this way raises the question of the Grey Zone ("the limit form of relation"). For us, then, the interdiction must always be provocative rather than paralyzing, showing by virtue of its exclusion just what it must include as intrinsic to the symbolic order. As we expect, this very ambiguity must remain to haunt the system and not to disappear, reflected in the exchanges between medicine and its clients and in the varied and volatile discussions circulating over the question of the quality of medicine and the rights of patients. Indeed, the ban and its upholding, fortification, protection and transgression become the primary loci of collectivization in the health care system, the discursive foci animating its vitality. We might even offer from the perspective of the travesty of the city of pigs that it is the ban and its discursive centrality and not knowledge and research (regardless of their import, which is undeniable) that is the locus of collectivization with respect to health and illness.

Of course the ban invites and requires sacrifice, for if one is to do the right thing, this means going against the grain (personal, irrational) not only in civilization as Stinchcombe says, but in science and particularly in medicine. Medicine must not only take pride in reason, but in prohibiting the personal, the irrational and all that necessitates the ban on weakness. Here might be the basic split that underlies everything: accepting the system or not, being a good or bad patient, doctor, nurse or practitioner, in fact, reason and its other, can all be said tentatively to originate in the idea of a split between strength and weakness. The maxim seems to be that one must exercise strength towards one's very own weakness if one is to sacrifice oneself to care for the weaknesses of other.

In order to advance an interlocutor to the idea of science as a system, we might consider this sociological version (despite the author's inflection) as a corpus of knowledge that is embodied (institutionalized or routinized) in practices, sanctions, codes and laws. This brings us into contact with the work of Parsons, later Foucault, and even Lacan (this because any view of system is structured in its way by an imaginary relationship that grounds it and makes it intelligible, the desire that Stinchcombe above calls "irrational").

> The state of exception [...] is not external to the *nomos* but rather, even in its clear delineation, included in the *nomos* as a moment that is in every sense fundamental. (Agamben, 1998, p. 37)

What Agamben means is that the irrational context of any rational endeavor (such as medicine) is not external to (so-called) reason but intrinsic to it, perhaps in the way that the will to ban the personal (whatever that means) is fundamental to the impersonal. This enables Agamben to reiterate a variety of sociological clichés that confirm the Grey Zone as a practice: the law (reason) depends upon violence (the irrational), which it also intends to exclude (in the sense that law emerges in an effort to master and control the irrational); similarly the constitution of medicine (its official code and bureaucratic rationality) depends upon the irrational passion invested in its nascent moment (perhaps enlightenment) and now forgotten (by the biomedical practice) in the way Benjamin's (1971) constituted power interpenetrates with constituting power: "the power from which constituting power is born is increasingly dismissed as a prejudice or purely factual matter"(Agamben, 1998, p. 40). Agamben summarizes his sense of the Grey Zone as follows:

> The state of exception is thus not so much a spatiotemporal suspension as a complex topological figure in which not only the exception and the rule, but also the state of nature and law, outside and inside, pass through one another. It is precisely this topological zone of indistinction [...].
> (Agamben, 1998, p. 37)

Thus, the nascent, violent, constituting and irrational element in any social formation exposes the ambiguity essential to the practice as the exception that its effort to prohibit must include in this very work of orienting and relating to it *as* the prohibition it is. The usage for the Grey Zone here: everything we exclude must be included by virtue of this gesture, that is, it must be oriented to and so, must exist in this sense as a social fact. What we can begin to appreciate is how the ban alerts us to the condition of medical science itself as the subject, not simply as the conscious ego who personifies Stinchcombe's "rationality" but as the one in the grip of forces that exceed such determination. This demonstrates again the idea of the subject as being two-in-one or split between consciousness and the forces in excess of that. The so-called irrational element signaled by the ban and the state of exception simply makes reference to the force of seeing-as as the imaginary connection animating any representation, or the unconscious, as if to say that science bans the unconscious or treats it as an exception to the rule, that it wants to ban talk of the unconscious, taking an exception to the talk of the unconscious while still speaking about irrational elements.

> In science, the subject is only sustained, in the end, on the plane of consciousness, since the subject x in science is in fact the scientist. It is whoever possesses the system of the science that sustains the dimension of the subject. He is the subject insofar as he is the reflection, the mirror, the support of the objectal world. In contrast Freud shows us that in the human subject there is something which speaks, which speaks in the full sense of the word, that is to say something which knowingly lies and without the contribution of consciousness, that restores [...] the dimension of the subject [...] this dimension is no longer confused with the ego. The ego is deprived of its absolute position in the subject. The ego acquires the status of a mirage, a residue, it is only one element in the objectal relations of the subject.
>
> Are you with me? (Lacan, 1988, p. 194)

> A system is often described as a harmony. Maybe it's the same word, the same thing. In fact, what use is it to discuss matters, what use is it to be concerned with a system in disequilibrium, a system that does not function right? Yet we know of no system that functions perfectly, that is to say without losses, flights, wear and tear, accidents, opacity—a system whose return is one for one, where the yield is maximal and so forth. Even the world itself does not work quite perfectly. The distance from equality, from perfect agreement, is history. (Serres, 1982, pp. 12–13)

Serres identifies life with history. The harmony imagined by the system needs to be contrasted with life in the way perfect equality should be contrasted with inequality. In life, any image or object is animated through its being used and applied in many different ways, ways that become sanctified in usage and distinctions as legitimate. The formless *jouissance* marking the unconscious as a multitude of forces can be inflected and given form in many different ways. Because what Lacan calls law, or Weber (1947) calls a legitimate or valid order, is necessarily conventional, any social order can betray to a discerning eye a degree of incommensurability intrinsic to this tension between the unequal distribution and the equality that it wrongs (Rancière, 1999), an equality that inheres in the equal opportunity to be marked, used and oriented to the *jouissance* that any distinction (object, image) offers for life itself before it materializes as significant and oriented action. The equivalence of equality with plurality, as noted by Arendt as the foundation of the human condition (2005) as the bottom line or image of the primal scene, is relevant here. This is the deceit of life, translated into noise when life is conceived as a system, but only significant as a difference that makes a difference, that exists, when recognized as empty or wronging the order of names. Life or history describes the process whereby humans work out and accomplish any social order as contingent and so as a distribution of inequalities. In other words, in working out plurality and trying to create a reasonable accord or unity, inequality is inevitable and coexists with temptations towards tyranny and resignation within the context of a dialogical imaginary and all of the excesses released by politics, the excesses identified by Rancière and Serres as "life." Serres identifies such imperfections as noise, losses, flight, wear and tear, accidents, opacity, all as figures of speech for the occasions where the Grey Zone can be expected to materialize and to become visible, and so to be an object of demonstration in itself.

> The speech that the subject emits, goes beyond, without his knowing it, his limits as a discoursing subject—all the while remaining, to be sure, within his limits as speaking subject [...]. (Lacan, 1988, p. 266)

> [...] So here we are presented with a question—what is the structure of this speech which is beyond discourse? [...]. (p. 267)

> If it is a discourse like the other, why isn't it in just the same way, immersed in error? (p. 266)

Let us say with these spokespeople that there is no rationality without irrationality, no rule without exception, no law without violence, but with a somewhat different inflection and more fundamentally, that there is no irrationality without rationality, no exception without rule, no violence without law (that is, without representation, without the symbolic order), and if there is no something without nothing (no Same without Other), then there is still no nothing without something. If there is no either/or without the Grey Zone, could it be that there is no Grey Zone without an either/or?

Agamben's notion of the ban or exception simply substitutes it as if a mechanism oriented to do exclusion and exemption (just as his notion of apparatus or disposition) for the idea of "trained incapacity" that Kenneth Burke developed from Veblen (1965, p. 489) concerning the method of discipline that any artifact imposes upon the user as the course of action entailed by its use as a necessary aspect of the artifact itself. If any symbolic order requires its own interpellation of a subject as a feature of the intelligibility of the order in ways that have always marked the Grey Zone, this convention (Foucault, Agamben) always risks travestying the Grey Zone as a site for the concealed exercise of sovereign power. Yet, if the symbolic order must get the subject it requires as the facsimile of its user, that user as such must be factored into the question of the kind of life she makes possible in ways that bring travesty and the likely story together. To paraphrase Baudrillard, this seems a more radical way of challenging the system, for instead of saying that it is bad or in error, we put it on the spot by disclosing its distinctions to lack vitality, to have no life (see Baudrillard [2006] on the difference between Nietzsche's challenge to God and atheism in *The evil demon of images*). Travesty describes the Real as if a symbolic order, taking form as the likely story that serves as if a script for performing realistically at life under the auspices of such an order, showing the user as engaged only and exclusively by the problems it makes possible.

Parsons' travesty of health and illness in modern society

In this context, we can understand Talcott Parsons' (1951) various writings on health and illness less as a testimony to his conservatism or structural-functional bias than a reflection of his desire to represent from the inside (so to speak) the symbolic order of modern society through the way it views and acts upon health and illness. Moreover, this allows him to use the relationship to health and illness as a quintessential sign of modernity, particularly in the shape it assumes as an enlightenment model. Here, he mimics the enlightenment society's aspiration to achieve a degree of self-understanding, showing how theorizing always begins by impersonating the voice of the collective it analyzes before transforming that voice through "objective irony" (Baudrillard, 2006, p. 39). Thus, to understand health and illness we must start with the ways in which our collective seems to grasp the problem in its undeliberated characterizations and categories. This initial camouflage reflects the effort of an insider to that society to make himself strange to its practices in order to represent that society to and for itself. Parsons' travesty lies in his exaggeration of the necessity for theorizing to be strange to its society and for the theorist to be a stranger. In such a gesture theorizing can always risk looking as if it accepts what it is describing without further ado. Here, the theorist in describing how the game is played and how the generalized other functions to regulate that play seems comic in appearing unaware of the limits of the game, as if in identifying the format of the collective he accepts it by virtue of the description, seeming to conceal its ambiguity as an object seen as it is. Understanding this gesture allows us to appreciate the way Parsons can dramatize the Grey Zone as a research opportunity in ways that the anthropological analogy can intimate but not develop. In this sense, the problem raised by health and illness as a symbolic order for social inquiry is twofold.

First, the object of such analysis now is not just health and illness but the modern enlightenment conception of health and illness as seen by a theorist who is committed to the very practices being described, i.e., who is intermediate between stranger and insider and who needs to represent that intermediacy in theorizing that exaggerates the position of theorist as both inside and outside such a society at one and the same time (this accounts for the awkward structural-functional method of representation).

Secondly, the agent of such a representation is neither philosopher nor common man, but sociologist, i.e., one who will represent the self-understanding of such a society as quintessentially social. In this sense, the topic of such a society is not health and illness as a natural order but as cultural, i.e., as meaningful practices which raise questions of evaluation and appraisal that are fundamental. What Parsons permits us to appreciate is the way in which health and illness as cultural object is the site of interpretive conflict between body and mind insofar as the physical is always treated as implicitly normative. In this way, Parsons' work is intended to confirm the place of sociology as that art which establishes the status of the science and therapy of the body (Descartes' [1960] exemplary knowledge) as a symbolic order.

The symbolic order of health and illness, then, is discerned in the fact that being healthy and ill is treated as desirable or not in terms of contestable standards that are constantly debatable and open to deliberation, and that any description of health and illness is itself a position within such a symbolic order and so, both partial (inside) and reflective (outside) upon itself. In such ways, Parsons' description of health and illness (in light of American values), should be read as a critique of the modern enlightenment conception of health and illness as (re)written by one inside that collective who aspires to represent its self-knowledge to and for itself. This beginning of the travesty limits theorizing to ventriloquism. The idea that health and illness is intelligible, as deviant and undesirable vis-à-vis a normative standard of health as conformity and of medicine as a process of social control, is not an invention for describing some (collective) object external to him, but an insider's representation of what an enlightenment conception of health and illness seems to require and imply within the context of the very terms which it lays down for itself.

According to Parsons, that the enlightenment society conceives of health and illness as conformity and deviance means not that health is normal and sickness is deviant, but that healthfulness is a model of normalcy and sickness is a model of deviance, a stipulation which itself suggests that this society is unable to comprehend deeply how even good or evil is anything other than capacity or incapacity, and so how it always is tempted to lose a grasp of any conception of value as other than functional or in relation to productivity. This type of society (personified in the figure of the modern enlightenment society) is reputed to operationalize value by equating it with capacity and, further, to identify capacity with work (productive labor). In this sense, the particular experience (the so-called life-world) is divested of its vitality and interest, i.e., of its relevance, in a way which makes it a continuously repressed and problematic underside to the question of health and illness.

Parsons says that according to sociology, the repressed and hence open question of the relation of real health and illness to capacity and incapacity is an aspect of the collective relation to health and illness that is both a persistent and problematic consequence of the category and its use, providing a model of what is normal and exceptional in a way that deprives the normal of its integral link to excellence and the exceptional of its essential link to particularity at best, or at worst, evil. That is, in this type of society, value as good and bad is treated functionally as capacity or incapacity in a way that has traditionally repelled critics of the enlightenment. Here, Parsons dramatizes the place of the Grey Zone in a society such as this: the symbolic order of health and illness locates a site wherein an essential interpretive conflict over the question of value is raised as an integral feature of the collective self-understanding.

Parsons permits us to begin to identify the symbolic order, not as an undifferentiated and seamless body of knowledge often typified in sociology vacuously as "culture," but as a site of interpretive conflict where any collective interest, e.g., health and illness, by virtue of the open-ended and fertile character of its problem as an aspect of the Grey Zone, is a place where conflict over alternative resolutions constitutes itself as part of the material of collective self-understanding. In this way Parsons permits us to understand the social conception of culture as a fertile site of interpretive conflict and so as the implicit home of a conception of the symbolic order. That the enlightenment society overlooks the particular in order to obtain a degree of control in its repossessive grasp of nature means that the relation between what is included and what is excluded is a continuous topic for members of that society when represented by one who would sociologize it (this is how the ban and the exception become such useful conventions). Sociology then achieves its place by virtue of representing such collective self-understanding to and for that society itself.

In the first place, what appears as natural can always be questioned in a way that means the so-called mind-body problem is quintessentially social, i.e., a site of interpretive conflict for the society. Social research always seeks to identify how and in what forms such conflict appears as a phenomenon in and for the society itself by identifying the relationships that are formed in connection to that problem itself. According to Parsons, the form assumed by this problem of the relation of body to mind is expressed in the (sociological) representation of the issue of health and illness as "secondary gain" in such a way as to show the essentially motivated (and potentially political) character of any conception of health and illness. Secondary gain is intended to describe either/or the use of health and illness to achieve (gratuitous) satisfaction in relation to health and illness, i.e., to use illness in order to maximize dependency or to use health and illness in order to maximize control over others, making hypochondria and power, vestiges of masochism and sadism, the two extreme fears haunting the imaginary. Secondary gain expresses the continuously problematic relation of objectivity to self-interest in the use of health and illness. In the second place, that what appears as illness by virtue of capacity and incapacity always shows its problematic relation to real health and illness means that this too is a site of interpretive conflict in such a way as to make the undesirability of such a relation a phenomenon in and for the collective itself.

The sick role

Finally, note how Parsons' conception of the sick role also serves the function of producing, for anyone desiring to sociologize, a representation of the collective interest in health and illness as an interest in achieving solutions to collective problems. Though the sick role is commonly taken as an inventory of aspects or criteria of what it means to be sick as exemption from responsibility, commitment to seek help and the obligation to cooperate in getting well, etc., we read these criteria as Parsons' way of representing how the enlightenment society orients to the problem of health and illness as a symbolic order.

What the sick role means, then, is that whenever the question of health and illness is raised to and for this collective, it is raised in such a way as to make observable the need to achieve solutions to problems of the exemption of responsibility, the willingness of all parties to seek help, to undertake obligations to speed recovery and to participate in systematic cooperative projects that will achieve solutions. These criteria are occasions to develop aesthetic relations to each as seeing-as, a pointing out of differences between what is essential and inessential. Each criterion then is not so much a matter to be decided by a disinterested observer in a propositional declaration of action, being this rather that, as if this observer is to determine whether what the proposition proposes is true or false, present or absent, widespread or rare, but more likely it is a way of representing how a collective interest is essentially provocative and fertile of interpretive problems that are continuously undividable. That is, from the conception of the symbolic order, the sick role does not identify descriptive properties but formulates for us how it is that we use and orient to the conception of sickness developed in such a society.

The sick role is a grammar that develops and makes explicit the ideal social relationship to health and illness typified in and by a society such as this. Arguing with its factual status misrecognizes the symbolic order as an empirical description (as in Whitehead's [1967] fallacy of misplaced concreteness). In Lacanian, the sick role does not depict a signifier to be interpreted (e.g., sickness) but makes reference to signification as a social fact in Durkheim's sense, the way being sick collectivizes interest and fascination around questions pertaining to its credibility, justification and management. This means, for example, that our task is not to determine whether or not the sick are exempt from responsibility as the first criterion might have it, but rather to ask, whenever the question of health and illness is raised in this society, how the task of deciding upon the relation between sickness and its exemption from responsibility is raised as a problem for members for which they must achieve some solution.

Note how this first criterion of Parsons' sick role, which refers to the exemption of sickness from responsibility, becomes an observable interpretive problem in the society. One of the ways in which the exemption from responsibility functions, not as a description of objective aspects of a role but as a site of interpretive conflict, can be understood in part as the question of its relationship to capacity and incapacity and the need to produce observable responses to the task of making observable claims to exemption. For example, some societies promise to provide those who are disabled or who claim disability from an illness exemption from tax under certain conditions, or subsidies or compensation for illness and injury. In such cases, members are required to produce solutions to the problem of what constitutes adequate criteria for being exempt from responsibility even though they may participate and show capacity in normal work situations. On these occasions and many others, sickness and health always raise the question of the extent to which it is involved in problems of justifying exemption from responsibility and the varieties of methods and procedures that the society offers to members for making observable such claims. In these cases, the sick role becomes a method of viewing which allows us to orient to the practices that the society uses to raise interpretive issues.

Secondary gain

Parsons' conception of the symbolic order of health and illness makes reference to the continuous possibility of raising the question of secondary gain or of the motivated character of health, illness and its treatment whenever related questions arise. In part, this means that the sick role produces solutions to problems in the form of intended interpretive resolutions of questions that can always be raised with respect to the motivated character of health and illness.

121

In the first instance, such questions follow from the relation of mind and body, reflected in the question of whether capacity and incapacity is a true indicator of real health or illness. In this sense, the relationship between capacity and incapacity and true or real illness and health is a continuous interpretive concern of members who seek to produce or provide solutions to it that are visible and observable in a variety of settings. For example, one problem that constantly arises in the discursive systems of health and illness concerns the complaints of the ill about their treatment and the suspiciousness of those charged with treating them towards their claims. Thus, the problem of malingering becomes an issue raised not by virtue of the personalities of participants but because of the essentially problematic relationship between capacity and incapacity and real health and illness. In the way that chronic complaining patients are produced by the need to make observable the real illness of those who cannot satisfy the criterion of incapacity, so also does the suspiciousness of medical personnel reflect the unstable relationship between signs of illness and health and methods of confirming them. In this sense, both complaints and suspiciousness are produced by the essentially problematic relationship between capacity, incapacity and real illness and health, and in this way, they are structurally induced by the symbolic order of health and illness.

Similarly, each social formation faces this problem in a different form insofar as age, gender, race and class each express in different shape the topic of normalizing, making observable and resolving the relationship between capacity and incapacity. Verification is continuously developed by patients and medical personnel in order to establish and confirm the fact of the claim of real illness in the system insofar as this question can never be unequivocally settled without reference to local culture. Similarly, normalcy is itself, i.e., health in the absence of signs of incapacity, is a task that regularly needs to be produced and made demonstrable. In the same way, different diseases present different problems of normalization and of making real illness observable, just as they produce different solutions to problems of concealing or making visible health and illness.

What Parsons' work begins to suggest is that the sick role formulates the collective interest in addressing certain tensions raised by the very grammar of health and illness, insofar as such tensions can be enumerated by Parsons in terms of his various criteria of the sick role. These criteria, then, are less descriptive aspects than ways of understanding how the collective finds health and illness problematic on each and every occasion when it becomes a topic. The sick role functions as a method which allows us to identify practices in a variety of settings that are addressed to problems, such as the exemption of responsibility, cooperation in getting well, etc., as if a set of collective concerns that are constantly disputed and raised on occasions when health and illness become topicalized. This focus, in turn, permits us to clarify the relation of incapacity to illness, particularly the ways in which this relation animates the cultivation and invention of capacity as the desire for the desirability of "normal" life.

Conclusion

Parsons' discussion actually makes a space for the ideal speaker since the reflection upon the limits of the practice in full recognition of its necessary artifice must develop the fluency of what Baudrillard (2006) calls "objective irony" to use the system against itself. To see the limit as a limit invites appreciating the relationship to a phenomenon such as health and illness as resting upon the formula as such and the formula as deserving the status of a necessary fiction and so as a necessity that can only be engaged playfully, avowed as equipment for living and disavowed as more than that.

We begin to appreciate the struggle of the subject as such, as a way of working through transference relations to what seems to belong to oneself (the symbolic order, the game and the generalized other) as the material conditions of opinions, beliefs and attachments to others, as the conditions that belong to one and yet need the touch of an aesthetic relation, which has to be supplied with form even at risk, giving form to speech in a way that resists temptations of hysteria and obsession, comic in its incipient awareness of its own limits (as the way hysterical and obsessive propensities coexist as part of discursive potential, making even this a struggle within between oneself and her weaker parts). Here, self and other are joined but not reconciled through the sensitivity to seeing-as: the otherness of material conditions is put into question as part of the development of self as seeing-as or of taking a perspective which strives to place this relationship as an opportunity for transposition. We tried to show through Mead (1967) that the very creation of the self is conceived as occurring though a struggle with inertia towards such conditions. We see desire reflected in songs of suffering and of being stunned with sorrow and in relation to this condition as such for oneself, for others, for Other; we imagine the magic of self-reflection and its various expressions as parts of a trajectory of desire, shaping aesthetics, ethics, eventually the inward calling of science, as efforts to heal the anxiety of the Grey Zone, seeing these gestures through a desire to theorize collective relations to health and illness, to suffering, affliction and life and its management.

Throughout this book, we have discussed from various angles how the Grey Zone of health and illness can be seen as making reference to a situation of fundamental ambiguity, and we have explored such a relationship by "piling up ambiguities," (in the words of Burke [1969]) through exaggeration, first by observing the collective speech as if a discourse, then by depicting the division within each and any subject as if a division within desire, and finally by constructing narratives that make a collective appear to desire more rather than less of itself and of its magic. While we cannot describe "down to the last detail" (to paraphrase Socrates [Plato, 1945]) the health care system and the public for health, we have been representing it in a way that shows its two-sidedness as if it has capacities to be both better and worse than it often seems to be. In this chapter we have continued to use the method of travesty as a formula.

7

Health and the City

Introduction

Basic ways of addressing the relationship of health and the city tend to assume the unquestioned meaning of each term in order to calculate the reciprocal influences between them statistically. But even statisticians and urban planners who participate in this enterprise tend to confess:

> The reason for which the evidence reviewed here is mixed and possibly confusing is two-fold: 1) There are many ways to define and measure health. […] [M]easures range from disease prevalence, LEB (life expectancy at birth), age-specific mortality rates, and indicators of self-assessed health; 2) There are many ways to define and measure cities. (Rodwin, 2001, p. 6)

Of course, he does not permit this ambiguity to infect his own work, recognizing in his way that this two-sidedness of the relation—"The city is, at once, a center for disease and poor health and also a place for hope, cures and good health" (Rodwin, 2001, p. 1)—poses a problem and a challenge for us. The challenge is not so much one of addressing just what it is to which the notions of city and health make reference, as the primordial *ti estin* question (what is it to which this term makes reference?), but a challenge posed by the question of deciding whether cities are healthy or not—"[T]here is already widespread belief that urban health is not as good as that of the population as a whole. Those who disagree point to contrary evidence. Strangely enough, there is insufficient evidence to provide strong support for either view" (Rodwin, 2001, p. 2). Yet, deciding upon a proper answer to this question is not really possible because of the absence of decisive evidence for the reason that "we have no routine information systems for monitoring the health of populations living in cities" (Rodwin, 2001, p. 2). Nevertheless, he will heroically march ahead despite this vacuum to "present a case for both sides of the urban health controversy—the city is sick and the city is healthy—summarizing highly selective evidence for each view" (Rodwin, 2001, p. 2).

There are many moves made in this expository structure, beginning with the recognition of a relationship between distinctions admitted to be too obscure to pin down with assurance, necessitating in this way the risk of improvisation, then imposing as a challenge an either/or question concerning the relationship for which his means of answering do not seem adequate. The exposition that begins in the wake of such a lack or deficiency thus offers in its way to apply a remedy in the dark, so to speak, without knowing what it is that is being queried and, because of this, lacking not just evidence or further information but any wherewithal to measure what it is that would constitute adequate evidence or information since his approach to the relationship is not grounded in any reflection upon whatever it is that he proposes to study. This two-sidedness of the relation of city to health is expressed in the disagreement he notes *and* in the lack of evidence for resolving this question in one way or the other. This type of talk treats the relationship of city to health not as a matter for theorizing but as an issue made visible by the disagreement. Here we begin to discern the grammar of the issue as a methodology for reinstating (re: marking) a belief in the form of an either/or question (are cities healthy or sick?), presumably of some urgency and requiring a response for which resources are not adequate. Note that the relationship between city and health does not *have* to be expressed through the form of this question, which seems to guarantee both the compromise of the selective evidence and the deficiency of any solution whose fate is to come up short. Yet, posing the problem in this way, in this shape of an interrogative that is fated to leave such a remainder (inconclusive evidence) not only guarantees coming up short but perhaps its enjoyment, i.e., the *jouissance* of coming up short as an instance of a death drive. The grammar of the issue begins to dramatize this unhappy compromise of the study of urban health and its empiricism as the gratifying discursivity of public life in the very fertility of formlessness, of the talkativeness making possible the proliferation of beliefs and opinions that circulate in ways capable of mobilizing a collective. What is enjoyable is having an opinion about the irresolute question, i.e., having something to say in a way that need not be committed. If Kierkegaard calls this talkativeness, then we might venture that the issue *makes* a public by virtue of this capacity to create irresolute talkativeness as a locus of satisfaction, perhaps by making opinions themselves into goods like commodities.

This structure becomes most apparent when the author confesses that the very question he posed to acknowledge the public and its interest—the issue of a healthy or sick city—is not "pertinent," presumably because it cannot be resolved with the evidence at hand, proposing to shift to another question:

> I suggest that the more pertinent question is not whether the city is unhealthy or healthy but rather the extent to which we can alleviate the problems posed by inequalities of income and wealth—in the city as well as outside of it. (Rodwin, 2001, p. 1)

The violence of substituting this question for the first is both ungrounded (why assume the relation of health to city to be as such?) and denied in this gesture because he has already proposed to continue to address the question of sick and healthy cities—"to present a case for both sides." So, although he does not seem to know what he is speaking for, he shows that the issue remains in place because the either/or question of the sick and healthy city is identified now with the question of "the extent to which we can alleviate the problems posed by inequalities of income and wealth," as if it is these specific conditions that are linked inextricably to the question of urban health (and remember, he proceeds as one in the dark and indifferent to what either and both the city and health mean!).

Yet there is something interesting in such a proposal if we read it carefully. First, he recommends that the locus of collectivization for a public is not simply reflected in the substantive content of some matter (health, education, welfare or voting), for this content might only mirror for a collective its own vanishing point as something or nothing, the inescapable link of its existence to inequalities of income and wealth as the conditions that, if left unalleviated, would condemn it to oblivion. On the other hand, if the absence of alleviation can make the collective nothing rather than something, the lack of alleviation does still make problems from such differences that constantly need to be addressed and discussed. Such a public is animated or brought to life by an issue that emerges through the destructive diversity of the collective, a diversity that is actually productive insofar as it creates many problems that require alleviation, that of all of the many differences in collective life, those of income and wealth supersede the others by virtue of the dependency of any content or commonplace on such differences. What comes into focus is not the two-sidedness of the issue (the question of the city as sick or healthy) but the two-sidedness of alleviation, the absence of which can conjure up the death of extinction (from inequalities of wealth and income) or the public life (or death) of irresolute talkativeness.

Herein lies the power of the passage for suggesting on the one hand that the relation of city to health creates or produces the question of alleviation and how it is oriented to the mark itself of urban health and sickness, making the difference between healthy and sick city appear in the imaginative relations to alleviating differences of income and wealth. This permits us to understand the relation of city to health as a political problem in the classical sense, specifically the problem of relating to differences and of reflecting upon the notion of alleviation as one position in this discursive economy.

Unexamined question

This leads to another interesting usage in relation to which we may take from Rancière (1999) to pose for consideration. He says that whenever a choice is involved (and it could be not just between actions to take but over different positions, theories, methods or evidence) and discussion hinges on that kind of opposition, interests always prevail that determine the talk to take shape in a format that calculates costs and consequences in the way that we might consider different interpretations, beliefs or opinions by adding up advantages and disadvantages as if profits and losses. The approach to the health of the city which asks whether the city is one or the other without thinking through either the notion of city or of health is such a strategy, and the evidence that it seeks, lacks and then selects is meant to tally up the powers of each position (each side).

Rancière calls such an approach apolitical because it is determined only by what is countable and excludes the uncounted (which we might treat as the indeterminate, ineffable, invisible, spirit or, in our case, the question of what the city or health each in its way can be taken to mean and to be), making the very question of choice a problem. In other words, how can one even conclude that a city is healthy or sick if he does not reflect upon what it is that is called a city or health and illness? Saying it otherwise, the question of whatness, of what something is, is always uncounted and a missing part of the conversation that only becomes political (dialogic) when it is brought into contact with the counted parts (interests, etc). Let us take this uncounted or missing part, memorialized by Plato as the Good, to be translated in Lacan's notion of the *object a* and in the enigma of Wittgenstein's seeing-as, registered in that effect on speech and in life that seems far because it is so near. This contact between the counted and uncountable is the space in which this relation (of what Rancière calls "demonstration") in which freedom (the freedom to say of anything what it is) comes into contact with the contingency of naming and classification that makes the social order a conventional distribution of inequalities resting on an ultimate incommensurability. A political approach to discourse in this sense does not simply inventory or add beliefs and opinions under the auspices of some standard of majority rule because this must assume and presuppose unexamined notions as variables "for all practical purposes."

What we must keep in mind as we proceed at this point is the limit of this unexamined conception of health as externally related to frequencies. For example, even life expectancy is assumed as a meaningful translation of the health of a collective by inferences that might always be challenged because it is simply affirmed in isolation from any deliberation upon the question of how it is true to the notion of health, remaining in this way unmeasured by the notion to which it assumes fidelity. For example, such data on death not only assume a connection of death to health which is arguable, but condense different types of death in unexamined ways and make assumptions about the quality of life and so of health and its variation. Moreover, before asking how death and dying relate to health and how a reported rate makes reference to the meaning it purports to imagine, we are entitled and indeed required to ask after the relationship of health to itself, how the usage and conceptualization of health that we manage to track and explore remains true to a notion of health. Part of our work here will be to expand the notion of health by exploring the kinds of relationship to life it both presupposes and anticipates.

The connection of health to death

Notice how Rodwin speaks about health and illness *through* death, providing death with a self-evidence simply by virtue of its statistics. Not really caring for death as it is engaged in life, he does depend upon the connection he imagines between the expectation of life as a kind of quantity and the disappointment that an untimely death brings, the very important and resonant notion that death can be at the right or wrong time and so can itself be an event that wrongs the person as if unlawful in its own way despite its universality. Here, though, he speaks not at all about the life of death, how it is lived and differentiated, experienced, and to whom and where and leaving what remains, what remainder. The excess of death, not the lack or hole in Being to which it points in the idiom of, say, philosophy and art, is the excess of its unlawfulness as it happens too much to the wrong persons and at the wrong times, that if death must be encountered by all alike, this pretense of its equality masks the wrong of its incidence, its capacity to strike us at our weakest moments, or to strike those of us who are weakest, or even if strong, to surprise us in ways for which we are never prepared. But then again, what is this event of death, this relationship we so name and to which we are so attached? And why is it so apparent that death is the barometer of our health and illness? Why is life healthy if it has perpetuity and why is it sick if it expires in an untimely way?

Note that the specialist tends to identify sick and healthy cities by reference to a death rate, and not even that, but in terms of life expectancies. This is interesting because a city ravaged by war or disaster is not *eo ipso* sick but perhaps simply innocent, defenseless or unlucky. Health, much like a capacity to ward off and minimize death, or to fortify us from death in great numbers and at certain times, is not addressed as a quality or a positive relationship except as a defensive encounter with death. Thus, health is not only defined in terms of what it is not, such as disease (which is wrong since not being sick is not the same as being healthy), but disease itself is simply equated with death. For a reflective approach, this all seems unsatisfying, for if death is a universal, an inevitable condition, then even if it results from disease at various points, this weakens the notion of disease by absorbing it into a condition such as death that makes life itself a disease, and disease a material condition without form. Health, as an image of whatever keeps us from death, maintaining survival, longevity and the like, is much like the tyrannical or dictatorial force that keeps us from perishing at the hands of our enemies. Confusing health with its force in enabling our survival is like praising Mussolini for making the trains run on time (while not being bad is not the same as being good, if we fear the subjectivity of value judgments, perhaps for many it seems the only way of addressing matters of value).

The formulation of a healthy life begins to take shape on the model of a master plan organized around the expectation of a normal length of life based on actuarial calculation. The value of health—its good—is that it is said to empower, enable and contribute to the lengthening of life. Health has value as a means to the end of lengthening life and to keep us fortified against contingencies, irregularities and disturbances that would disrupt such expectations. We see that healthfulness is implicated in an imaginative structure organized around visions of expectation and its disappointment in striking ways. Moreover, since the idea of a norm for length of life is based on a collective statistic, the eventfulness of health is invariably grounded comparatively in ways that induce any subject to accept the relativism of health as it applies to her.

Extending the sense of health

The normative character of the relation of health to illness is typically expressed through the ideas of self-governance, planning and taking care, and an image of prudence or moderation represented as a formula for the course of self-management designed to ward off disease and death. This vision of the relation of health to illness as a social relationship, of action oriented to an order and governed thereby in its course (Weber, 1947), links healthfulness to death and disease, conceptualizing health as a defense as such. In this formulation, what is self-evident is the use of health as a measure of the success of a strategy for self-defense, stripping health of any connection to the quality of the life lived. For practical purposes, a healthy life becomes a successful life in such a way. It would be interesting to examine obituaries to see how they pursue this connection in praising a life and lamenting its death, and particularly in inventorying achievements, for it very well might be that good health is reckoned among the good and virtuous achievements of a life (and why should we get special credit for health as if it is a considerable achievement marking us a being of high quality?).

Most important, this vision of healthfulness has to be undermined by a vision of its opposite or the conditions under which it fails to materialize, an image of the relation of health to illness not as normative but as a result of the fortuitous and unpredictable movement of disease and time of death, whether incoherent or patterned but occasioned by chance. Thus, the master plan for healthful self-governance, unlike the pedagogy for dentistry, can never guarantee the limitation and control of the irrational occurrence of disease and the capricious timing of death. Therefore, if the occurrence and incidence of disease and the timing of death are truly elements of a healthy life in the epidemiological and actuarial vision of health, then these elements become the definitive condition of health, the difference that brings to view the limits of health, as if health sees itself in the mirror of such an opposition, the conditions without which it would not be. Health then confronts its eventfulness as an idea in conjuring up an image of its own death, of the random play of disease and mortality, suggesting that the death of the notion itself, or of any notion, is not simply signified by chance and randomness, but by the view of the world as such matter, as an object for computation and calculation. This determination of health by one of its elements that should only be a part but is now made into its "structuring principle" is what Žižek (1997) calls antithetical determination. The universal (health or the relation of health to illness) is constituted by subtracting from a set some particular designed to embody the universal itself. The universal then arises, is posited as being-for-itself (health as such) in the act of splitting the wealth of particular diversity from this element in its midst that gives body to the universal (Žižek, 1997, p. 94). In other words, length of life, life expectancy, disease rates and the like, each and all come to embody health in the mirror of its opposite, an image of the death of health itself as a living notion as embodied in the failure to manage and plan for the inevitable attack of disease and death, the deficiency in self-governance marked in the failure to have a system for oneself.

The relativism of health due to the very nature of the rate as such means that anyone's health is measured by (because against or in reference to) the health of the many, linking health intrinsically to the question of justice and injustice and implicitly to the law. This is because death that strikes at the wrong time, or really at any time, is necessarily compared to the normative expectation in ways that can make of any one particular death an occasion for citing the injustice of this particular in relation to the universal (the normative). Moreover, if health imagines a trajectory that is expected to harmonize with a statistical expectation that is assumed as normative, then any disruption or departure appears as deviant, as an offense or infraction that transgresses the normal.

As the unanticipated noise that disrupts the expectation, death begins to dramatize the model of health in the primordial connection of harmony and homeostasis that Plato (1945, II.IX.398c–403c, pp. 85–88) envisioned as its rudimentary shape, the image of collectedness resisting disorder and dispersion. It is here that health comes to view through this very opposition as the desire to rectify the imbalance created by excitation that Freud (1961) discussed under the rubric of the pleasure principle. That is, death stands as a figure for the excitation that life seeks to overcome in reinstating its balance in ways that make healthfulness, pleasure and harmony synonymous. Here, though, Freud challenged himself and us to understand this very desire, this pleasure, as itself a kind of death (the deadly redemption of harmony) which recoils in the face of excitation to create a living death. Finally though, Freud urges us to move "beyond the pleasure principle" in order to explore the need for something other than harmony (pleasure), the drive of *jouissance* to maintain the excitation itself as part of the meaning of life (and of health). In this way, Freud reveals the tension in the very notion of health between its harmonic and erotic aspects, imagining the healthful life as continuously exercised by the challenge offered by the conflict between stability and restlessness, between desire (for finality) and drive (for vitality). What we might begin to appreciate is that a long life is not necessarily healthy if it is not vital, and a shorter life that is less successful in keeping death at bay, suffering excitation in its manner, is not necessarily diseased. Further, we see that the value of health is not simply to function as a means of defending against death because, as a notion, health enables us to put into play the question of what is a good life as if it might be such questioning and the relationships it makes possible and demands is a better sign of the healthy life than its length. The most popular epidemiological indicators of health in a population, infant mortality and length of life, point to the unspoken relation of birth to death as the beginning and end of any human story in Arendt's sense, but always as only a tentative framework for revising what is in between these chapters, the life that is lived.

Birth, death and the in-between

The self-evidence of birth as a commonsense phenomenon has been exposed over time by anthropologists such as Malinowski (1955), who showed the problematic character of the relationship of sex to the event of procreation, always revealed in a range of solutions to the problem of reconciling unlike ideas (sex and the event) through thinking that assigned responsibility for paternity in various ways. That is, the relationship between sex and birth does not necessarily have to be resolved through causal accounts that follow the trajectory of sperm because the enigma of birth can and has persisted in various ways. After all, the source of birth is attributable to love, a relationship, *techne* or any number of conditions that may not necessarily require a specific intervention, or as we appreciate now, even a notion of the erotic imaginary.

We could use Piaget's discovery of the perplexities of birth, and the question of how we enter the world, as a sign of the primordial concern for origin in Western philosophy, such as in Plato's *Meno* (s1949c), where the mystery of the origin and indestructibility of idea, usage and notion was raised. The discourse around the question of origin, marked by the voices of Plato's vision of soul in collision with the deconstructive unmasking of the illusion of such a position, becomes part of the phenomenon of the discourse itself, part of what natality expresses in collective life, perhaps in the shape of Lacan's empty word that invites a more demanding formulation.

Here we begin to appreciate how the question of natality marks the collective fascination with origin and, more particularly, with the relation between unlike ideas; for example, the exchange between sex and birth stands in for the relation between any apparently unlike events in ways that express an interest in the notion of a relationship (if in the case of birth this is a relationship between before and after, or between an act and its consequences, the focus remains on relatedness). In this sense, it is difficult to imagine any society that has not been exercised by the question of the relation between unlike events as even the simplest society has always seemed to connect the rising of the sun with consequences for growth and vegetation.

Creativity and corruption

Birth, on the surface expressed in the jubilation over a new arrival, always masks concerns over time, over the inexplicability of source, the consequentiality of present and the indeterminacy of effects and influences upon an unknown future, concerns that pose riveting problems of action and interpretation for those who would desire not to leave well enough alone. Birth has always engaged us as a focus of creativity, the trope of natality serving as a sign of the eventfulness of the source *and* of the beginning of an inexorable decline. The idea that what comes to be must perish, of ashes to ashes and dust to dust, bring birth and death together in the figure of life as decline and amnesia, typically in ways that Lacan and those such as Agamben discuss the progress in enlightenment that tends to forget its moment of inception, its creative origin (e.g., in the way Benjamin spoke of parliamentary democracy forgetting its origin in violence), or as sociology has spoken of institutionalization or the routinization of charisma. On the other hand, since life mediates the in-between period between birth and death, corruption is often reputed to follow from the inability to be accountable, the forgetfulness of productivity that allows its influences to dissolve without acknowledgment, emerging in the shape of indifference that Arendt identifies in the lack of care of any present for its past. In this sense, what is arresting about birth is both the violence of its emergence and the corruption that must follow in its wake in the form of its amnesia for its own history, often taking shape in the resistances that accumulate. This anxiety, captured in the formula of life as preparation for death, can be almost comic in its implication that life causes death or pathetic in its suggestion that only engaging our death can arouse us to think about the dimensions of a vital life.

In Hesiod's (1953) *Theogony* and Plato's (1949b) *Timaeus*, the creative violence of birth was recognized in ways that tended to mask the decline of life, displacing this collision through the figure of parental self-governance necessarily linked to a reflection upon origins and to the negative consequences of maintaining its violence through mechanical domination. Here birth can (and should) become an incentive, or at least an opportunity, to develop a good life through an understanding of human relationships to material conditions such as death. Thus, if birth makes death possible, then it also makes possible that reflection upon life that must coexist with the haunting immanence of death as a sign of the two-sidedness of human existence at its best.

Border crossings

The exchanges between birth and death are vividly dramatized in the typical use of infant mortality rates as an indicator of a healthy community, as if the mark of disease is the failure of life to materialize as expected, the failure of the promise to be fulfilled. Despite the force of this indicator, it appears to rest upon a notion of sterility that annuls the claim of productivity, almost as if the death of the infant reveals the limits of such an aspiration towards mastery. To better grasp the imaginary placement of birth and its failure to persist as an indicator of disease, we might contemplate the failure of death to persist in the reappearance of the dead in life, of the dead coming to life, whether as ghosts, spirits or the aura of those who are gone. If a sick society is one where the living die unexpectedly, then what of the society where the dead might reappear in life? Would such a society be sick by virtue of its saturation by superstition? Empiricism might say so. Perhaps the reappearance of the dead in life is a necessity in contrast to the unexpected reversal of life into death as reflected in the statistic of infant mortality. Both infant mortality and ghostliness reflect the dissolution of the boundary between life and death and so the fact that it is not one or the other that is irrevocable (birth, death) but the border itself. Here we can ask how the boundary between life and death is imagined in infant mortality and in concerns for the afterlife of the dead in vital traces. The work of de Coulanges (1955) on perpetuity and of Durkheim (1961) on ancestral influences become opportune occasions for exploring such border crossings.

Analogical thinking

We should appreciate now that a concern for birth as a collective representation must be a concern for the relationship between unlike ideas typically identified as analogical thinking. Birth first identifies the problem of the relationship in an approach to the event and its consequences, because the relation between procreation and what follows remains as enigmatic as the relationship between the event and its sources. Whereas empirical thinking reflects causally, necessarily treating any such relationship as probabilistic at best, the analogical approach to unlike ideas sees any relationship as a feature of the desire to master the effects of action (the absence of care of birth for what it creates forever immortalized in the myth of abandonment of Oedipus for the Greeks and in the modern myth of the monster of Frankenstein and its abandonment by the scientist).

Yet the primary feature of the analogy as a figure for birth seems to concern its status as a figure of desire for mediating the relation of thing to word and back again, the translation of the complexity of experience into a common conception, constantly seeking to maintain the life of the word by remembering its border with death, making the disciplined care for what is created in the life force of discourse, an engagement with the soul of human things that are made and circulated among us. We care, then, for what is created by speaking well, i.e., by thinking being (and so, nonbeing, death for us) in ways attuned to the soul of the relation between word and thing, to that intuition of form meant to intimately mediate the external and the internal that we imagine as the weaving of discourse as we aspire to inhabit its garb. Now we should recognize that the content of analogical thinking is nothing other than form itself, the need and desire to give form to material conditions (to the thing via the word, to the word via the thing) in the relationship Weber (1947) prosaically called "mutually oriented action."

The epidemic

Media representations of the spread of disease increasingly link prevalence to community; for example, in the case of diabetes, it is said that while it was once regarded as a middle-aged disease, it now affects every age group, anticipating according to the World Health Organization a 39% increase worldwide by 2030 (Dalby, 2007, p. Y1). In Toronto, such a rise is seen to coincide with what is called "suburbanization" and a landscape of fragmentation, including separation from stores, transit and services, a car culture and the decline of a street life and of public spaces. In addition to the ugly, resourceless environment, the *Toronto Star* mentions lack of access to nutritional food (and the prevalence of fast food outlets) and opportunities for exercise (walking and bicycle paths).

> Toronto's inner suburbs are the urban epicenter of an obesity and diabetes epidemic that is shortening lives and threatens to overwhelm our health-care system, says a groundbreaking study [...] The report's most startling finding is that urban sprawl—not just poverty and an immigrant population at greater risk—is contributing to diabetes rates in the city's poorest neighbourhoods that are almost triple those in more densely populated areas downtown. "This is a story about social disadvantage," said Dr. Rick Glazier, co-author of the report [...] "If you are not living in poverty and disadvantage, it doesn't matter what your neighbourhood looks like." (Monsebraaten and Daly, 2007, p. A1)

This is a curious conclusion, almost as if poverty is competing with the "look" of a community to determine where the guilt lies in disease. Yet, it is not as if poverty causes the diabetes rate as much as it weakens the abilities of residents to defend themselves from ugliness in the environment. This complex exchange between influences such as social class and beauty is simplified by such a rhetoric that reaches its verdict by computing a diabetes rate in areas with characteristics called:

> "Activity Friendliness" [which] indicates whether the area encourages daily physical activity such as walking and bicycling. Factors include crime and car ownership rates, and proximity to stores [...] [and] "Healthy

Resources" captures residents' proximity to things such as healthy food, places to exercise and health-care providers. (Monsebraaten and Daly, 2007, p.A1, sidebar ["Ailing Toronto neighbourhoods"])

What Rancière (1999) calls the counted parts—sprawl and its resourcelessness, ugliness and isolation—coexists with healthful factors enabling nutrition in eating, and exercise, and with poverty. The researchers want to know how sprawl, healthfulness and income interact in a causal format that can account for the variance. The interactions between these three factors are impossible to disentangle (if we could create a divine design for an experimental matrix controlling for each factor in relation to the other, we might prove to our satisfaction that one factor is guilty of causing diabetes), but unfortunately we humans have to live with the ambiguity of unexplained variance despite the willpower and assurances of ideologues. Note then that the interaction between neighborhood and poverty creates a surplus exceeding any one verdict about the cause of disease, an interaction reflected in the figure of desire. For neither condition, whether poverty (low income) or communality (friendliness and access), makes anyone sick, functioning instead as conduits or mechanisms through which demoralization is expressed. This is obliquely recognized as follows:

> "If their neighbourhood is just completely unsafe and we're telling them they have to walk a half an hour every day and there's nothing to walk to—there are no sidewalks, the lighting is poor, the snowdrifts pile up— it's not that people are not motivated, it's just that they can't," said Glazier. (Monsebraaten and Daly, 2007, p. A11)

He thinks that calling this a function of motivation is assigning blame to victims as if to say that the victims are weak-willed. This simplifies the question of desire by reducing it to motive and choice or agency over against determinism. However, it reinstates vividly the question of what drives those living in ugly and resourceless environments. So, if one asserts that, "Living conditions need to change," and another replies that, "It's more about raising people's incomes than razing buildings," then this leads us to ask after what Rancière calls the missing part or uncounted element in the discourse, a part that exceeds either poverty or access, or even nutrition and exercise potential. What is this uncounted element in diabetes other than the imaginary of health and illness? Is it part of the desire for life itself?

One might say that the epidemic is only on the surface diabetes, but that it is really demoralization itself reflected in the collective inability to overcome bad conditions (in this case, disparities in income and in the ugliness of an environment). Both income and ugliness are conceived as variations distributed unequally throughout collective life. This leads us to reflect upon the symbolic order of such distributions.

Variation as a communal problem

If experiences are distributed unequally, then dealing with any one condition is simultaneously dealing with all since the distribution of variations means that comparison is built into the problem of accepting one's lot. Even if differences occur in everyday life, this occurrence is oriented to as a common fate to which all must adapt. In terms of the symbolic order animated by the problem of health and illness, we note first the mystery of the cause, registered in the enigma of the determinant of health and illness as a question of the unfathomable surplus that exceeds representations of cause and effect. This discourse, organized as it is around an adversarial exchange between positions arguing for the relative import of different kinds of deprivation, of income, access and beauty, can only count such effects as having the import they do because of a concerted imaginary view of the impact of environment upon persons and of a mysterious intervening force that mediates these influences, too little income and too little beauty tending to crush persons and in some inexplicable way manage to produce specific symptoms through such a force. In this case, the person and the environment are wedded together as the same, whether shadowed by ugliness or by low income, both conditions having the effect of the same, that is, to determine the person by inflicting her. No matter what the environment is reputed to distribute, from the perspective of the imaginary relation to the distribution as an oriented material condition and as an object of desire (what sociology calls a social fact), the variation in experience is as a relationship, a variation in the capacity to separate oneself from the environment. In this way, the real danger appears to be the contagiousness of an environment and its capacity to infect people with a kind of deficiency that prevents them from separating themselves from its effects. At this level at least, health and illness depend upon the capacity of residents for objectification, for representing their environment as an occasion to develop rather than as a sealed fate that is part and parcel of anyone's identity.

Returning to Rancière, we note that the problem is not one of adjudicating the question of whether income or beauty is more important to this relationship, but that we must use this wrong revealed in the discourse in ways that might redeem the political question which it presupposes and yet, by which it is animated, the question of the city, the good city, as an uncounted part of the discourse. At this point, we take this question to address the problem of the collective relationship to variation in the distribution of good and bad conditions, as a question that is missing and yet needs to be posed, redeemed and discussed as the missing part of the discourse, its political engagement.

Polis

The relationship between the city and health and illness can be heard as addressing the question of the *polis* and its limits. This follows from the primordial notion of city as *polis,* as a collective that works out and on its differences and in this respect (since difference is not an exception to the rule but normal), needs to suffer ambiguity as continuous and not simply as an interim state of affairs.

> The city is not primarily a "community" any more than it is primarily "public space." The city is at least as much the bringing to light of being-in-common as the dis-position (dispersal or disparity) of the community represented as founded in interiority or transcendence. It is "community" without common origin. That being the case, and as long as philosophy is an appeal to the origin, the city, far from being philosophy's subject or space, is its problem. (Nancy, 1991, p. 23)

What he means is that the city as a figure brings to view "being-in-common" as a condition of fundamental ambiguity, as the unspoken commitment to the "we" that simultaneously pervades us in our dispersal and escapes our capacity to determine it as this-or-that in a common origin (whether consensus, state of nature, jungle or war). This appeal and its aura that haunts all representation is expressed as the *polis* (the fundamental ambiguity of the "we").

The *polis* is defined historically and essentially as grounded in an unspoken sense of "we" in ways that come to personify speech (at its best) as both mimetic and diversified, both together and apart, and so, as continuously oriented to its discursive character. The commitment to being-in-common, neither self-evident, unitary or indivisible, is *imagined* as an inescapable necessity of co-speakers anywhere (this is Nancy's "problem"), a necessity forever in excess of what can be determined and so, fundamentally other, as that beginning (in the idiom of Hegel) always in need of development, explication and actualization. This trajectory or graph of desire in Hegel's *Logic* (1968) recognizes the whole (absolute or Other) as a necessity that is both and at once a source of imagination and frustration. In this case, the hole in the signifier is registered in the hole in the We as an inescapable site of signification, always intimating the indeterminate to the whole that exceeds it. That is, even those denying being-in-common as a problem by calling it logocentric, essentialist, fantasy or delusional always appeal to such an imperative in their speech, invariably revealed in its desire for recognition marked by the transference relation of speaking to an auditor (Lacan's big Other). Thus, the relationship of *polis* to city is not empirical but grammatical, making reference to the dream of a fusion between speech and action assumed to be intrinsic to any notion, to a course of desiring that only appears when instabilities in various interpretive solutions to problems become visible. That is, anarchy, war, corruption, selfishness, power and utilitarianism do not refute the *polis* but materialize as part of its discourse, always occasioning in specific ways the need to make use of whatever the notion of *polis* recommends.

The dialogical character of *polis* as the unthought bond of intersubjective desire to say more than can be determined is made visible in practices of interpretation and action such as in questioning the relation of city to health, where these practices bring to view irresolution as itself the social phenomenon centering the vitality of collective life. Since the relationship of the city to the Good is long-standing, we can understand the question of the Good of the *polis* along these lines, but with the caveat that we imagine this relationship as grounded to some extent in a relationship to ambiguity. This is to say prospectively that a good *polis* is one that *suffers* the necessary ambiguity of its bond rather than be victimized by it (or insulted, injured or threatened by it). The question of the "we" comes to view in the conventional equation of the good community with the healthy community in a way that automatically equates health with the Good (in ways that both Parsons and Foucault famously criticized). Of course, this assumption is subverted in this text by impersonating the voice that conceives of the good community as the collective exercised by the question of this very relationship of health to the city, the collective imagined as being true to its desire to be reflective about its practices, inviting all inquiry on health and the city to be accountable in some way to this measure. This is the exaggeration that is forced upon the narrative. While it might be accurate to say in certain cases that a good city is a healthy city in the strong senses of both city and health, we could begin to disturb the notion that a good city is *eo ipso* a healthy city in the conventional sense by making some trouble for the convention of identifying the Good with health and by implication, the typical use of cooperation and malingering as medicalized versions of the ethical and unethical respectively. We should appreciate today that there are many ways of discussing the relation of health to the city and that most of these ways do not set out to make problematic the notions of "health" and "the city" that function as crucial signifiers in the relationship. Note how the concern for "being-in-common" expressed by Nancy as a reflection of the communal is proportionate to the relationship to the distribution of variations in experience of the environment. In part, the city is envisioned as a relationship to variation in such a way, the best relationship to the distribution of bad conditions, to the contagiousness of the environment and its capacity to extinguish the strongest prospect of human desire.

Infection

The city, then, can be understood here as a scene that produces variations in conditions that always threaten to make bad conditions superabundant in the same way that the body can be said to produce bad cholesterol or inflammation or multiplication of cells that endanger health. Part of the imaginary of the *polis* is the fear of infection, the fear that the purity of distinctions (definitions, methods, conclusions or agreements) will be annulled by the forceful mixing and matching of incommensurable terms and interests, by what it fears as an incoherent circuit of signifiers without any basis in nature, conventional and arbitrary, that can deprive the collective of the unitary resolve it requires of itself. Because the desire to interrupt this circuit always originates from its midst, *en medias res*, any intervention can only be a sacrifice, a leap in the idiom of Kierkegaard, that is ethical by nature of its refusal (in the words of Lacan[1992, pp. 311–325]) to give ground in relation to its desire, the desire to represent what is fundamentally ambiguous, not as a cure or a final solution to meaning, but as part of the healing touch. Or, in the words of Wittgenstein (1965), ethics begins to describe the collision when, in trying to say what is, we run up against the limits of language, when we encounter this limit in the spirit of *jouissance* rather than as a moment of pain. The struggle against indistinction in language in the service of an attentiveness to discrimination is often seen as unnatural enough to warrant being treated as if self-inflicted punishment, taking on discipline in ways that unnecessarily give one pain. This is similar to ways in which regimes of healthfulness counsel (indeed demand) punishing, self-inflicted disciplining of the body in defense against the overproduction of its bad conditions. Thus, balancing the pain of bad conditions against the pain of self-renunciation is an analogy permitting us to appreciate one tacit effect of enlightened society, applying both to body and city, making the relation to both a continuous balancing act always in need of new information, expert intervention, advice and possibly reeducation.

If purity is seen to be infected by ambiguity, then standing up for purity seems to make demands of self-renunciation that can only be painful. Indeed, one could follow Scarry (1985) in personifying such a fear in the figure of the one in pain (for example, the torture victim), the one deprived of sentience in a state overcome by intense self-absorption (for example, with the body) that makes objectification and mediation impossible because the condition for developing a relationship outside of oneself seems to be extinguished. Extending this usage, infection by ambiguity could be feared as a kind of disease that strikes speakers silent, that renders them mute, depriving them of voice. More prosaically, when silence is of this nature in everyday life (think of the characters we typically engage in leisure and workplaces), when it does not seem thoughtful and oriented but painful in the way of one who appears almost as if he is being tortured by having to speak, we can identify our colleague as being in pain. Yet if some suggest that the silence of pain means that it does not signify, Scarry demonstrates that pain as the relation it is must be significant in that sense, confirming reflection upon pain as such in ways that require the kind of distance or spacing antithetical to self-absorption, as the sort of "making" of the world and culture that pain unmakes. In this sense, the *polis* and its requirement of sentience is not refuted by pain, but brought to view as necessary and desirable on such occasions because pain as silent must still speak in its way.

This leads some like Lyon (2005) to concretize pain, as thought to be exemplary in German idealism and in notions such as *bildung* (and presumably Heidegger) by attributing its glorification to theorists such as Schiller, who is assumed to make necessary the pain of aesthetic education. The usage from which Lyon recoils treats pain as a disciplined relation to conversation, a demand to work on one's speech along the lines of the psychoanalytic model of abreaction or working through resistance, making pain into the sensitivity of any subject to talk that approaches her repressed core or center. In this way, any discursive challenge to formulaic talk would be construed as painful, perhaps as a simplified caricature of the notion of a "poisoned environment." So the uprooting of distinctions that we identify as the undeveloped beginning of any speech always identifies pain as a figure for the anxiety that is released by the dialectical engagement of the subject with language.

If pain has such a place in this discourse (perhaps as a misrecognition of the necessary experience of "going against the grain" in dialogue), then such criticism accuses it of being used as a euphemistic strategy to distract us from the negative consequences it inflicts under cover of its pretension of discipline as necessary. Even such critics as Sontag (1978), in her polemic against metaphor, obliquely recognize the tension here as intrinsic to the aesthetic subversion of usage. In this respect, Radley (1999) too tries to develop an appreciation for what he calls the aesthetic relation to narrative as opposed to content, but this, while good-spirited, is much too concrete in its sorting, making the aesthetic relation to content an example of the either/or and reducing the aesthetic to a simple opposition to content. Most concerns revolving around the pain of speech seem to base their accusation upon a sense of the labor or travail they imagine involved in reflection in ways that have a degree of truth, and indeed any symbolic order presupposes a speaker needing to accept a degree of restraint upon herself in submitting to the rule of some standardized format, in the way objectification remains necessary and even desirable to some extent (an acceptance that seems to some as if a self-infliction of pain). Yet negative images of such pain can only imagine it on the model of a punishing superego, as if there is a possibility for what they call "anti-mimesis" as the pleasure of effortless ease and convenience that can only transgress the constraint of mimesis. In contrast, the Grey Zone must acknowledge the ground of speaking to reside in the potential of an improvisational and creative mimetic relationship and its character as a fluctuating mix of pleasure and pain (Plato's *Philebus*).

Immunization as the strategy for resisting such infection seems to require a sterilization of language structurally similar to the requirements of the body, and by implication, the spaces of the city where the diversity of new arrangements seems to threaten long-standing agreements and boundaries. This tension at the heart of the discourse of the *polis*, forever pitting immunization against infection as if an either/or choice, leaves open the question of the Grey Zone, the in-between zone in which ambiguity is mediated as the possibility for creating an improvisational relationship to this opposition between immunization and infection just as infection must be risked and immunization must be relaxed. That is, in the language of Plato (1960), the Same must open itself to its otherness just as the Other must be alive to its grounds (in the idiom of this work: the *polis* must be alive to its own intrinsic diversity, the many ways in which it is represented, just as these many ways of making reference to the *polis* must be bound together by the concerted desire that co-speakers must share in being mutually oriented).

If pain, as if being compelled or forced into silence, is an omnipresent material condition, then suffering tries to reflect upon the inevitability of such a condition and on strategies of composing oneself as such. It is in such ways that we might appreciate both pain and suffering as part of the *polis* and its discourse, for as pain points to the kind of inflexibility or speechlessness suggested by either extreme of immunization and infection, it is expressed by relating to this opposition as if fatal, or at least, as a binding normative order, whereas healing begins to address the possibility of a prosthetic relation to such an opposition as these extremes are placed by reflecting upon the question of influence as a healthy rather than sick relationship to language and life. Thus, these remarks make central to any relationship the condition of mediation as both topic and resource, as discussed in Chapters 1 and 2. As topic, in the words of Scarry, mediation is a condition of sentience and so, of the *polis*, and as a resource, mediation envisions a practice or method for engaging the conditions in which we experience the relationship of language to the world as a living relationship. Yet, mediation can only *fantasize* its own absence, just as life can only fantasize the inner spirit of death from the outside, so to speak, making mediation forever imaginary and ambiguous.

Such an investigation could begin with certain common conceptions, and these conceptions begin to lay grounds for understanding the relation of language to the *polis* and of both to health and illness. What is sick in the idiom of Wittgenstein (1953) is fixation on abstract visions of language and life, which inflict upon us a relentless and painful hermeneutic distress, making ambiguity an occasion for what Arendt calls hatred of the world and its symptoms of reductionism, privatization, rage or perhaps Plato's (1955) vision of *misology* as a pain which can only be rectified by conversion into healing, the *modus vivendi* with ambiguity as the signifier begins to appear as a relationship in a living language, taken up, in the words of Benjamin (1971, pp. 155–194), as booty for the poet to plunder. The grammatical investigation suggests that urbanity has the capacity to produce both the coexisting temptations of freedom and evil. The sickness against which we must take precautions refers to ways in which we who are drawn to the city must inoculate ourselves from its effervescence and from the temptation to inflate the present moment as eternal and our selves as free and sufficient.

This is to say that it is not metaphor, figuration or poetry that makes Socratic ignorance (I know that I do not know) a paradox, but the fundamental ambiguity of the desire for knowledge, of the need and desire to speak about what is presupposed and given, i.e., what is already accepted. That this impossible position can yet be inspiring, while neither soluble nor something from which we can escape, is a gesture always appearing inefficient, immature or untimely, because the material conditions of speaking seem like an iron cage. It is in such examples that we might note the primordial force of the image of a Grey Zone as a zone of ambiguity, enabling us to begin to recover what is undeveloped in the modern enlightenment recognition. Yet to appreciate this, we must grasp the pacification of discourse not simply through its more obvious manifestation in the transaction between co-speakers (so-called intersubjectivity) but as an aspect that resides in the very bowels of the word itself.

Ambiguity regarding pain and suffering, our own and that of the other, is an inevitability according to Mead's (1967) conception of the self as divided between its twin capacities to be subject and objectified in the same way as toe, table or cow, that the body never vanishes because it is correlative with the self and the omnirelevance of seeing-as as the human way. Thus, the body recurs as a feature of the power of humans to imagine themselves as if mere objects (toes, tables and cows). This is why the power of humanity remains a blessing and a curse, for the advantage of seeing-as is at the same time a burden reflected in being able to see oneself as nothing, as objectified, as mute.

Pain and suffering are good examples here, no longer simply metaphoric implications of speaking as we suggested previously, but in the case of pain, the actual injury experienced in the conception of fateful silence is a sign of the mute inarticulate impotence expressed in our reduction to objecthood experienced as pain. Pain helps remind us that our not being a body in Mead's sense can only coexist with our similarity to the body, always bringing to view for us that border when pain makes our inexpressibility vivid. Pain then brings us back to the difference that Mead tended to gloss in the eventful engagement of this self with its nonbeing in silence.

It would be important then to contrast the reflective silence integral to the self and its necessary solitude, to the silence in being overcome by or with grief, which might still seek space to negotiate the experience, with the mute response Scarry and others have described in pain. The silence of pain seems a reduction isolating and mute in the sense that one can only compose herself to pray for an end in the form of relief from the experience, seeking at best the method or *techne* that might make what is unendurable pass away. In this way, too, pain does make a place for the virtue of *techne* in a world that is unmade, a world in which there are no spices and nothing better can be expected than escaping the worst. It is in this manner that having the self enables us to imagine its extinction and all of the atrocities that can and do befall those such as us. This also shows us the ambiguity in rhapsodies over technical progress, limited as they often are to the relief of pain, which we need and long for and anticipate prayerfully but often misidentify as the Good rather than as the relief of what is bad. Discriminating relief of pain from the Good is not ungrateful, but it does reveal its knowing that while a painless life is better than a painful one, it is not the good life by virtue of this alone and, as Plato (1945) implied, could be a dog's life.

Having the self also enables us to imagine the pain of others, not as our pain to be shared but as the condition we need suffer and develop in relation to this difference by recovering a voice that can measure this for us as self-formative, and so less as an external experience that we have but as an experience we need repossess as part of our struggle to know ourselves. If in pain the body recurs in the visibility and drama of our sense of extinction, in the sense that we are, after all, a body as well, then in the pain of the other it recurs as our experience of this difference between one and the other as the sameness of our mortality that must be shared, whether acted upon or denied, as the common fate.

Doxa as sickness and the city

If we understand life affirmation as the *doxa* of healthfulness, we can eventually inquire into the uses of health and sickness in the city. First, we can begin with certain common conceptions, and these conceptions begin to lay grounds for understanding the relation of language to the *polis* and of both to health and illness. For example, Wittgenstein (1953, p. 19) identifies sickness as the condition when "language goes on holiday," which means that the speaker resists the work of examining ambiguous notions in use as symptoms of collective problems because they are treated as notions to be cured rather than healed. For Wittgenstein, healing notions means taking them up, finding their use strange or odd and so trying to redeem them in their way as moments in problem-solving sequences that make sense when understood as imaginative positions. Here, inquiry is active and works rather than goes on holiday, because it is not lulled into sleep by speech that it accepts as formulaic and makes into its own as if a second nature. Today we might say that language goes on holiday when we treat it as a usable databank, when we forget the "creative function of truth in its nascent form'" (Lacan, 1991, p. 19). Benjamin (1998) identifies this state with the "shock" of contact with the masses where the masses serve as his figure for the amorphous crowd of passers-by imprinted on the soul of the creative person. The masses are the figure of speech for the crowd of words or fragments from which the poet begins, the images or data of remembrance that would continue to paralyze him until he could begin to work on its mechanistic appearances. Both language and the *polis* require the space of mediation, the creative distancing of separation where habituation and sanctification are neither simply accepted nor in contrast simply rejected, but represented and publicized: the public realm. The space of mediation is invariably the space of solitude, giving us a glimpse of an image of the healthfulness of the city as residing in its capacity to make room for ambiguity (for the opportunity to develop a capacity for seeing-as).

Excess as a social force

So what is reputed to be sick about the modern city is, in part, its freedom, or its capacity to release desire from its fetters, to unchain *eros* as a force that is essentially two-sided, because unchained desire, *eros* at its best, can lead to good or evil, requiring, as Plato (1960) says, an intelligence that is capable of measuring desire (and is modern medicine not aiming to play the part of such an intelligence in its offer to moderate desire, understanding itself almost competitively as a vision of self-understanding or of intelligence equivalent to philosophy?). Arendt (1971) develops this tension as the work of thinking that operates as an influence upon judgment and will. And this is how those like Foucault (1965) can suggest that the science of medicine has corrupted the Good by making it into health (even though Foucault distrusted any notion of the Good). Then, just as the modern city is typified as unhealthy, so is the medical practice that arises to defend us against the body's violence, now defined as the *sine qua non* of intelligence (in ways that could influence us to treat health as the highest and most comprehensive human Good because it is the only Good that can produce accord). Most importantly, if the excess of *eros* takes shape in a way that is distinctively modern, then it must show in a way true to the notion of the modern how the need for the antidote of intelligence exists in this form, then such an intelligence must expertly discern the relation of mind to body (implied in hyperbolic desire); in other words, it must not be simply a science of body or a science of mind but something like a reflection on judgment or on the thinking that enters into excess (into satisfaction, pleasure and enjoyment). Can we venture a difference between modern and classical images of how intelligence can limit *eros* without repressing or destroying its force?

We need here to begin to explore the meaning of the contagiousness of social life, because modernity is typically treated as that situation when the force of indistinction dissolves clear-cut distinctions and borders in a way by shocking individuals and overcoming their defenses, weakening them in the idiom of Nietzsche (1956). In speaking of such forces, Durkheim (1961, p. 280) says: "Does an individual come into contact with them without having taken precautions? He receives a shock which might be compared to the effects of an electric discharge […] If they are introduced into an organism not made to receive them, they produce sickness and death." This "sickness" is described by Santner (2001, p. 22) as an "uncanny sort of surplus animation" through which the fullness of life can affect us. If the desire to be in the city, to be where the action is, is deep, then it can be understood as the desire to become immersed in the effervescence of the social, to give oneself to the intoxicating contagiousness of the social.

That we can become ill in the city (become mad with the intoxicating excess of its effervescence, or more conventionally, "hysterical") suggests that urbanity has the capacity to produce both the coexisting temptations of freedom and evil. The sickness against which we must take precautions refers to ways in which we who are drawn to the city must inoculate ourselves from its effervescence and from the temptation to inflate the present moment as eternal and ourselves as free and sufficient. This extremism in response to conditions is, according to Durkheim, a feature of the vitality of social life and its forces; such prompting into opposite directions is part of the overstimulating character of the social, bringing us together by pulling us in all sorts of different directions (part of the dangerous *eros* Plato [1945] noted in his likely story).

Inoculation is connected to both space and time. In relation to space or social distance, the fear of being infected by the diverse and unruly influences to which we can be exposed was dramatized in Plato's (1945) representation of the character of Socrates in the *Republic* (particularly in Book 3 where Socrates was made to defend the segregation of the man of virtue from unsavory or unruly influences such as in the education of judges, and in Book 6 where he discusses the corruption of philosophers by the marketplace and implicitly popular culture). Plato uses Socrates to dramatize the extremist temptation to immunize virtue from influences that have the potential for corruption because of their overstimulating character. The interlocutor to Socrates is Plato himself, who engages the unsavory influences against which his Socrates seeks to inoculate himself, showing an art that is neither fearful like Socrates, nor reckless like the fool, but prudent. That inoculation is often impotent in the face of the unsavory influences it seeks to expurgate is shown not only through the figure of the return of the repressed but in the way the war against evil has to imitate the very evil which it contests, an age-old proverbial version of the Grey Zone that recurs in liberal headshaking, popular culture and its media, in politics and in most instrumental doctrine.

Inoculation is connected to time by seeking to defend itself from the demanding aura of any present that invariably appears as overstimulating in that our existence in time creates experiences of loss or disjunction that at any moment can occur as challenge or as an occasion of lament. What is overstimulating is the two-sided destructive and opportunistic relevance of temporality for desire: "the world in gross and in detail, is irrevocably delivered up to the ruin of time unless human beings are determined to intervene, to alter, to create what is new. Hamlet's words 'The times are out of joint [...] I was born to set it right,' are more or less true for every generation" (Arendt, 1954, p. 192). I suggest that the lure of the city and of its social effervescence lives off its capacity to empower the present moment, any present, as a period of the highest expectations, the period in any life when the consequentiality of action and the contagiousness of the social comes to view as decisive, as fateful. In part, social life is overstimulating because it can arouse us to extremes, to action or inaction, always enticing us with the prospect that our choices at present can make a difference and so with the prospect that the present has an aura of decisiveness about it if we can take heed. In any present, the drama of taking heed or not is infectious, stimulating us to exceed our limits, perhaps to imagine an eternal present.

In this way, Durkheim put his finger on the normalcy of ambiguity in social life when he modeled it on the crossing of boundaries and borders and thus on the interpenetration and mixing of signifiers, as if language is expressed in the figure of metaphor that bridges distinctions conventionally sanctified, representing the threat of contagion and infection when distinct terms appear to become indistinct. In the language of Durkheim, the contagiousness of a dense and volatile social life is reflected as threatening indistinction, as the pain of being unable to determine and differentiate, of being unable to discriminate, the fear of being the subject who is powerless to influence the language in use. That power is marshaled by imagining that a grammatical investigation, as Wittgenstein (1953) calls it, can make a difference, that it will not be a cure but can and should apply the healing touch to ambiguity (which, as we might see by now, is just a confirmation of the vitality of the social and so a condition to bear and not to lament).

Durkheim might say that the characterization of the modern city as sick makes not only modernity out to be essentially corrupt (and so loses the phenomenon) but it makes the social corrupt as well, misrecognizing the effervescence of social life as if it is hysterical and pathological instead of seeing its vitality as normal and intrinsic to the meaning and measure of the social. Durkheim supposes the vitality of social life to always and everywhere have this effect of being overstimulating. The problem is then not so much a choice between health and illness but one of developing a reflective relationship to the overstimulating character of the social (to excess or to the surplus as Bataille originated and as Lacanians like to say). Overstimulation itself becomes a material condition when the unruliness of the emotions manifests itself with the solidity and weight of unalterable matter, causing us typically to misrecognize such inflammatory aspirations as desire incarnated. The problem discussed in this chapter is a version of the relation between life and form that Simmel (1971, pp. 351–393) so deftly discussed, in ways that anticipate each and all of these speakers, including myself, who try to identify the Grey Zone as that very distinction, not as an abstract notation but as a continuous and opportune occasion for research because members have to engage and try impossibly to reconcile such ambiguity in varied and specific ways.

8

On Being Old

Introduction

It might seem strange that the problem of age and aging brings to view the tensions in the relationship of enlightenment progress and the Grey Zone. We can see this in the commonplace representation of age as a public issue, for example as discussed in the *Globe and Mail* (Miller and Scoffield, 2009). Here it is reported that age is and promises to become a major problem for "G20 nations" because of the threatening "dependency ratio" that predicts "[o]ver the next 20 years the number of Canadians over the age of 65 will rise to 40% of the population from 20% today" (Miller and Scoffield, 2009, para. 3). The implications of this Malthusian nightmare is the alarm over increasing debt needed to support such growing dependency, new stimulus packages that strain the collective capacity to distribute resources and the like. What remains fascinating, though, is how what is thought good and beneficial can produce what seems bad. That is, if enlightened medicine succeeded in conquering collective maladies that were signified typically in lower life expectancy rates and higher infant mortality rates, not to mention the conquest of diseases, then such gains have not liberated society but have produced instead disadvantages that are even more problematic.

If conquering disease has created the problem of chronic disease or of living with the disease, then conquering early death has created the problem of living with old age. Certainly the alarmists are not proposing that the aged and the diseased be exterminated, but then we might wonder that when push comes to shove (e.g., time for resource allocation) whether or not such a fantasy might haunt even good-hearted liberals. The gains of enlightened medicine have produced the consequences of living with these effects; that is to say, making disease livable has created the problem of living with disease as a problem not simply for the sick but for all who are touched by them. We want to explore how this representation of the Grey Zone helps us think about the reinstatement of the patient experience because such an experience now can be seen to apply not simply to the aged and diseased but to their caretakers and the experts who must deal with them, and neither caretakers nor experts can be expected to know what it is to live under such conditions.

This shows that a medical version of the problem and its solution, even as it succeeds in realizing its medical objectives, cannot anticipate the consequences of such action as contributing to anything more than the abstract survival of a category. This glosses the life of the sick or of the aged that would always need to be engaged as a result of even the most successful actions taken towards their health and illness. Medicine tends to view living as sick and living as old as an upshot of medical procedures that keep the old and the sick alive, where the only consequences of import to follow in the aftermath of such successes is the expectation of cooperation with expertise that sanctions the impersonal formulation of what the patient experience is and treatment in accord with such.

This can be noted in the alarm expressed in the media over the new dependency, for this focuses only on the right of dependents for resources that must be shared in a society such as ours. Once the medical problem is relieved, then, the important problem of both sick and aged, of any dependent, refers to the partitioning of resources and to rights of the different categories now treated as political in this sense, i.e., the problem of justice. This avoidance of the question of how to conceptualize the life of dependency as the weaker party, and so as an ethical question connected to a debate on justice, avoids asking how the collective need orient to living with dependency now that the medical problem has been reduced to one of cooperation with expertise and of negotiating the institutional framework organizing such relations as service delivery. I believe that this is the best version of Agamben's (1998) notion of bare life as living in a way that is subject to the political calculation of resource allocation, that the achievements of the system actually produce the need to endure (and survive) a life of dependency, where each and every one is treated as a member of a category governed by instrumental inventories of resource allocation.

(Thus, in Rancière's [1999] sense, the uncounted part refers to the question of what is a good society, or a just relationship to the weaker party, that remains the genuine and repressed political focus glossed in the attempts to calculate consequences of positions.)

> In Rhode Island, which is also wrestling with high unemployment and severe budget shortfalls, Gov. Don Carcieri proposed cutting his state's prescription drug program for seniors. "It was a very difficult decision, and it's strictly a budget decision," said Corrine Russo, director of the state Department of Elderly Affairs, which runs the program. [...] "[W]e're at the point where we need to ask everybody to sacrifice on this budget [...]" (Henry, 2009, paras. 21–22, 29)

In this astonishing revelation, the aged are treated as if an interest group, reluctantly required to sacrifice just like every other constituency, showing us how the progress of enlightenment that has sustained their very longevity is two-sided, creating a vision of living death as bare life, living with age or sickness as if a member of a category dependent on the largesse of sovereign others who are in position to accept or take exception to such ambiguity (the ambiguity separating person from category or that differentiates between categories in terms of their "equality"). Here then might be another version of the patient's experience, capitalizing on the difference between being treated statistically (stereotypically) in this way or as one with qualifications that exceed such determination. In the kind of society we are examining, there seems to be nothing particular about the aged or about aging except its inevitable destiny as an object of care and dependency in relation to scarce resources and so an inevitable burden upon both self and others. Plato (1945) tried to make some trouble for such a notion.

Note in the opening of the dialogue in the *Republic* at the home of the elder Cephalus, how Socrates does not assume that he knows Cephalus' experience of old age but puts that question to him, and it is Cephalus' answer that begins to frame the discussion as a first approach to the collective representation.

> To tell the truth, Cephalus [...] I enjoy talking with very old people. They have gone before us on a road by which we too may have to travel, and I think we do well to learn from them what it is like, easy or difficult, rough or smooth. And now that you have reached an age when your foot, as the poets say, is on the threshold, I should like to hear what report you can give and whether you find it a painful time of life. (Plato, 1945, I.I.328, p. 4)

Socrates makes it possible to hear the experience of the aged as instructive, showing in this way that the one who deals with the aged or the sick must desire to speak with them as such, on the grounds of the expectation that the talk makes a difference. Is this not a precondition for reinstating the experience of the patient (of the aged, the sick) as a matter of relevance for those who are touched by them? And we see the desire as twofold, as the induction of desire in Cephalus, to speak and converse, and in Socrates' commitment to arouse himself to find his voice in the talk. In response to what he views as the misguided complaints against old age by the elderly who "regret losing the pleasures of their younger days," Cephalus cites the alternative he attributes to Sophocles; when asked if he missed the pleasure "of enjoying a woman," he replied "I am only too glad to be free of all that; it is like escaping from bondage to a raging madman" (Plato, 1945, I.I.329, p. 5). In contrast to the conventional nostalgia for the loss of youth and its erotic powers, and regret for the unhappiness and misery of old age, Cephalus imitates the poet who is relieved at being old and escaping *eros*.

This reply begins to enable us to appreciate the ambiguity surrounding the idea of decline in old age: Cephalus claims that the reputation of the misery of old age is a result of lamenting and misrecognizing the loss of bodily powers and erotic aspirations and capacities as a major condition instead of seeing old age as a path opening towards relief from "the raging madman" of *eros* on the road to tranquility. The status of this contrast of raving *eros* and serenity is unclear, and the status of the body in this imaginary is yet an open question. If he seems to want to balance the aching distress of lost *eros* with the opportunity for respite, it is based on a utilitarian vision of old age as if it needs to compensate for such a dispossession. If the decline of the body and its evacuation of *eros* leads to the serenity of monastic old age, then, as Socrates implies, old age has nothing positive of and for itself as a relationship (and indeed, Cephalus' tranquility seems a mask, as Socrates suggests, for his particular advantage in having money). Most important for the dialogue on justice, though, is that Cephalus exposes the possibility that the reputation of decline in old age can be used as a pretext for privatization and for "doing your own thing," away from the demands of conversation; in other words, the reputation of old age can be used as a pretext for withdrawing from public life in the same way that the reputation of illness will come to be used in malingering. The discourse will then include a permanent skepticism towards both conditions, agedness and disease, as either or both wanting to be privatized or needing to be privatized.

The status of the body is important, for on one account, if its dominance seems to be left behind ("the raging madman"), then the regret for its decline and memories of past powers seem to make it as dominant a condition of any present. In other words, the preoccupation with the body is omnipresent, making its dominance everlasting. Even as Cephalus claims himself to be free from such bondage, unlike his contemporaries whom he belittles, the need to reflectively monitor the body in old age seems inescapable. Freedom from the body as a raging madman is still constrained by the limits posed by such irregularity, by the need for such an escape. If the body is omnipresent rather than a lost object, then just what place does it occupy in the life of the aged (not to mention the sick)? What this section raises as the surface of the representation of old age is the relation between physical decline and insularity that the status of the body as an image seems to provoke. We anticipate that Cephalus separates youth from old age by virtue of his ascribing the possibility of an intelligent relation to the body in old age. This can be made problematic, as Plato suggests and as Freud comes to do. Questioning the intelligence of the relationship to the body requires resuscitating the body as an image and not simply as a natural fact of life, i.e., it requires returning to such basics. Let us begin to explore such images routinely circulating in the discourse.

Physical decline/passing time

> Because the question of aging is bound up with end of life, there is
> resistance to reflecting upon it. Idea of incapacities suggests that human
> life is transformed into a more pathogenic development of *ad pejus*.
> (Vischer, 1966, p. 11)

If conventions say that aging is simply a stage of physical/mental decline, then this
identifies it with a limiting case that does not begin to formulate its character as a relationship.
Even if physical deterioration is a frequent effect of aging, so might be a cranky disposition
or many other such consequences as incidentals that accompany aging as it occurs. But
then again, what kind of "occurrence" is aging, for it seems so amorphous that it is difficult
to distinguish from life in general. The subject of aging must be conceived as oriented to
what it means to age, to the kind of relationship aging is rather than is not. This can be
thought of as the ideal speaker, the one imagined as theorizing aging. For example, in the
most rudimentary sense, aging can be formulated as a relationship to passing time that
could include everyone and anyone since all can be noted as oriented to the experience of
passing time. Could we venture, in order to supplement this beginning, that aging must
specify the condition when passing time is conceived as decisive, dramatic or even fatal?
The ideal speaker, one who orients to recover impossibly the unthought whatness in the
different views of aging, is conceived as one engaged by the notion of aging.

If aging is treated as equivalent to life itself, then it becomes simple endurance or growing
up, as if aging is just adding years, increasing, quantity, longevity, in a way that seems
equivalent to growth. It is plausible to treat aging as simple growth, but this invites us to
ask what needs to be added to growth as a relationship (in the formulation) to make it into
aging? (Here is a funny thought: if aging is adding years on, then it might be seen as hoarding
or in the practice of the collector who safeguards his years in a miserly spirit, connecting
to both Benjamin's [1971] Collector and Simmel's [1971] Miser.) We often treat the aged
in this way by asking, "Just what are you holding on to?" or by bemusedly commenting on
their not wanting to let go, as if living for the aged is like hanging around.

If aging is simply passing time, or even living and growing, as in the way a plant grows,
then this reductionism disregards reflecting upon whatever seems to make aging the
social phenomenon it is. Of course, what aging is and is not is always an open question,
but it is the desire to engage such openness in the face of its impossible resolution
that marks the ideal speaker as the implicit focus of the narrative trajectory. If aging is
identified with growth as living, then the narrative tends to be indistinct from biography
of any kind. In this case, aging is not informative specifically about the environment,
simply noting the fact that it is historical and that it changes. The rhetorical burden upon
the aged to tell a good story is heavy because patience for platitudinous reconstruction
tends to be short-lived.

If aging is treated as living in the manner of undifferentiated growth, then the difference it makes for memory, reminiscing and the correlative experience of such a process can be simply translated into an awareness (or not) of being historical, of being in position to reflect upon changes, for nostalgia, for recording alterations in the environment (as a tribal elder functions as an anthropological informant recalling the history of his tribe), in the way the survivor compares what was the city then with what it is now. If aging is the narrative of passing time, then its ideal speaker seems to be the historical informant who passes on some sense of that to which she was privy, almost in the way of arcane or secret testimony. Aging could be revitalized as data, redone and used as an archive, a curriculum, even as knowledge transfer or translation, as material for art such as documentaries and for techniques such as Twitter and all such gestures of information enhancement. Aging is viewed as a capacity to produce material that stands to be lost and the experience is typically presented in a narrative that is conventionally historical in the ways old people talk about their past, and about changes, to their audiences, who are required to listen respectfully.

When the narrative of aging is identified with the historical informant, the tendency to equate it with biography makes it difficult to separate the experience of the informant from that of a witness to her time in ways that can always undermine the claim to individuality. We might venture that a true individual needs to reclaim her life as both the same and other than the history in which it participates or else her voice simply reiterates the collective script. On the other hand, without such a faceless sacrifice there would be no history. Although this is a thin line, the individuality of the informant is probably marked by the way her testimony not only provides for historical information but in a way that includes her testimony and its inevitable distortion as part of what such a history is.

As a derivative of this, if age is identified with minority group status, then the historical narrative will be fashioned as such, experience typically reported in terms of fads and fashions in power and its succession in generational climaxes, golden ages, atrocities, events of various magnitude and selected trends and their surpassing. The conception of age as an experience of marginalization of a minority might correlate with covert senses of inclusion and exclusion that differ from simple historical testimony. Age would not be a report on living as life and its history but as witnessing the spectacle of a succession of age groups and their peculiar stylistic configurations that begin and end, emphasizing inclusion, exclusion, mortality and the like.

If the narrative defines the environment by generational power, as if the storyteller acquires the identity of one who suffered such decisive changes as participant, witness, victim or some other role, then the translation of aging into such a mode, perhaps modeled on the succession of one generation of immigrant after another (to their children), always could make the narrative a lesson for the younger, something informative or of useful value. The aged will be listened to especially when their stories seem convertible into material by those who listen and who might treat these experiences of use and value. This raises the question of what the aged are supposed to know.

If maturity, experience and wisdom are the typical answers, then what the aged in any present know is the past that was a present once for them but not necessarily in a way that is significant unless it can be translated into their life at present. That is, maturity, experience or wisdom is not the same as piling up information about the past that was once their present, for information must be made over into knowledge. The problem seems more interesting because of the connection of aging to the corpus of knowledge, to the social legacy, to the literacy of the collective. In this sense, the aged, often denigrated as having an unfair advantage over the generation of newcomers, can be easily lampooned as obsolete and restrictive fetters upon each generation. Many popular doctrines, such as Richard Florida's (2002) book, base their special appeal on their claims to eliminate the "burden of strong ties" of the past, and demagogues routinely have been engaged by the kind of ambivalence the relationship to the past creates, on the one hand as a source of sacred mythology that needs to be revitalized (the destiny of the people) and on the other as a seat of prejudices that need to be eliminated (the constraint of bad opinions and ideologies).

The aged as a minority group

The aged are typically viewed as a minority group whether they are statistically prevalent or not. This is because being a minority as a social and not a statistical phenomenon means that the aged are viewed as excluded from full scale participation in collective life. Or better, the ruling expectation is that the aged withdraw and renounce some part of their share as if holding on, as mentioned earlier, is selfish or miserly. But this privative view of the minority, whether as excluded or voluntary, can apply to blacks, Jews, those with disabilities, women and even to youth (among the many other possible minority groups that could be identified) since any category can be seen as such. In this way, comparable to the incidental character of growth to aging, minority status seems external to age.

The connection of aging to marginalization has many resonances that are obvious but also unthought, as in the monopoly exercised over information of their past by the aged in any present. If the aged are a minority, then this is less important because what they know of the past might be officially ruled irrelevant or obsolete, but it can still be a cleavage between young and old in any present over the monopoly of the old over memory and information of the past. Dependent on the statistical prevalence of aged as minority or majority, this ban on memory could always be a resource for the invidious comparison of aged with youth. If collective tenacity clings to the view that the old want to withdraw and to be with their own, want to be both privatized and insular, then this self-interested view of the aged is often held with reservation as if it is a question that could be/should be put to them despite both legal (retirement) and medical (for their own good) justifications.

Such views are often medicalized in the image of aging as represented in ads, stories, news and on the internet as an experience affecting selected parts of the population, typically identified as a period of physical decline in which those so categorized as old or aging are seen as needing and wanting to belong together on such a basis and usually wanting to be together, preferably in freedom from work and at sites where they can cultivate leisure. So a television channel specializing in film classics recognizes the appeal of its content to older folks by having advertisements on idyllic habituation of the homogeneous aged in retirement homes (ads incidentally mimicking the homoerotic scenes of beer commercials for younger adults). Such images only apply to those imagined as resourceful, for they coexist with selected representations of the aged who live in demoralization at the edge, poor and forlorn, as if the period constitutes an emergency, the desperation of physical decline in the absence of support displaying bare life that needs intervention.

At this level, the exploitation of the image is typical, whether in human interest stories of old survivors of life (specialists in longevity being acclaimed and praised, probably for endurance) or those shown as potential victims for commercial ends (nursing homes, relatives or predators). The images, whatever their substance, tend to focus on age as a concern for an undifferentiated collective, almost as if age and aging constitute a spectacle noteworthy for that alone. Aging, then, tends to be identified with the old, rather than with the evolution or growth of a life as registered in birthdays, and the old as a minority group, pictured as enthusiastic or desperate on the basis of isolation or in contrast, access to resources and support.

The defining feature, then, of the old and of any age group is that their likeness seems to endow them with a desire to be together (like-like), the collective picturing how those ruled by a category can only endorse that rule by accepting it as their own and as their choice as if what determines them is chosen by them, both privileging such as freedom and showing its possible limit. This seems to work for all age groups, represented as loving being with their own and intermittently looking at outsiders as nuisances (except in cases of those seen as needy members of an age group who are supposed to want the attention and company of outsiders).

At another level, these images of the old as dependent, isolated and/or exploited conjure up their picture as a minority group whose weakness divides the collective by the topic of responsibility around the issue of intervention, precisely in terms of the ways in which responsibility for the aged is formulated. The question here asks implicitly to whom the aged belong—family, society, private sphere or public—and if their position and the difference between their weakness and strength reflects bad luck (no resources of their own, no social support, no family and so no use value) and the kind of regard they can expect from a collective needing to be forced to care for them (the model here might be Simmel's [1971] article on the Poor).

The division in age

The reason the issue divides a collective is due to the division in the category itself, for the aged are not necessarily desperate; they also appear as insular and exclusive in cases where their resources permit control of political bodies, faculties, governing and administrative relations of corporate groups or even families, wherever their perpetuity is viewed as a sign of injustice (as in the celebrated canon of dead white males). Where the aged are strong and repulsive, their dependents are pictured as waiting for their death; where the aged are strong and nice, the dependents are pictured as affectionate; where the aged are weak and nice, they are pictured with sadness, regret, guilt; and where weak and repulsive, they are pictured with indifference.

This points to the issue of the insularity of the aged, whether strong or weak, in that their common interests, typically viewed as arising from helplessness, can also be treated as a means of enforcing dependency upon others (heirs or juniors) in ways seen as limiting opportunity and development. That the experience attributed to aging can be viewed as a sign of dependency or tyranny, whether strength or weakness, revolves around the question of rights, representation, exclusion and the problem of dealing with the relation of age to stratification, whether advantages such as seniority or disadvantages such as retirement or disqualification. Thus, as the issue binding public life, it appears as if aging and the aged reflect the problem of special interests and the difficulty of abridging the homoeroticism imaginable for any category defined by age (adolescence, young adulthood or agedness) as an inequity that is two-sided, capable of fertilizing not only isolation but constituencies, markets, amenities, arts and an expanding sense of diversity that accompanies such insularity (the idea of multiple identities).

Trajectories, graph of desire

We have discussed the way various images reveal emphases on uniformity, homogeneity around recognition of common interests and the status of the old age group as minority group, whether rich or poor, creating issues, such as retirement vs. the neediness of deprivation, much as if the category is seen as indivisible and the problem one of adjusting to conditions of whatever kind, e.g., excessive free time, that can result in either leisure or desperation, leading to perceptions of polarities between abandonment, or inner isolation vs. insularity, or at least wanting to be with one's own, and an aura of homoeroticism with which any age group is endowed. For the collective, an ideal seeming to be striven for makes reference to some vision of justice for a minority group and the burden of falling short in this. The good imagined is something like best practices, a policy vision of doing the right thing.

At one level, we have discussed the way this interest stimulates the collective, creating fascination for the minority group (whether to leave it alone or to intervene) even if it is one's own parent (i.e., what is it that they want, autonomy or companionship?). The aged can be weak or strong in ways that connect aging to the problem of justice (c.f. Plato's *Republic* re: weaker party), and if they are strong, it raises questions of moderating influence and advantages in intergenerational relations, e.g., seniority and patrimony.

At another level, age refers to creative destruction (c.f. Schumpeter, 1992) and what is envisioned as the ideal is the need to discover a stationary position in the midst of social change and dismemberment. Thus, age is not only a problem for a category that divides a collective, whether weak or strong, but a universal relation that binds a society, not simply with respect to differential treatment but regarding the problem of inevitability in relation to changing customs, usage and, despite differential advantages, posing in the way the problem of accommodation for all.

To this point then, the relation between different levels in the discourse mirrors Plato's model in the figure of the Divided Line (see the *Republic*) between what he called images and beliefs: first, the collective focus on the homoeroticism of the aged, whether strong or weak, as the defining feature, whereas in public life the issue concerns the status of the aged as a minority group; and second, a contentious debate about how to act with respect to this issue. At the level of what Plato calls *thinking* above the Divided Line (i.e., above squabbling over beliefs), in response to the confusion of usage, the collective can be seen to show an interest in giving form to this mix of images and beliefs by reflecting upon the discourse as if it is organized by the question of the relation between generations as an *aufheben* that is not simply instrumental.

Of course, the public life organized around the issue of age can only be divisive and irreconcilable until a collective is able to represent the division itself as mutually beneficial and so to display itself as community (in the way the relation between generations needs to be reformulated in educational practice as a relation of teaching to learning). This means that the homoeroticism imaginable for any category (its relation of like to like) *could* be a virtue (in the way separatism has historically argued whether for same sex education, Quebec nationalism, Black separatism or special education) but will be a fetter upon development unless it is overcome through a notion of shared being (Nancy, 1991; McHugh, 2005) that focuses not upon exchange value but on what can be learned from one another. In this sense, the debate on autonomy and heteronomy, on separatism vs. the mixed life, accentuated in the confrontation between Stalin and Trotsky over the best path to take for communism, always marks the collective problem of the aged as an occasion of action and reflection.

Thus, changes in a collective regarding fluctuations in values, interests or power as a problem of social change are inevitably linked to generation, obsolescence, redefinition of priorities and the like. Under such conditions, the inevitability of change and the need to survive it raises issues of succession, renewal, metabolism and generational relations.

Such concerns begin to open up the discussion in relation to renewal and perpetuity, inviting work on imitation and mimesis, posterity and dissemination, the canon, oeuvre and so forth. One version of the fate of age is that the aged are condemned to raise the problem of a difference between speech that is obsolete and speech that is timely, that the function of aging and the fascination with the aged is connected to the question of how and to what extent the fate of aging is connected to obsolescence. Why this is interesting can be appreciated by recalling Benjamin's (1999, p. 544) comment on the enthusiasm of each generation towards the up-to-date and timely, for it is by virtue of the enthusiasm which each generation ascribes to its present that Benjamin defines modernity itself, raising as the dialectical challenge in each generation the tension between detachment as difference and enthusiasm.

The body of common culture

Recall in Plato's *Republic* Cephalus' contention that an intelligent relationship to the body (and to old age) is one no longer tyrannized by the "raging madman," that is, by *eros*. Supposedly, one has matured to the point of being in position to treat the body as the servant rather than the lord. *Eros* then, less a source of vitality than a menace, threatens all humans by luring them to self-destructive actions. If Sophocles (Plato 1945, I.I.329a–331d, pp. 5–7) was used to voice a desire to be free of enjoyable sex, then we now appreciate that it was an aspiration to be free of the body as a source of bondage.

Thus, it is neither women nor sex that he wants to escape but self-destruction. Presumably with old age, one can be reflective about the self-destructive temptations released by the tyrannical body. It was Freud (Freud and Breuer, 1952) who said that this desire to repress the volatility of *eros* recurs as a constant for the species and is only attainable through what Hegel (1967) describes as a mechanization of self-feeling, or a kind of hardening of the heart that seeks to dominate the domineering body. Freud describes this as a process of abreaction in which the mind and body collaborate to ward off the evil elicited by unwelcome impulses and the guilt and self-reproach typically associated with such, where "excitations are converted into somatic symptoms" (Freud, 1952, p. 146) and correlatively such an experience can also be linguistic as in a translation that "gets rid of it by turning it into words" (Freud, 1952, p. 365). In this way, speech too becomes a formulaic defense or form of resistance analogous to the symptom. The subject develops a symptom whose pleasure substitutes for the pleasure of self-destructive *eros* in the way that wheezing in asthma or bronchitis might substitute for the cry for help in abandonment or scratching in psoriasis for the desire to tear oneself apart. If repression is achieved through substituting the symptom and its pleasure for the satisfaction of erotic self-destruction, then *eros* the raging madman is the source of vitality *and* morbidity, of life *and* death, that coexists in the enjoyment of any self-destructive gesture, the pleasure in its pain and the pain in its pleasure. According to Freud, the Grey Zone as the joy of self-destruction and thus, the seat of guilt, is typically displaced through the formation of the symptom to which the subject attaches herself and which makes transparent her identity. If it is the symptom that expresses the fate of the subject, her agency as a recurrent causal force in life, then the person and symptom are mutually implicated. The intelligence celebrated by Cephalus is then a prayer that he will be able to develop a reflective relationship in his old age to the symptomatology that marks him as the particular type he is.

This is to say that the "raging madman" as a figure for *eros* can be nothing other than the tendency of each modern moment to absorb the enthusiasm of its subject, creating the neediness that creative destruction requires to replace its objects of desire in favor of the new and up-to-date. In line with Plato's conception of the connection of beauty to procreation and inspiration, we could say that the beauty of the modern moment (in any period) lies in its power to inspire its subject to replace that with which she is already satisfied, i.e., to want to make a place in her life for the new simply because of its newness.

This is how we can say that modernity inspires the subject to renew through replacement what is perfectly satisfying and so both creates and surpasses dissatisfaction. But the exaggeration of modernity means that the fate of any satisfaction lies in its vulnerability to the dismemberment that renders any and all object of desire always open to replacement. Most critics know that capitalism creates need and stimulates consumption, but the implication is more interesting than this gloss. Every thing faces its becoming obsolete as its destiny. Especially when we consider the succession of styles in the arts and letters, we can note how modernism exacerbates a permanent human restlessness on the grounds that it is necessary and desirable to have and hold (to esteem) this object because its very existence makes all objects before it obsolete.

Thus, the logic of the modern points to the inexorable appeal of the up-to-date because in some (yet to be determined) way it makes everything comparable appear outmoded. Therefore, the modern object does not have to be more efficient than its predecessor (empirically) because it only has to create the appearance of contemporaneity. Some have said that the modern resonates with fad, but this is a misleading gloss. Bauhaus, Surrealism, the Beat Generation, Deconstruction, Conceptual Art, Critical Rationality and the like may have had specific generational appeal, but only because this appeal was grounded in the capacity of each of these to surpass the past by affirming the present in their very negations. These doctrinaire gestures may or may not be more efficient representations of the problems of their predecessors (whatever that means), but their success lies in being more vivid affirmations of the exemplary ways in which the present appears to master its past at any current moment.

Therefore, the capacity of the modern to overstimulate enthusiasm for its unprecedented character is the condition (the body of collective speech as the raging madman) to which the aged have to develop intelligent relations. What the *Republic* shows is that this temptation can be corrupted, taking the shape of privatization, unless the aged rethink it as detachment in the strongest sense. The ideal speaker for the aged that Cephalus could not acknowledge and Socrates sought to develop is engaged by this difference between privatization (withdrawal) and detachment in relation to the enthusiasm of any present for its own unprecedented precedence (the raging madman). This allows us to appreciate how the present is always self-aggrandizing and voracious at the expense of the past and how its rhetoric, inescapably powerful, must always mock the past as part of its extremism.

The body as the figure of *eros* in the metaphor of the raging madman helps explain the self-destructive absorption of the subject in the enthusiasm of any present for the imaginary unprecedented advance that it seems to signify. The modern moment makes visible the inexorable fate of man-made things as a cycle of obsolescence and replacement, and it centers such a collision most vividly in the city. Cities are monstrous in part because their identification of newness with innovation (of movement with change) dramatizes obsolescence as the condition of being both old and sick (glossed as "rationalisation" by Weber [1930], and "*anomie*" by Durkheim [1961]), assuming shape(s) that collide so dramatically with what is described as new and up-to-date that they can only render such vestiges silent remains without the power to voice resistance that could be intelligible. Obsolescence can only weep at progress.

> Whence this dangerous result: the properly cultural interest, powerfully creative, is often—not always—inversely proportional to the passions of the moment, and sometimes—not always—corresponds to what holds no interest. This analysis holds as much for the work of art as for scientific research (Serres, 2008b, p. 105).

This gives renewed sense to Baudelaire's (1972) notion of cities as "capitals of the civilised world" that must create both joy and sorrow, sorrow for what passes away and joy for its replacement. In this way, obsolete objects, people and spaces become grotesque in the exact sense used by Sherwood Anderson (1996) in *Winesburg, Ohio*, for this revocation of value leaves behind in its very gesture of renewal vestiges of narratives that are deposited at these sites as fragmentary remains. Thus, renewal is not a uniform line of progress, for it creates in its very making of obsolescence a secret lore or treasury of remains to be picked at and often recovered in the everyday archaeology of city life. Freud hints that the enthusiasms of any present (and of any tribe, community or city) can be read as an archive of object choices that remain formulaic masks of the excitations aroused by the traumatic intuition of the groundlessness of Being, of the recognition that any conversion of experience into word is just that, a symptom that the category, even of the collective as a "we," is a symptom and nothing more. In this sense, the raging madman is desire and the force of its formlessness, joined through the association of body and crowd to the corporeal character of language and its capacity to defend against excitation through standardization and typification.

Perhaps what needs being said, and what Cephalus hints at, is that the loss in old age which he welcomes is not the loss of *eros* conventionally understood but of that time of the self-absorbed acceptance of incidentals as if essential, making the gain appear now as a power to discriminate, which seemed to be lacking in retrospect (as if the raging madman was something like a tyrannical impulse within the soul leading to its submission to the rule of incidentals). Aging would then make reference to the increased power to discriminate and to the subtle erosion of an ignorant absorption in the incidental enthusiasm ruling the environment at each and every moment, seen from the present as if a history of progress.

Justice: corporeal and aesthetic

Now we can return, in conclusion, to that vision of the social order as bare life ruled by a symbolic order calculating interest groups according to a grammar for the quantitative adjudication of the allocation of resources. In that social order, the defenselessness of the individual, in relation to the rule of enumerative priorities misrecognizing this limited and partial relation as just, can be expected to characterize the young of each generation who lose their heads in enthusiastic self-absorption to their present. But this is misleading, for if the old lose their heads to the young, then the problem is losing one's head to whatever way the enthusiasms of any present are defined. If neither young nor old are immune in this respect, then the problem requires formulating the nature of immunity to enthusiasm of any group in ways that might point to its mean and extreme shapes. The mean of immunity would be the detachment that stands between privatization and devotion, extremes that seem to reflect the force of the raging madman. The raging madman is a kind of extremism towards speech.

This Platonic view of the corrupted just speech as analogous to language going on holiday in the idiom of Wittgenstein (1953, p. 19) shows how the severing of language from its qualitative roots, its holidaying in that respect, is proportionate to speech that loses its bearings in relation to its own possibilities, accepting in any present the body of opinion and belief enthusiastically embraced as the doctrine of the moment, necessarily banning as obsolete any sense of other because of its fear of being unable to control the raging madman that is the ostensible body of public opinion. Language going on holiday is the growing indistinction of distinctions, blurring the boundaries between words and things in ways that make each and any distinction vulnerable to destruction. Thus, the raging madman seems nothing but a figure for the crowd (of words or of people) into which the poet (according to Benjamin [1971]) can venture with reservation and the theorist (according to Socrates[Plato, 1945, III.XXI.489e–496e, pp. 196–204]) with trepidation, the crowd standing for the overstimulating and absorbing enthusiasm of each and any present for itself and its own (narcissism). The raging madman is somewhat like the self-destructive self-love of the collective, raging with the enthusiasm of a crowd towards which intelligence must always develop distance (rather than withdrawal or resignation).

Plato's travesty is based upon using the old man Cephalus as a mouthpiece for that very youthful view in a way that shows how it is not age that differentiates between such opinions or positions but the wealth of Cephalus. Thus, the disembodied view of justice as resource allocation is not the monopoly of old or young but a mask of the strong in ways that lead to treating the parts of a population as interests, their rights and liabilities as quantitatively accessible, and the formulation of all burdens as limitations that can only be rectified through the largesse of a benefactor or the self-improvement of those expected to be grateful. Justice is, then, viewed as such an exchange of favors between strong and weak. That the sick, the aged, nor anyone else might have a problem if they are strong does not alleviate the problem of the collective in dealing with the weaker party. This seems to require the kind of disengagement celebrated in Kant's (2007) aesthetics as the desire for form and developed in Benjamin's (1971, pp. 155–164) conception of the aura and Simmel's (1971) aristocratic notion of distance. Plato's *Republic* creates the dialogue between distance and enthusiasm as the problem of the aged but, as we should note, in ways that promise to absorb age into theorizing itself as if the old is the quintessential theorist and so potentially disregarding the interest in form that we have advanced throughout.

Fate, symptom, caricature

Is aging a fate? This is a provocative misnomer because, despite its inevitability, aging is not a fate in the same way that death is not a fate. Fate makes reference to the causal force of agency as in coming to terms with its consequences, the causality connected to the being of the agent and not the action. Here, we could speak of the way the causal force of agency repeats itself as a recurrence in the condition of aging, posing as a problem to be solved the appearance of every intended solution as problematic in the same idiom. For example, though there are many consequences of having a child or of being a parent (c.f. Bonner, 1998), fatefulness would always identify the link of consequences to the agent and her signature in ways that are marked and not universal. In fate, the consequences seem correlative with the singular manner of the agent because fate makes reference to the causal force or recurrence (including its unanticipated consequences) that is connected to an identity. The misnomer reveals that fate belongs to the person and not to the category, as Benjamin showed in his distinction between fate and character, or better, belongs to the stylization of the relation of person to category that shows both sides powerless to escape the other. This is how Benjamin can say in fate that misfortune is elevated to the status of a law, that it becomes binding (Benjamin, 1978, pp. 124–131).

Basically, the causal force of agency is both inescapable and overstimulating in ways tempting us to imagine it being otherwise. That is our fate. If aging is not our fate, overestimating our powers to influence conditions such as aging occurs with the causal power of a recurrence that seems almost second nature because of its apparent inextricable link to our identity. It is this link between fate and identity that is our problem.

If age plays the part of the symptom, the conversion of our self-love into a category that seems almost somatic, then our identity will always occupy a space of ambiguity in relation to the category, making the old both true to age (to the category or to being old) and something other or intimate. The category as the body of the experience (the signifier or the word) always converts it in a way that leaves a remainder. What remains after the conversion (so to speak) is the intimacy that it traverses and reduces (displaces, condenses in the category). Thus, being typified is less our fate (though a situation that we all inherit universally) than the condition of developing a dialectic between the intimacy and externality of the category. The experience of the category is the intimate ways in which we receive it and it receives us, reciprocally reshaping each other in mutually oriented action. What marks the aged (and possibly the sick to some extent) is not then the universal condition of being categorized in ways that put intimacy into jeopardy but the problem of addressing this dialectic in terms of its local detail or content, i.e., the dialectic suppressed and yet assumed in the caricature of being old or sick. For example, for age we ask what kind of remainder does the conversion displace, that is, what kind of fundamental trauma does it mask?

> We win by capitalizing on our debts, by turning our liabilities into assets, by using our burdens as a basis of insight. And so the poet may come to have a "vested" interest: in his handicaps; these handicaps may become an integral part of his method; and in so far as his style grows out of a disease, his loyalty to it may reinforce the disease. […] with the poet's burdens symbolic of his style and his style symbolic of his burdens […] The disease, seen from this point of view, is hardly more than the caricature of the man, the oversimplification of his act […] deceptive unless its obviousness as a caricature is discounted. (Burke, 1957, p. 16)

If disease and age are treated as handicaps that become stylistic in Burke's sense, then the functional or utilitarian aura that he invests in the caricature minimizes the aesthetics of the desire to poeticize bad conditions (burdens and handicaps) by revitalizing them in word and deed. Bad conditions, like the raging madman, can tempt extremist responses, but what Burke makes clear is that whatever contingencies they elicit in this way, it is unalterable for any such adjustment to become a caricature. In relation to the caricature of old age, Serres states, "The creator is born old and dies young, the opposite of those who are realistic, and, as they say, have their feet on the ground, know how to be infants and die senile just like everyone else" (Serres, 2008, p. 122).

Being young while old or old while young is part of an either/or economy that risks making the old immature (the California mom who wants to be like her daughter) and the young stodgy (the stick-in-the-mud child who copies elders), whereas the mandate of the duck-rabbit requires old to be young while holding on to what they are, and young to be old while holding on to what they are. Here, instead of the portentous notion of wisdom, we might need a vision of maturity and then perhaps wisdom might come to view as a way of understanding this. These reflections permit us to approach old age as a struggle between the temptation of caricature embodied in the category in its prosaic sense (generalized other) and the opportunity for inventiveness in relation to this and any category as such. The handicap of the category as a burden always invites rewriting. At least in this respect, the exchange with Cephalus might invite us to consider the relation of maturity to *eros* as the interpretive landscape of old age. Again, the challenge of the category is the demand it imposes on the relation of togetherness and apartness, how the individual must be both together and apart in relation to being old.

9

THE FORMULA: MEDICALIZATION AND ITS GUISES

Introduction

This chapter will treat medicalization in different ways but always as a collective representation in Durkheim's (1961) sense, as a relationship to language and action. In this chapter, I propose simply to open up the discussion around the most basic usages connected to the understanding and application of this notion, eventually intending to amplify it in several ways. At this point, we will ask what is being done in such conceptualization, how it comes to exercise such an appeal in everyday life, and how we might begin to think of resuscitating the usage in order to grasp elementary problems it is addressing.

Advance or infantilization?

If the period of enlightenment is used as a figure of speech extolling progress and a historical vision of the modern moment in all of its glory, then this achievement must remain two-sided since its very advance intensifies our encounter with the limits of what we know. For example, just as enlightened thinking permits us to colonize many dark areas, this increased intelligibility often only enables us to relate the area generically to general conditions in ways that leave untouched the particular and/or intimate connection of the area to everyday practice as a problem of collective life that invites a reflective existential engagement and struggle. The problem materializes as one of making familiar that which had been treated as strange. Think of how the advance from considering mental illness superstitiously, perhaps as a result of witchcraft, to the point of construing it as disease, does not simply conquer the condition or eliminate it but heightens its ambiguity by dramatizing all of the tensions that inhere in its use. Even before Foucault, many have resisted the medicalization reflected in treating any conduct as disease. So it has typically been reputed that the advance in intelligibility from applying the category of disease to conduct is gained at the expense of a kind of normative imposition that makes health into the *sine qua non* of the Good. To grasp how domesticating conduct through the use of disease might not be a self-evident case of progress, we might only think of talk in the media where pundits regularly make an event familiar by a repetitious reiteration of what anyone knows. Thus, there *is* a degree of progress in such talk that increasingly offers us assurance about the unknown and leaves the intimate collective engagement with the enigmatic conduct untouched.

Along these lines, I was recently exposed to a discussion about obesity in the media, with advocates for obesity expressing delight that the condition was finally being recognized as a disease rather than a lifestyle or choice. This example can be thought of as a way of working through the ambiguity discussed here as Grey Zone, by using the notion of disease in this specific case as a prop, trying to understand how this concern could be meant and what sorts of problems this kind of speech and interpretation was trying to solve or situate. As a start, the advance registered in thinking of obesity as disease rather than lifestyle might appear as an improvement by being treated as something perhaps involuntary and not freely chosen, some condition for which the person is not responsible and should not be blamed, supposedly making us more caring, enlightened and tolerant towards obesity while still repressing not only the ambiguity of this question (the question of disease for example) but the truly repressed question of how we need and/or desire to speak about such a condition.

On one level, reputing disease to be an advance reflects an opinion that, as a bona fide disease, the condition might be appreciated and made more intelligible as a field for causal inquiry and thus seems progressive because it rationalizes and makes researchable the condition in contrast to archaic views. This leads many to appreciate the use of disease as a category since it appears to improve upon more primitive understandings that attribute the condition to mysterious factors or to willfulness because the idea of disease tends to normalize the condition, making it intelligible, perhaps by seeing it as part of a circuit of causal relations. So it is typically treated as an advance when conditions such as depression or obesity, or problems in reading or even learning, or problems called sleep disorders, or being listless and without energy, are recognized as certifiable diseases, since prior to this recognition, people might have been blamed for what was involuntary or treated as if it was part of or a result of beliefs that made these conditions permissible. Note that this is not to say that such conditions lack any somatic sources but rather to try to raise the question of what the stakes are in treating such conditions as diseases.

The medical shape of an enlightenment vision of disease suggests that as reason advances, the fight against disease is increasingly successful. Reason in its medical form rationalizes disease by locating causes, formulating conditions and calculating probabilities but always in ways that both announce and expose the limits of such mastery as only part of the story of disease in collective life. This achievement can make disease transparent as something about which many can have information in ways that make the domestication of disease a focus of collectivization or a badge of being well-informed in collective life. Thus, much talk and methodology circulates around the question of disease and its relief. The "progress" so welcome here means nothing else than that the category is topical, some matter increasingly attended to and for those subject to the condition this can always be good (as a matter of pride as in "that's my condition that everyone is talking about!") or bad (as a matter of shame as in "don't tell anyone who cannot see that this is my condition, my secret!"). When we treat disease as a phenomenon in this sense, as an image circulating in collective life, its status as topic makes it resemble many other kinds of concerns (food, sex, fashion and war) in ways that make the advance progressive because it treats the notion as a topic and so opens it up to and for all of us.

What this advance suggests is not only an increase in talkativeness or volubility about the condition and the overcoming of a kind of silence, (in ways spoken about as the "advance" registered by Freud's work on sexuality, the unspoken topic), but that a uniform and indivisible sense of the notion as one thing and one thing only is treated as broken down because it is no longer seen as a thing but as a construct and so is to be treated neither as external nor innate but as divisible according to interests. If disease or any notion is seen as divisible according to the interests of the one who orients to it, then this suggests that it is a construct that can be used in many and different ways and is not simply tied to one ruling use, permitting a kind of flexibility and freedom always to our advantage. Yet, according to Plato (1945), this is an advance only insofar as treating the notion as a construct, or what he calls an image, must advance upon views of the notion as a brute fact or "thing." Because disease is treated as an image, it exists as a plurality, as many views developed according to different interests, such as medicine, patient, family, society and the like. This is the lowest region of Plato's Divided Line, reflecting an advance that is still only a beginning, always requiring of those who want to pursue the matter that they remain somewhat dissatisfied (but not in the sense of unhappy). In this way, progress is reflected in the transformation of the category of disease into a *topos*, or place that centers and founds a public.

It is an advance in the sense that people seem to treat it seriously, talk about it and might even be willing to invest resources for studying it. But recall Kierkegaard's (1962, pp. 68–69) hesitation towards the advance reputed by enlarging the scope of what is talked about: "By comparison with a passionate age, an age without passion gains in scope what it loses in intensity [...] where mere scope is concerned, talkativeness wins the day, it jabbers on incessantly about everything and nothing." Using this controversy between the status of medicalization as advanced or not, as a starting point, whether it enhances or infantilizes the one to whom it is applied and the one who applies it, let us proceed a bit further.

What is medicalization?

> *Medicalization.* A concept made fashionable by Ivan Illich and Michel Foucault, the term commonly denotes the spread of the medical profession's activities, such as their increasing involvement in the processes of birth and dying. (Gordon and Marshall, 2005)

Though many others have contributed to this usage (Parsons, 1951; Freidson, 1988), it tends to identify the expansion and regulation of organized medicine over conduct as a distinguishing feature, though this leaves as implicit but unspoken the influence of "somatization" and of views influenced by medicine that saturate common culture. In this sense, Freidson has emphasized, along with such medical redefinitions of human conduct, the reclassification of (so-called) deviant behavior from being seen as bad or immoral to its status as illness. The focus of the conception is then directed to the increased power of medicine as a profession along with the influence of its nomenclature. But, unless described in detail, this simply reinforces the sociological cliché that power rules life and that the professions are simple expressions of self-aggrandizing territoriality or, in other words, as biomedical weapons in the colonization of everyday life. Medicalization is described as a means (almost as a tool or technology) for expanding the jurisdiction of medicine by redefining social issues as problems that require medical intervention and regulation or, at least, official consultation and use of medical expertise.

Here, several points need be made. First, the conception of medicalization as an instance of colonization (of the biomedical model) is seen by sociology (another profession) to be part of the desire to enforce and control deviant conduct, and in this way it can be used by us as data that displays the self-understanding of sociology itself as an expression of the manner in which sociology addresses itself to human conduct, presenting itself in part through its view of the pervasiveness of self-assertive power in every area of life. Thus, the interpretation functions as a *symptom* of the imaginary of sociology and its appeal to the view that life is invariably colonized by knowledge through some pretense to a higher purpose that always needs be unmasked. In this guise, at least sociology speaks for an unhappy and pervasive skepticism in everyday life that views rip-offs and spins as the law of the land. The first point then is that the interpretation is simply a symptom of the phenomenon it means to describe and so at best can only serve as a beginning for exploring the discourse. This further confirms how the authority of interpretation does not depend upon its referential accuracy but rather lies in its capacity to disclose the necessity of the symptom particular to it and, indeed, of any symptom as "equipment for living" (Burke, 1957).

Second, this particular interpretation does not help us address medicalization as a feature of the Grey Zone, because its view of colonization cuts off analysis of the phenomenon itself in highlighting as essential the limited case of the empirical practice of the profession (to which, of course, many opposites could be cited). Third, the interpretation treats as exemplary the normalization of deviance instead of providing for the ways in which this is done in practice as something other than simple classification (labeling). So we would have to ask how medicalization is done in ways that permit us to formulate its omnirelevance in everyday life as not just an aspect of social control, of the regulation of deviance, of professionalization and the like, or better, how such usages make reference to a more fundamental problem, connected to health as well as illness, and to many practices other than medicine.

For example, in thinking of medicalization as a practice, we might first explore the standard ruling medicine, so that we might examine ways in which these are translated in everyday life, permitting us to inquire into the kinds of ordinary actions they seek to accomplish. For this experience we might think of practices such as diagnosis, prescribing and testing as such important features of medicine in order to appreciate the hold upon us that medicine exercises.

To describe in a way that diagnoses is to produce a description that identifies its object (e.g., a patient or even a target for policy advice) in ways that make the failure to take action a noticeable absence because diagnosis identifies a condition that seems imperative to act on. Such description is intended to be prescriptive by showing the remedial character of the condition described where the specificity of the description is intended to confront the other with an either/or choice where inaction can be confirmed as uncooperative, listless or unintelligent. In this sense, diagnosis makes describing prescriptive rather than, say, the way in which Freud (1963, pp. 273–286) treats interpretations as provocative constructions designed to stimulate reflection and "work" rather than to compel a specific course of action. This interest, of course, leads to prescribing as an offer of technical advice conveyed by the prescription that, in its way, puts the medical practitioner on the spot for exposing what she is presumed to know and, particularly, how she might stand in relation to the corpus of research. But diagnosis can also put the practitioner on the spot for her artfulness in sizing up the situation that the symptom presents. The influence of diagnosing and prescribing as conventional signs of know-how and intelligence and of efficacy and problem-solving, become pervasive examples of the influence of medicine in the appraisal of actions in all areas of life and in the development of standards for evaluating discourse, taking shape in formulaic ways often institutionalized in organizations and relationships. Of course, medicalization also makes its influence felt in the notion of testing and needing and desiring to confirm with conclusiveness speculations in many areas. Though testing derives from a venerable convention (e.g., the mathematical emphasis of Plato's academy) where one needs to see for oneself and experience for oneself what is reputed to be (and so is a staple of empiricism in the best sense), it makes reference deeply to Kenneth Burke's (1957, p. 298) notion of "sizing up the situation" and to the desire for self-knowledge that we have discussed positively in this work. However, the medical transformation of this notion for developing a technology of self-management can only translate testing into the ideal of a progress report, to which anyone and everyone must be chained in the expectation of being able to constantly audit fluctuations in behavior, making the testing of the patient more transparent by virtue of this travesty that exposes it as if a performance measure, job review or report card. Yet testing in such cases always seems a substitute for the absence (and the presumed impossibility) of any dialogical relation to the symptom, permitting the test result to stand as the best we can expect under such less than perfect conditions.

Being classified

If medicalization can be understood as making reference to the application of categories of health and illness to conduct, then it implies in such a gesture that the authority of the somatic serves to impose a normativity upon whatever it describes. Here, the designation of illness presupposes an unassailable standard from which it is supposed to depart in the way sickness is assumed to depart from health as aberrant from (assumed) normal. This has long been recognized and criticized as if designations such as illness make vivid the socially constructed character of any distinction. This is uninteresting, a starting point and nothing more. Developing this "something more" invites a formulation of what it is to designate someone as sick. For example, think of how classifying someone as ill seems to deprive him of agency in a way that exempts him from responsibility for untoward behavior. Yet at the same time, we note that illness as such a designation frees the actor at the same time as it shows him to be determined. In its way, then, the category liberates someone from responsibility, and hence guilt, by showing him to be determined by forces outside of his control as if he is victimized by whatever makes him act as he does. This is one place where the ambiguity of medicalization appears as a feature of the subject in the space between agency and determination, responsibility and freedom, but always as a matter of interpretation and judgment for an observer.

Talcott Parsons' (1951) conception of the sick role and Foucault's (1973) work on social regulation have contributed to this modern attempt to show the interpretive consequences of diagnosis, revealing in their ways the link of the diagnostic and interpretive in a hermeneutic gesture that tries to unravel some part of the mystery of conduct. Regardless of whatever we think of this work, it shows how the treatment of interpretation as diagnostic in this sense (our preliminary use of medicalization) is a way of exempting the behavior and actor of guilt. In other words, if the ascription of causation assigns guilt (as in Wittgenstein's [1953] translation of "cause": "he is the one!"), then in the case of medicalization it seems to assign guilt to impersonal conditions over which the actor has no control. This is as if the world and its chance workings are somehow found guilty of victimizing the actor through *fortuna*, which just happens to position her to be its subject. Although this seems a laugh, it might be the final word of suicides (and perhaps of all dark moods, realism and misanthropy) when it takes upon itself the *persona* of the judge who must come to a verdict on causation (e.g., World, I find *you* guilty of making me a victim even though in that gesture you free me from guilt! World, you are killing me with kindness! World, you are guilty of making me too confused about whether to thank or hate you because my innocence in conjunction with your guilt makes the injustice of *our* life too painful to endure!). So one of the things medicalization seems to do is reveal the thin line between guilt and victim, suggesting in its way that if the victim is now free from guilt, being a victim is still painful and unhappy, or conversely that being guilty might be a way of beginning to be reflective and to improve oneself, whereas the victim is fated to accept this beginning as an end. The opening here to Freud (Freud and Breuer, 1952) is instructive: paraphrasing he who says, we think you enjoy being the victim and you might begin to experience guilt (and agency) in relation to that so as to reflect upon how the guilty mechanism of world (trauma) has succeeded in converting you into such a posture. Freud: guilt is ambiguous and it can be the start of something better as in the taking of responsibility for agency.

Weakness

We want to ask how the collective orients to disease as itself a collective problem. We remain skirting around the edges of medicalization because we do not yet grasp what kind of message the collective might be said to deliver with its talk on disease. As a symptom, medicalization makes reference to what is unspoken and unthought in the collective representation of medicalizing as a practice, first by pointing to the work the collective must do to overcome the lack of complete assurance in making decisions about conditions as such and reaching conclusions about responsibility (guilt and innocence), cause and effect, black and white, while wallowing around in a Grey Zone of indeterminacy. On this level, medicalization reveals a sign of collective distress at being unable to distinguish victim from cause.

Here, Nietzsche's (1956) opinion that metaphysics is a disease is interesting because he gives us a new twist on disease not simply by making it familiar but by identifying the condition as a symptom of desire. Nietzsche's thought takes the shape of asserting that only one in a weakened state would turn to metaphysics. Whether we agree with him on metaphysics or not, he provides an important inflection on the status of disease as a symptom of strength and weakness that reflects a collective approach to disease in these terms. Because he equates metaphysics with idealism, the refusal to face reality, a turning away, he develops the notion of disease as grounding action and inaction because what is strong or weak(ened) is really human desire, a figure for a condition of internal resourcelessness when the individual seeks stronger and stronger stimulation.

Thus, despite its heterogeneous images and beliefs, disease seems to be bound together in collective life as a representation of the problem of the ambiguity of desire and its development in relation to the weakened state. Hegel (1970, pp. 440–441) sharpens the figure of disease in this respect: "In disease the individual is entangled with an external (non organic) power and is held fast in one of its particular organs in opposition to the unity of its vitality." So in disease we say that the individual is determined because the inability to respond as a whole permits one particular part (one condition) to take possession of the whole and to affirm itself as the whole. In disease, one seems to be seen as possessed by the condition rather than self-possessive towards it. Disease depicts the one subject to such separation from what Hegel calls her "inner sides"—her wholeness or experience of unified vitality. Here Hegel put flesh on Nietzsche's weakened state as a kind of externalization or self-separating distance from one's own highest capacities and powers.

What these thinkers do is make the subject's position in relation to desire intrinsic to disease. Plato might be uncomfortable with Nietzsche's hyperbole but not with the unspoken thought in the image: that the modernization of the city, with its freedom, flexibility and abundance of choices, shapes desire by making overstimulation, and so calculation, an important factor. As we noted earlier, health, then, is formulated not in opposition to illness but as a relationship to such conditions and so as a way of living life under such conditions. What is diseased in this sense is not the presence or absence of bad conditions but deadly relations to any conditions. This is the implication of calling metaphysics a disease, that it is not good for life and so unhealthy in that respect. Theorizing then offers to measure any account by its relationship to life or in Plato what it does for the soul (a strong version of what is perhaps lamely called the life world).

What Plato calls *eros* or procreative desire as a life-affirming drive is two-sided, capable of good and evil and so always in need of reflection. Plato uses the relation to spices as a model for such calculation and discrimination. That is, when thought through in modern life, health and illness invite us to calculate strong and weak relations to our priorities and needs. This means that the desire of the subject will forever be a parameter of the collective representation of disease, releasing juridical and ethical implications that can never be disregarded. Above the Divided Line, the question of self-monitoring desire and its limitations becomes central to disease. Therefore, if thinking does advance in this respect, it does not simplify disease as a problem but makes the complex dialectical resonances of the relation compelling and perhaps, insoluble.

Now, the question posed by the Grey Zone is what Plato calls dialectical, not one of choosing between the opinions that disease is an advanced or primitive way of thinking, but rather of finding one's way through the oppositions, making observable the phenomenon itself, the phenomenon of disease as a situation of action materializing in ethical collisions over the monitoring of desire in relation to inescapable conditions.

Influences, fate, chance, taking hope

Note that what remains interesting for us here is that when any condition such as obesity is conceded to be a disease, this is tantamount to passing its interpretive control to medicine and to giving medicine the right to treat this condition technically. While these implications are not fully understood, they do suggest that it is the fate of obesity to be formulated technically according to criteria that always risk preserving its weakness, as if the effort to survive it at any cost is the strongest relationship imaginable.

Treating the disease as an advance amounts to talking and thinking in certain ways that can be applied to any condition. It is not uncommon in collective life to regard many of our influences or conditions as weakened states (involuntary, irrational, something we inherited but did not choose, something unwanted, unlucky or, in contrast, our good fortune) in ways that apply to place, gender, class, race, physiognomy, money, family and the like. Note the ambiguity here: our inheritance of conditions that we did not choose could license us to rightfully disregard them. In this sense, any condition raises the question of whether or not we chose it or were chosen (so to speak) and whether or not it can be seen as belonging to us. Here is the fundamental ambiguity of any condition or mark: is it to be disavowed because it was not chosen or is it to be cared for because it belongs to us and so is part of us? We can ask this about life itself, rejecting it because we did not choose to be born (we did not vote on it) or to take care of life because we inherited it and are charged with dealing with it as best as we can.

This permits us to understand the ways involved in treating the thought of obesity as disease as an advance or form of progress. The turn to medicine tends to legitimize the condition as medical and something for which we will not be blamed, a category that can elicit support, even treatment and the expectation of a cure around the corner, a prospect linked mainly to the hope of technical progress. Because the condition does not and should not be seen as really and truly belonging to me, I can transfer all rights to medicine; I can give medicine rights over my disease. The category of disease legitimizes the condition as an unwanted guest from which its subject seeks relief, promising resources for influencing the condition or eliminating it. Disease then has an imaginary in the idiom of Lacan, marking a condition that we inherit involuntarily and so a condition outside of our control in *that* sense (as not our fault, as needing relief and that can be studied and acted upon), but only with my cooperation. Yet, the ambiguity resides in disease still being under our control as a matter to constantly address and to explore experimentally within the limits of our inheritance, because our having the disease means that it is part of our intimate history and a mark of what and who we are in life.

On the other hand, if the condition is part of my inheritance, it *does* belong to me as part of my intimate history. Or to put it otherwise, the condition must be a part of myself with which I am intimate and to which others can only be external, distant and possibly intrusive. So in transferring to medicine the interpretive rights to my disease, we highlight the two-sided ambiguity of disease more dramatically, for even if medicine is most goodhearted and loving, it is fated to trespass on what I know of myself. In this way, we can begin to appreciate the two-sided character of any notion and, in this case, of disease: on the one hand, the imaginative structure of disease can legitimize our right and duty to put ourselves in the hands of a qualified expertise, an expertise offering to control an area and a body of knowledge that might provide attention and relief and certainly some promise of care rather than neglect or contempt. On the other hand, if this gives us some pleasure to be certified as having a legitimate medical condition (as if we are now entitled to speak of ourselves as sick), such confirmation never ends our problems but only marks their ongoing presence in everyday life, the problem of working out and in this particular condition.

The reassurance of the mark

One of the ways of thinking of the category of disease as an advance is that it suggests an area for work, evoking some promise of future action that might be possible, if only for the attention, sympathy and investment of resources that such a category promises. We see this in the power of naming conditions as diseases. For example, in Kieran Bonner's (2007a) research on alcoholism, he finds people spending an inordinate amount of attention devoted to calculating how much drink per day or week makes one a certifiable alcoholic. We might begin to anticipate how the conditions of drinking, pregnancy and aging can be affected by being medicalized, how the advances in sympathy and attention might be weighed against the violence of external interventions and the demands to cooperate by transferring interpretive rights over the body to outsiders, even ones who are skilled in certain important ways. The advance in naming is something like this: when the person is told that what she is suffering is what is called depression, she is introduced into the ways of a body of knowledge and its imaginary protocols and prospects as now belonging to her. In one sense, the name tells us that we are not alone and in this way functions as a kind of advance.

The label of disease can serve in many ways as reassuring in the face of behavior that is perplexing. The very fact of the label imparts a diagnostic function to the condition that can exempt all parties from responsibility and so from the fear that the condition is a matter of their own making. Not guilty by reason of insanity verdicts are a good example of this (and there exists some material on the implications of calling an incestuous fireman sick rather than a criminal [Blum, 1970, pp. 39–45]). Besides the precedent of alcoholism, Freud's (Freud and Breuer, 1952) list of examples of neurasthenia and the anxiety neuroses, reflected in symptoms such as fatigue, irritability and, now, sleep disorder or even anger, can be treated in ways that give those involved great reassurance. Victims of anger or even road rage or abuse can use the diagnostic category as a way of understanding the action as directed to them impersonally, and not really as specific and contributing targets, in ways that give more relief to the victim than the culprit. The model of the longsuffering wife of the alcoholic, whose understanding of the condition as a disease frees her from personal responsibility ("He still loves me, after all!"), is not only a model for the victim of abuse or intimate anger but also makes reference to a generic cliché in popular culture and even the best literature where the intimate of the diseased one always seeks to know if the disease accounted for the response to her or not. We say medicalization can help members deal with situations that confuse them and that they cannot easily resolve in either/or formulae. Sociologists have long asserted that the husbands of women categorized as mentally ill get relief from the categorization in such reassuring ways, but also use the category to "read" their wife in such a way after the fact and in this gesture, can drive them crazy as if making the category a self-fulfilling prophecy. Calling people diseased can get everyone off the hook, but then, not really; hence, the Grey Zone. One of the most interesting moments in the enlightened conquest of superstition in medicine is marked by the "advance" in conceiving of enuresis or bedwetting as a disease rather than a childish act of indolence or malice, a decisive turning point in the enlightenment of incredulous parents; and yet, the disease does become part of a domestic archive and of a person's personal history. Think of how the idea of the makeover, so popular in television shows, flirts with the thin line supplied by the prosthetic imaginary between disease and disorder, pointing to the possibility of being noisy, loudmouth, gossipy, disorganized, lazy, tired or unkempt as a medical problem.

To counteract the one-sided sociological view of medicalization as professional dominance, and of disability activism as stereotyping, we must reflect on the great advance of Freud in treating melancholy as a medical problem. Laplanche rightly calls this an "extraordinary invention" (Laplanche, 1976, p. 248) because the analogy permits us to treat what seems the "normal prototype" of depression as a medical problem reflecting the work following the loss (whether death or abandonment) of another. Of melancholia, Freud says that "it never occurs to us to refer it to medical treatment because it does not seem to us pathological" (cited in Laplanche, 1999, pp. 248–249). In this gesture, Freud identifies what we have called the weakness of disease with "pathology," investing medicine with the capacity to recognize the pathological element in conduct. Freud's genius differentiates him from everyone else in that he treats the recognition of pathology as amoral, as a descriptive problem organized around a grammar of object choice. We might use Freud's approach here to weakness to identify its specific character as pathology.

Towards a grammar for public health

We can use a method borrowed in part from Wittgenstein's "thought experiments" in which we select examples out of an interest in discovering whether and/or how we might reproduce the very phenomenon we are studying, in this case, medicalization, by imagining elementary conditions that are necessary for it to emerge as an eventful action or distinction. Thus, we ask what we need to see in a usage, action, example and the like in order to begin to understand it as doing and showing medicalization, or what a world might look like in which all actions and actors are ruled by a discursive interest in seeing health and disease everywhere. It is through such examples that I try to recover an elementary scene of representation for the phenomenon in such a method. The drama of such examples is provided when they contrast with the usual understanding of what is medical or not because they then bring into focus, against all objections, the character of medicalization as a social form.

In *Canadian Living*, an article entitled "How to spot a psychopath" (Beun-Chown, 2007) identifies what it calls psychopathology as if an epidemic upon which it tries to warn its readers to reflect. Basically the article identifies some examples of women being exploited, usually financially, in relationships in which they had assumed good faith but on the basis of cursory, superficial knowledge that they inferred from external signs such as charm, manners, disposition, amiability and the like. These dashed expectations and disappointing relationships were rescued from being matters of self-reproach for those victimized by being reformulated in this article as a result of behavior called psychopathic that was perpetuated by their "significant others," aptly named in turn, psychopaths. Some experts were used to formulate the problem for the reader: "Most of us will bump into a psychopath every week. [...] they are willing to do something really nasty without any concern for what happens to you" (Beun-Chown, 2007 para. 4).

What is first interesting here is how bad conditions, or the ways in which we run into nasty and uncivil people or conditions and circumstances that bring this out, is formulated as an epidemic. This leads us to think about the ways in which diagnosis can be used to invest what might be routine characterization with the aura of disease and what this kind of work does for those who engage it. In other words, how does it help those who suffer fluctuations in the quality of relationships over the course of a life to have a diagnostic category for so representing the others in these relationships as psychopath or diseased, and how does it help them to think about themselves in such cases? Secondly, what is the additional value of representing such an experience as part of an epidemic? Finally, if the sexual marketplace is an occasion for such speculation, how does the diagnostic category of psychopath replace, say, capitalism as such a relevance? Note that psychopathology does not immediately exempt one from responsibility for her bad relationships if we can always ask why psychopaths are so appealing (a question the experts answer by citing charm and appearances that are deceitful, making the need for experts even more urgent).

In a certain sense, the epidemic is attributed to ignorance and the lack of information in the way diagnosis is reputed to require some discrimination or special skill.

Such questions seem to point to some elementary considerations in the formulation of public health as a Grey Zone. The article informs us that the psychopathological condition is carried by the sick who look healthy, suggesting the pervasiveness of the disease, invisible under a normal façade in the way of the terrorist or serial killer next door or the growth of cancer that is undetected, or of anything going on in the body or polity, anything that grows and remains undetectable. That the sick look healthy suggests that we need guidance in detecting symptoms unnoticed to the untrained eye. This is one way in which health and illness is formulated as a danger, creating a need for the expertise and action of public health to monitor and survey the life of the community in the name of safety, the environment in relation to pollution, tobacco in relation to health, nutrition and the like. This is not to argue against such initiatives but to try to show how they work as part of a process, and though all of these activities are different, this analogical approach allows us to see some common mechanisms; for example, informed diagnosis rather than causal speculation gives ground for the intervention of expertise; epidemic conveys the idea of a collectivity rather than the isolation of one victim with idiosyncratic character and so some vulnerability that might be impersonal in the sense of externally induced rather than an upshot of personal decision-making. Finally, the notion of danger suggests that steps need to be taken, that preparation and pedagogy is required, because the phenomenon is both prevalent and invisible.

The grammar of medicalization seems to point first to the condition of a deceptive carrier, the difference between appearance and reality, and its detection by a qualified expertise. Secondly, the idea of epidemic suggests not merely that there are many of them but that they breed and so that there are common and perhaps incalculable conditions that nurture this collective in ways that can only proliferate and worsen unless remedial action is taken and some forceful authority is delegated to enforcement agencies with the rights to regulate this growth. Finally, reeducation is typically offered in the form of a curriculum proposing rules, in this case, for identifying the psychopath. "[They have] an utterly empty hole in their psyche" and no conscience (Beun-Chown, 2007 para. 11), "traits [that] easily remain invisible until after the psychopath has already ensnared you with charisma, lies and glib chatter" (para. 7), but since such indicators offer no predictive validity (and cannot distinguish a media pundit, politician, professor or corporate executive from a psychopath), we are advised that we can only recognize one after he strikes. It is said by the experts that the traits of the psychopath are invisible until he strikes, traits possibly discernible in symptoms such as "charisma, lies, and glib chatter." The category can only be used after the fact to identify what was there all along.

In the article "Party's over: most students don't drink heavily but the problem is, they think everyone else does" in the *Toronto Star* (Gordon, 2007), the journalist claims that changes in the drinking behavior of college students leads many entering freshman who had anticipated heavy drinking in the environment to change their preconceptions on grounds similar to Constance Smelsky, who had figured "that alcohol would be the way of fitting in and making 'friends for life'" (Gordon, 2007, para. 3) and, upon discovering this was not so, felt relieved of "pressure" (para. 4): "I thought, okay, I don't have to do all these things that I thought I did. People could like me for who I am, and not from me trying to fit in by drinking" (para. 5). Or, as another says: "I feel good about this, I can be myself, I can do what I want to do" (para. 7). The article continues by saying that such students reject the "prevailing wisdom about today's wild student behaviour […] [that] creates a false picture of student life […] And [is] one of the biggest reasons some kids drink dangerously" (para. 8). The article says that these students have become leaders in an educational campaign fuelled by a "scientific approach known as 'social norms theory' […] aimed at eliminating misconceptions about alcohol consumption by educating youth with solid research on how most of their peers actually behave" (para. 9).

Can we use this representation of campus drinking behavior to begin to compare the fear of the psychopath next door and its danger with tobacco, pollution and environmental risks and dangers? Is there something common to second-hand smoke, pollution, alcoholism, and the prevalence of psychopathology? Most obviously, these are all occasions to imagine the danger of an epidemic that requires immediate remedial action.

The alcohol case here is interesting because it shows the bad behavior to be a kind of enticing "norm" in the sense that everyone is assumed to do it and this alone is interpreted as a temptation for anyone. Although this is not correlative with the object (alcohol, tobacco, polluting), in the sense that the object does not *make* everyone do it, in this particular case it is the fact of everyone doing it that is the danger. This danger (possibly shared with tobacco and sex) is pertinent particularly for those identified as young and gullible. The subject is conceived as weak, as drinking (or smoking or having sex) because everyone does it, but it is not self-evident that this majority rule could determine the subject's behavior (the ego ideal) unless she orients to doing whatever everyone does (ideal ego), i.e., desires to be at one with the many. The misconception would then help weak subjects who do whatever everyone does because they could find out otherwise. The "scientific research" can clear up these misconceptions and put norms on a secure footing. Here, following the rules is the "route to making friends," but there might be deeper auspices, as, for example, in locating oneself as normative or not in a population. For example, a respondent was quoted in the University of Chicago national sex survey who was relieved on discovering the data on sexual frequency in the population because it made him feel less atypical. Therefore, much of this kind of talk enables people to figure out how they stand with respect to the normal and abnormal, and they use statistics to achieve this kind of understanding.

Most relevant is that this kind of mapping operation is usually done when one enters a new situation, such as an organization, neighborhood or foreign country, and has to follow the rules to discover what is going on. This is similar to the model of wayfinding when we check out how people do things in certain ways in order to use such data as guidelines for ourselves. Besides visitors to a hospital, students entering university or high school, spectators in the courts, inductees in the military, tourists and such, this seems standard operating procedure in many domains of everyday life and, in addition, is related to notions such as suggestion or conformity that make reference to opinions or voting or consumption that is influenced by perceptions of such frequencies in the population. (In fact, this is the way many typically choose entertainments or restaurants or places to visit, by relying on reviews that serve as guides to best practices in the ways such types often say that if everyone likes it, then it must be alright.)

What we begin to appreciate in such examples, of special relevance for issues of public health and safety, is that the focus on misconceptions (on popular innocence) makes information and expertise necessary and desirable. We see this for the examples of the psychopath and of college drinking and, in both cases, in the face of the epidemic about which warning is given; it is less the activity that is central (psychopathology or drinking), although rules for identifying the psychopath are mentioned, than it is the normal recognition procedures operative in collective life. This is to say that "society" is the subject, the patient, in the case of women becoming involved in relations (vulnerable or at risk) and for the example of the entering university students. It seems that medicalization in some important sense is addressed to members who need to develop recognition procedures for sorting out their place as normal or not in an ambiguous environment.

Thus, we open a space for inquiry into the truth of weakness. Weakness could point either or both to such innocence and/or ignorance, or to one's resistance towards taking the risk of inhabiting an ambiguous environment, leading us to ask after the sense of weakness that is true to the notion. Weakness becomes transparent in the picture of the subject, in both examples, in the midst of a strange collective and being without resources; both the freshman and the exploited dating people are characterized as governed by expectations that are innocent, unrealistic, out of touch, dreamy and, in the absence of reliable information, lacking anything of their own to depend upon. This is part of the pathos of public health, its having to work with a population that it finds pathetic and always in need of remedial or preventive treatment: that this population seems to lack will or knowledge to prepare for emergency.

10

Introduction

Since the Enlightenment, prosthetic devices have occupied a special place in the medical sciences as a potent symbol of the power and perils of mechanist medicine. In the eighteenth and early nineteenth centuries, mechanist physicians and natural philosophers touted prosthetics and other corporeal simulacra—most famously the complex automata of Vauconson, Jacquet-Droz, and others—as a positive demonstration that mechanical explanation sufficed to account for all physiological phenomena. These claims were countered by Romantics and other anti-materialists in a body of literature that consistently portrayed prosthetics and automata as endowed with ghostly or spiritual qualities that escaped the understanding of their mechanistic creators. The problem of "the ghost in the machine" (Ryle, 1949)—the relationship between body and mind, but also between mechanism and nature—has been one of the central *topoi* of philosophical struggles at least since Descartes; prosthetics and simulacra bring these problems sharply to a head, insofar as their mimetic functions require their designers, prescribers and wearers to generate explicit and implicit theorizations of the body and its mechanical reproductions. Thus, when Sigmund Freud chose Hoffmann's "Sandmann" to explicate his notion of "the uncanny," he was only one of many seeking to claim the contested ground of simulacra as evidence for their own understandings of the relationships among reason, passion and corporeality. Prosthetic devices have long been a site for hotly-fought contestations over the enlightenment project to define selfhood in strictly rational terms. (This paragraph summarizes the conventional view of prosthetics in terms of which we approached it as an area of inquiry and was written by Matt Price for the Grey Zone in Health and Illness project.)

The conventional view of prosthetics as a situation involving replacement of a lost limb or of correcting a damaged or impaired condition needs rethinking, because the discourse has been obscured by its assimilation to a social issue or to deviance studies, and because replacement has come to be reconfigured within the context of new technologies and, most importantly, ways of reformulating replacement as an economy of desire in which loss comes to include not simply what was detached physically (as in amputation) or a result of misfortune (a burn victim or blindness) but what anyone can define herself as lacking. What is interpreted as lost is the capacity to be as satisfied as one might think possible and it is this lost capacity for satisfaction that the subject wants to repossess, even in the way of improving upon what is already possessed because at present it cannot produce the satisfaction to which she is entitled.

Thus we must modify the usage of prosthetics as has occasionally been done (Wills, 1995) in order to center its connection to enhancing or rectifying what appears unalterable (this also permits us to illuminate the second sailing itself as a method which is similar to and different from other approaches and so part of a discourse revealing the imaginary of enhancement in its various shapes).

Enhancement as the desire for rectification can be connected to the injustice of a mark (for example, in the way one can decide if he wants to treat his being marked ethnically as if it confirms the loss of an inalienable right to be otherwise, or if he decides that his curly hair shows the loss of his inalienable right to have straight hair), suggesting that any condition can be treated as the infringement of a right and so as a loss of entitlement, as an injury that might serve as the basis for a claim. Simmel (1971) shows how our conception of equality as a right, differing from what he claims to be the Renaissance notion of distinctiveness, empowers anyone to claim entitlement to anything and everything that he lacks as if it is a violation of his right. In this sense, prosthetic desire is grounded in a vision of equality and comparability that can produce in and for oneself under any condition a sense of injury that easily understands itself as being deprived of something (some quality), the loss of which requires rectification or enhancement.

This needs clarification in several ways because any number of methods might be construed as prosthetic (and in the most restricted sense, prosthetics refers to the insertion of material into the body): walking canes or guide dogs for the blind, eyeglasses and other enhancement devices, the window pane, elevator shoes, mirrors (enhance our capacity to see ourselves in ways that we might need and so express the condition of our lacking such power as if a loss, and our need for rectification) and, most importantly, pharmaceuticals (note how this can also connect to the study of alcoholism). Implants tend to raise the question of loss in the shape of the desire to enhance (improve) a condition that strikes its subject as an impairment (or an infraction of her entitlement).

Any technology can be said to enhance our powers as if our prior condition was one of deprivation or loss of what the technology offers, as if we *now* decide that we suffer from being dispossessed of what the technology promises to redeem. For example, in the hair or breast implant, the subject typically defines himself as needing rectification and so as lacking something desirable. The discourse seems to be about changing conditions or rectifying the injustice of having characteristics that undermine confidence and ways of thinking about oneself.

In interviewing such subjects about these dissatisfactions, we find that their choice to rectify or change is taken freely as their own choice even when they concede its dependence upon codes that they did not invent. Appearance modification or hormone replacement admits that the condition in question reflects a convention, a normative order that did not originate with the subject's misrecognizing it as her free choice, while yet resisting the notion of simply being determined by a normative view of appearance. Between these positions, the subject identifies with neither extreme of freedom nor of victim but with the middle ground of representing as one's own the norms inherited (if the modification makes one feel better it is because he *makes* the satisfactions and dissatisfactions aroused by the question of changing the condition into a perfect expression of his feelings). The subject typically contends anyway that all such matters are irrelevant with respect to the fact that he chooses to have the implant because he can. Here we appreciate the view of the disruptiveness of nature in the shape of the unwanted condition, the inequity that produces the sense of loss.

What seems unthought is the subject's disinterest in being reflective about her wants or needs (or even whether it is her choice in contrast to her being determined externally) because she simply wants to do what she is in position to do. Note that the idea of assimilating wants to can (of wanting to do something simply because we can) is historically a feature of the tyrannical discourse (or: for any reflective subject, we typically suppose the need for an interpretive space between want and can, and for acting on wants and acting on can). Prosthetic desire seems to operate in the space where conditions are accepted or rejected mechanically, perhaps treated as an opposition that needs to be reconciled rather than as a difference that needs to be developed. Typically a condition (a characteristic) expresses the overwhelming character of a limit inviting rectification, a mark of irregularity that (as Žižek might say) is produced only in its recognition. Certainly the hair might really and truly be thin or sparse in terms of some statistical measure of the normative hair in a population, but seeing it as a loss (Rancière would say a "wrong") requires recognizing and interpreting the condition as the sign of an infraction (i.e., even the claim that the "norm" makes it so or "made me do it" is undermined by the condition that it is the subject's interpretation of the "norm making it so" that is what makes it so).

As an approach, the *modus vivendi* of prosthetics could identify a true prosthetics as an analytic framework for an entire project insofar as it strives to create distance between nature and the social by overcoming and objectifying that absorption in and by the body that tends to render us mute, that produces what Scarry (1985) calls pain. The disruptiveness of nature has different analogues in each and all of the various studies on our Grey Zone project. In terms of prosthetics as an area rather than as a method, we might note that the modern city and its need to limit desire intelligently can be expressed in the capacity for a reflective engagement with the aspiration towards bodily change. Such a reflection would have to approach those conditions that seem to be inherited (such as hair, breast and nose) as conditions similar to many others which appear to preexist us as signs of something old and unalterable, something like the world as constructed before us, so to speak, in ways that impose upon us the body itself as a kind of incoherent inheritance. But then a true prosthetics might begin to show that we are speaking about the limitation of desire in ways that identify more conditions than the body, conditions such as the drinking of alcohol or planning for children or even watching television and being exposed to its information and images. These are all conditions we inherit in the sense that we are thrown into the midst of collective representations which (in a way) can be said to preexist us. In other words, the old refers to more than the body because it makes reference to our representations from which we take our bearings and in terms of which we begin all our projects. Can we then begin to think about the two-sided nature of desire in such cases and how a true prosthetics might try something other than reconciling the two sides as if opposites by instead trying to come to terms with a middle ground? This question assumes that, for inquiry, prosthetics at its best rejects the extremes of accepting the world as it is (or seems) or rejecting the world as it is (or seems) in favor of an improvisational relationship that in this chapter we are calling prosthetics (because instead of adding something new and external, it enhances and develops what we already have, modeled particularly after linguistic play in the arts and in humor). Note that the world is symbolized in our research as the collective representation(s) of the body in a way that stamps prosthetics as a relationship to such conditions (representations) that seeks to escape the extremes by developing a middle ground that can explore them as different expressions of an elementary problem.

This suggests that we can think of prosthetics as a method, a way of establishing relations to ambiguity that tries to develop ambiguity as a practical problem in selected cases. If the discourse on prosthetics leads us to rethink the notion of truth even as it is disseminated in discussion about the difference between a genuine and spurious limb, original or counterfeit body parts, then what we might appreciate is that it is not the "truth" of the object that is at issue (is this a true-to-life foot, breast or hair?), but the question of a true relationship to the part that is viewed as lost. A true relationship would reflect on the place of the body and its parts in our life, well-being and the like.

The imaginary of medicalization

As noted, in one sense, this is a result of the growth of science and technology, but it also refers to new ways of thinking and speaking, using medical categories and images to define all conduct, and especially those that have no apparent connection to medicine. Here are a couple of examples.

(A) Growing old has nothing to do with medicine except for our need to govern ourselves, take care of our own needs and so forth. Of course, the body changes during aging, and we must be careful and regulate ourselves, but it does not *have* to be seen as a significant medical problem and certainly not as a disease. Now, often, aging *is* seen as a disease and even as a condition so deficient that people try to cure it through cosmetic surgery. Instead of being viewed as a normal condition that people must pass through as part of living a life, it is often regarded as a sickness, which could lead to remedial action such as prosthetics or drugs, in order to relieve the condition.

(B) Similarly, a two- or three-year-old who is high-strung and excitable may be seen as suffering from bipolar disease as if she is sick, often justifying medical intervention. Between these extreme examples, normal troubles such as not being able to sleep well, fatigue, sexual listlessness and the like are often treated as reasons for medical intervention, and certainly as bases for medication. So, one kind of problem in which we have interest involves this type of interpretation, even comparatively in cities here and there, as gathered from media, the press and interviews with medical people. Is there an increased tendency to apply medical ways of thinking to normal conditions? In the idiom of sociology, we might think of this not only as a social trend or even fad but as a social fact, "external and coercive" in Durkheim's (1938b) idiom, and we could ask, what kind of symptom does this mode of interpreting conduct begin to reveal?

In this vein, it would be interesting to consider how such matters stand in a society that is not as completely modernized as North America, for example, in Argentina, China, Italy, and particularly in the city, and whether normal troubles and normal conditions are seen typically as occasions for medical intervention or classified as diagnostic problems. How are these matters talked about in family, media and organized medicine? In our media, every problem of health and every condition that is addressed seems to become an occasion for predicting an epidemic, as if the condition threatens to become so widespread that we as a society will be helpless to deal with it. In this sense, the condition is often treated in the same way as a crime wave or an impending nuclear catastrophe.

Here again we need to consider what goes into making (conceiving of) any condition a disease. Note that we are not searching for a final solution in the shape of one definitive interpretation, nor a complete sample of opinions, but usage that could provoke us to rethink the notion of medicalization, that could empower us, in the idiom of Wittgenstein, to make it strange, odd or queer. In this respect, we can ask just what goes into counting troubles such as sleeping, over-talking, feeling bored, dissatisfaction with one's appearance, overeating or not being punctual as diseased. This question allows us to appreciate how a conception of bad conditions creates the opportunity for imagining a prosthetic relation to the condition in ways that include not only so-called enhancement technologies and cosmetic surgery but drugs and any regime of self-improvement. In all such cases, the disease is akin to one's dissatisfaction with some condition, and the prosthetic *techne* seems to offer the promise of relief. In this sense, the imaginary is grounded in the expectation that the modification will make a difference. This suggests as a program for possible research the question of how the notion of medicalization and its "work," as they say, becomes most visible in the way the collective speaks in converting any and all conditions into deficiencies, including its methods for identifying conditions that one is assumed to lack and need, and then in anticipating such lacks as an epidemic that can only be redeemed through preparation and remedial action.

Instead of natural disasters here, to make it more vivid, we might think of exercise or nutrition or even a sustainable environment. In other words, making the condition into a lack and the lack into a collective deficiency that endangers the perpetuity of the collective itself not only *makes* the epidemic a social fact, but creates the opportunity for self-appointed specialists to explain and interpret this situation, and also creates the controversy fated to occur in its name as a political issue. So here, we seem to have an interpretive chain that invites research into an imaginary that includes assumptions and interpretations about conditions, their conversion into lack or deficiency, their image as requiring remedial action, as a possible source of impending danger in the shape of a catastrophe, and of a public collectivized around this as an issue. We need to appreciate the fertility of such an imaginary, its displacements and condensations in a range of usage open to analysis instead of treating these as opinions or matters of fact about which we need to take sides rather than analyze.

In this sense, the notion of Prosthetics has been criticized (Jain, 1999), first as a metaphor that collects a variety of different tools and activities under its name (e.g., airbag, cane, glasses and voice all seem to distinguish the activity differently) and then as based upon a normative standard for the user. This reasonable criticism ignores the imaginative structure and the symbolic order of any such tool. It should be clear by now that the otherness of the category is an intellectual opportunity that its sameness makes possible. Yet the insight that any tool is a site of the imaginary should not bewilder us if we recognize that the important question to ask is not what the tool does but to what need and desire does it seems to answer? As Jain implies, part of the analysis requires recognizing any tool (the white cane or the eyeglasses) as presupposing a user that is normative, and this must follow from the idea of an oriented actor for whom the tool (the key) is an intended solution. The symbolic order exists on the basis of the ban that takes exception to ambiguity as such (including the imaginable range of marginal uses). Thus, any artifact assumes a normative standard of user-friendliness, typicality and standardization that interpellates a subject and the symbolic order to which she is subject. Prosthetics is "normative" in the way the symbolic order must create a subject that meets its requirements and a body of knowledge which this subject is supposed to have (to know) in order to inhabit the regime legitimized by the order. Prosthetics simply helps us recognize the power of travesty by making explicit the ambiguity in any usage as problems to solve. In this way, Prosthetics helps make observable ambiguity itself as a problem to negotiate. What we begin to appreciate throughout is that ambiguity, whether as part of a transference, as the hole in the signifier (a word has many senses) or as the hole in Being (the incompatibility of part and whole, the excess or the remainder), tends to be treated as a limit or deficiency in and of life itself, as a recognition against which we need defend ourselves and rarely as an incentive for inquiry.

Prosthetic desire

Similarly, a condition such as aging can be interpreted as disease, just as the overactive child can be seen as suffering from a bipolar disease, but it is never self-evident that such conditions qualify unless they are given the inflection of pathology. If this investment is made (in seeing the condition as such), then it is not much of a step to seeing the city or nation *en toto* as suffering (or about to suffer) an epidemic. Pharmaceutical intervention is suggested. In a way, this is the model for the television makeover genre and also conjures up a vision of the collective per se (the city) as needing a makeover and a cadre of pundits to offer advice for such.

Policy becomes a solution when someone like Richard Florida (2002) is hired by a city to rescue it from whatever it seems to lack because of his reputed experience with cities that seem to resemble this one in ways that make them each indistinct from one another. Yet the epidemic is not simply reflected in the uniformity of all cities but in the innocence of any city (like the woman and her psychopath) that does not seem to know how to distinguish itself by using common conditions distinctively. What any one city lacks is a vision of applying knowledge that can only be supplied by a pundit. Thus, any one city is pathological if, in its innocent self-absorption, it cannot see the forest for the trees; that is, it does not know how to apply the knowledge that is out there to its own situation. Because such a city does not know to mark itself as distinctive (it does not know how it differs from any other or how it counts as a city that *is* rather than merely exists as a city in name only), it seems to require a makeover and a pundit to guide this transformation. The pundit, who does not himself know this one city from the others he has visited because they are each and all "creative," also must leave a mark (like the rescue team in New Orleans) to remind himself where he is and has been. Here, we can begin to address the relations between medicalization, epidemic, public health and punditry (policy).

Related to medicalization is a recurrent theme suggesting that medical practitioners need retraining in order to be compassionate towards patients and to be respectful of their dignity and autonomy. While this is a theme in every area, it is noteworthy in dealing with the aged and in long-term care, where it is not only medicine that is encouraged in this way but the family as well. The family (and "society") is often said to be disrespectful towards the aged and aging, inviting us to ask how this works in different cities and periods. If medicalization is thought of as a trend in the ways that have been suggested, then it can be factored into the popular or mass culture of collective life in the same way as any of its usages or categorizations (lifestyle such as fashion and food, celebrities, customs, consumption and object choices).

11

The Recurrence of the Body

Introduction

We have discussed the relationship of mind to body as a fundamental enigma for revealing the work of the Grey Zone as a phenomenon of everyday life. The constancy of the collective fascination with the body is a function of the division we have discussed throughout, between the fear of being objectified as if a body (because we share such corporeality) and the hope of differentiating ourselves from that with which we are comparable by virtue of our being able to see-as. We have discussed such problem solving through tropes for a dialectic relation to language such as the Same and the Other, the *aufheben*, togetherness and apartness, and other figures designed to narrate the struggle to be at home with such an irreconcilable division.

The capacity to represent ourselves and to divide ourselves into faculties or characteristics cannot be taken for granted, grounded as it is in notions of border, boundary, separation, characteristics and powers, both seemingly in and out of our possession, that we invent, attribute, assign and imagine as property both sovereign and dispossessible. Nevertheless, the body and its parts can serve for any and all who are attentive, and not just for its subject but for the collective at large, as an archive of object choices and of passages and transformations of desire. Thus, if *das Ding* makes reference, as Lacan (1991, pp. 243–326) says, to "the beyond of the signified," then we always can ask for the way the body discloses this trace as a problem (i.e., how we understand the "beyond of the signified" in reference to the body), or how collective representations of the body begin to disclose this "beyond" or unthought element in the discourse. It is here that notions of trauma and symptom help us to formulate the body in relation to mind.

> It is from that moment when we speak of our will and our understanding as distinct faculties that we have a preconscious, and that we are able in effect, to articulate in a discourse something of that chattering by means of which we articulate ourselves inside ourselves, or we rationalize for

ourselves with reference to this or that, the progress of our desire. It is definitely a discourse that is involved. (Lacan, 1992, pp. 61–62)

The materiality of language

In these ways, let us bring the so-called mind-body problem down to earth by developing its character as a discourse rather than as an exchange of arguments or opinions that only have to be adjudicated according to empirical or logical criteria by an observant or careful philosopher or medical scientist. I suggest that this discourse reveals for a reflective eye the desire to imagine and master the enigma of automation, that is, automated relations to speech and action that are learned as if a second skin, and that it proceeds through recourse to prosaic commonplace figures of speech of ordinary language. The brunt of this discussion will explore the uses of selected commonplace figures of speech almost as if they are formulae for abbreviating and condensing difficult thoughts in ways that seem to mark a struggle in collective life to determine and objectify the invisible movement of spirit in health and illness. We will explore the two-sidedness of such automated speech and the collisions that come to view as a Grey Zone capable of stereotyping human experience and yet opening itself to inquiry by exposing complex assumptions about the relations of mind to body. Instead of taking the mind-body problem as an interaction between two different substances, thought and matter, we will explore such a commonplace itself as in part a desire to speak about seemingly irreconcilable, ineffable and yet tangible influences, i.e., a problem of expressing the inexpressible.

We can think of language as a body insofar as it can be understood as a corpus of rules, practices, methods and procedures regulated by contestable ideals, aspirations and self-images. Language has a degree of materiality reflected in the word, the signifier and the letter. While there is nothing good or bad about the fact of the materiality of speech per se, if in speaking we can relate in different ways to such a body, then our speaking might be tied rigidly to formulae and scripts that render it relatively inflexible, or it can aspire to inventive and improvisational relationships to the script (the code) as such, still showing that even the most inventive relations to speech must be tied to formulae sanctioned by a symbolic order. It is in this space wherein the dialectic of freedom and constraint must materialize as a mode of common expression that the speaker can be both together and apart in relation to its language. As a corpus though, this linguistic body has appeared to many such as Blanchot (1982) as if a corpse or cadaver that always has to be animated and brought to life by psyche or at least, as depicted by the trope of *prosopopeia*, as a bringing of the dead to life. Here, the idea of speech bringing to life the dead word resonates with the notion that the image, like a cadaver, is brought to life by the ways in which it is oriented to and used.

The example of the materiality of speaking practices has been made visible in conventions of typification that standardize expectations and responses as in the normal formats of common sense and in generic usages such as proverbs, platitudes and clichés, often treated ambiguously as examples of automated speech. In sociology, George Homans once used the proverb as an example of the kind of inflexible slothful practice that science always needed to overcome in a conclusion that Harvey Sacks famously challenged by demonstrating the rationality intrinsic to the structure of the proverb (Sacks, 1992, pp. 419–429). Of course, Kenneth Burke has innovated in the use of the proverb as a frame of reference for making explicit the symbolic order itself in ways we have followed here (Burke, 1957, pp. 254–262). Alternatively, attempts to overcome such automation or to transgress it mechanically through linguistic subversiveness, or in tropes designed to surpass rigidity, still tend to sustain the automated character of such hyperbole. The need for speaking to be expressive in standardized ways in order for more creative relations to develop means that the proverbial or platitudinous expression is not good or bad on its face, but an aspect of the materiality of speaking that comes alive through the ways in which they are engaged and reinvented as dialogical seductions, as ironies that recurrently establish them both as phenomena for analysis (as data), and as resources for doing analysis, as part of the format of conversation, dialogue and of exposition.

In this view, the relation of speech to the body is invariably a relation of speaking to its own materiality, a recurrent attempt in the best sense to give form to the material conditions of speaking. Such giving form then introduces desire into speaking insofar as the desire to give form, to endow speech with something more, rests on the capacity to imagine that it could be otherwise and on the function of this ideal as both an incentive and a source of frustration. This sets up the notion of the imaginary as revealing the two-sidedness of desire and the necessary and overstimulating model of wholeness as an imperative human vision.

Lacan's (1991) use of the body as a figure to stand for an ideal or paradigm is interesting, first because by calling the body a paradigm, it divests it of its status as a kind of incorrigible, external condition in naming it as the standard that the subject orients to and emulates, tries to live up to, and so, is in some sense internal despite its apparent tangible externality. What this means is that corporeality as a standard of materialism is that ideal of tangibility and either/or that pervades representation, endowing it with its character as (what Hegel [cf. Birchall, 1981] calls) finite understanding and its capacity to do determination, identification in the most efficient way possible. What is suggested here is that the meaning of the signifier "body" is undergoing a modification, allowing it to serve on the one hand as a figure for paradigm, standard and image, and on the other hand, to apply to its typical usage as that corporeal bit of material we tend to call our bodies in ordinary language. Most important is that whatever we say about the body or take it to be must depend upon mind, since body as content of a representation remains an oriented object, meaning again that any talk about the precedence of the body as a causal force in life must by its very occurrence deny what it affirms because such a notation of precedence as mimetic can only be an example of mindedness.

As a paradigm, the body is intended here in the image of an intelligible container, as having a definitive beginning and end, with characteristics or properties that add up to a collection that is discrete and definite as if a set. This notion of closure, definitiveness and finality serves both as a construction within the subject and, at the same time, as if a foreign body within that has a degree of separation. The body then functions in this discourse within as both a motor of idealization and of frustration since the standard always exceeds any resolution. As has been said throughout, though, the tension between the body as a standard of language by virtue of its tendency to honor corporeality as the Good (the tendency to give body to speech by converting speaking into a body) coexists with the aspiration to give speech to the body or to give the body voice. This tension recurs in the struggle to subvert being objectified (being treated as table, toe or cow) by taking a perspective on such treatment. This tension of course recurs, as we noted, in the depersonalization experienced in pain and perhaps in any serious illness. But if this recurrence is accurate, it suggests that one task of medicine in relation to such vulnerability would always be to collaborate in resisting such objectification, seeking always to be in position to facilitate the capacity to take a perspective(to be a self) under such conditions. Let us try to set up this collision.

Thus, to take a perspective, to seek to repossess the selves we have, recurs as a problem of both medicine and its patients as a problem of the desire to rehabilitate vulnerability through the ways in which we encounter one another in speaking together. Here, if we think of art and poetry, rhetoric and its canon might first come to mind, in its inventory of tropes and methods of figuration, as ways and means of enlivening discursive contact. But this is not necessary as figuration itself can be banal, automated, robotic and, as we know from mass media at least, in no way guarantees a creative relation to speech. We might tentatively ask: how do we speak in a way that gives voice to the body of speech?

Stepping over

So we must be careful if we assume that theorizing or poetry or speech rich in figuration is the avenue of escape from mechanical relations to speaking. Heidegger (1962) provides, perhaps unwittingly, another perspective on this by socializing or making over the notion of transcendence in such a way that, on the one hand, seems to suggest its opposition to automated speech and, on the other, brings it into view as automated in its own way. He talks about transcendence as a mode of human being in the world that orients to what he calls stepping over.

> The world is transcendent because, belonging to the structure of being-in-the world, it constitutes stepping over to as such [...] the transcending beings are not the objects—things cannot transcend or be transcendent; rather, it is the "subjects" —in the rightly understood sense of the Dasein— which transcend, step through and step over themselves. (Heidegger, 1962, p. 299)

I am interested in the ways stepping through and stepping over the conditions of a common language is a struggle, within language so to speak, with the normal temptations to be ruled by robotic and automated relations to commonplaces, in order to get us to think about how we might be innovative in relation to a code, i.e., how we might participate in and reflect upon what is called the symbolic order and how the recurrent force of the body of language might be subverted mindfully. While Heidegger seems to oppose desire (for stepping over as he says) to mechanical relations to speaking, Lacan (1991, pp. 242–326) noted that such desire is automated in its own way, calling it the imaginary (the desire Heidegger described as stepping over), identifying its emergence early in the development of the infant through the example of the mirror image as a source of idealization and of frustration. So the body recurs as two-sided, making reference to the automated character of speech that is disclosed both in its banality *and* in the desire to overcome it by using speech against itself in ways that seem both necessary, desirable and yet standardized in repetitive ways.

To paraphrase Sartre (1968), speech is a good example of freedom within limits, that it is not unlimitedness that is the prize, problem or possibility, but improvisation. Note two things this excludes: being inventive cannot mean qualifying everything said pedantically by noting the fact that it could be said otherwise, for this is simply an obsessive strategy of continuous qualification that evades action; yet, speech cannot simply transgress the code hysterically on the grounds of its opposition because this exemplifies the case of being determined by what we oppose. As we noted earlier, Baudrillard speaks here of the strategy of "objective irony":

> One is compelled to produce meaning in the text, and one produces this meaning *as if* it arises from the system (even if in fact the system lacks meaning) in order precisely to play that meaning against the system itself as one reaches the end [...] so as to make the system reveal itself more clearly [...] This ambiguity probably remains throughout the text at every point. (Baudrillard, 2006, pp. 40–41)

Baudrillard's rhetoric (often maligned by academics) trumps everyone here: we take exception to the system by challenging it in this way, by developing, accentuating and exaggerating the system, "playing it against itself," "playing on the logic" itself to make the system reveal itself, refining the method of subversion in a performance designed to reveal the limits of the order in the voice of one feigning being an insider in order to expose its outside, the provocative method of travesty (Blum, 1993) that he calls the seduction of "objective irony."

In this sense, obsessive and hysterical relations to language are robotic, automated or banal insofar as they externalize speaking by acting as if they do not participate in the very ambiguity from which they recoil. (In my travesty paper [Blum, 1993], I used transsexuals playfully as a hysterical reply to the constraint of gender, the overbearing straight-gendered world as obsessive, and transvestism as a primitive and somewhat generic attempt to explore boundaries in the absence of a strong androgynous relation that had neither to destroy nor mechanically accept such conditions. Androgyny then figured as the improvisational alter to an automated relation to gender.) The interlocutor to the automated relation to speech is not then freedom or spontaneity but what Stanislavski (1989) calls mechanical relations to the type or to the characterization, i.e., bad acting or action transparent for its undialectical mechanism.

As noted, this expresses the tactic of theorizing that aspires to destabilize the commonplace in the way of the second sailing and the canonical strategy of this work, from Plato though Lacan and beyond. This two-sided relationship to usage appears as both a necessity and a convention that, in using what it inquires into and inquiring into what it uses (e.g., Meno and Theaetetus), always risks appearing in contradiction and as if it is unaware. This important qualifier "and" expresses the difference between Baudelaire's notion of absolute humor (reflective comedy) and Bergson's conception of ordinary humor (being laughable).

Disfiguration

As a beginning Freud (Freud and Breuer, 1952) is best here, for in anticipating Wittgenstein's advice to treat the commonplace as "odd," he advises us to resist its apparent intelligibility and its ingratiating offers of self-disclosure or self-reporting in order to discover its rituals of avoidance and, by virtue of this, just what it is trying to say. Freud dramatizes the problem not simply as one of overcoming a generic relation to speech but of having a degree of command over its ambiguity shown in the will to take risks in speaking that would create a scene of mutually oriented action in which participants could begin to lay down their arms by using the transference constructively rather than for self-aggrandizement. The spell of language as a body is not broken by the subject in such cases. Listen to Freud on the hysteric in therapy:

> As far as the physician was concerned, the patient's confession was
> at first sight a great disappointment. It was a case history made up of

commonplace emotional upheavals, and there was nothing about it to explain why it was from hysteria that she fell ill. (Freud and Breuer, 1952, p. 212)

Her use of commonplace formulae to describe her history in ways that begin to reveal to him something about her (regardless of whether her case history checks out, is true to the facts or not) alerts him to a kind of resistance that she is giving to avoid addressing something that matters to her. Here, whereas a mechanical relationship to speech on the subject's part might seem habitual as if unoriented, Freud sees it as disclosing that she does not want to expose herself, or in the best sense, her inability to find her voice in the narrative in a way that is intimate or a singular expression of who she is. This applies to any speech that seeks to describe itself, showing, as Lacan (1988, pp. 247–260; 1992) says, that the ego, far from being an executive function or overseer, is a symptom used by the subject to handle other problems, making consciousness, the self-report, the survey and the narrative, always expressive bits and pieces of construction work, to be interrogated, diagnosed and not simply applauded. For example, think of our stance towards surveys and opinion polls, or of the talk of pundits, if we treated any and every response as a hallucination. Obviously the distortion is only a beginning in order to develop ways and means of rethinking the notion of disfiguration. Here in another example Freud comments on Hamlet, showing again how overtalking or reticence, honesty or deceit is not the issue but the way in which it is done.

When in his heightened self-criticism he describes himself as petty, egoistic, dishonest, lacking in independence, one whose sole aim has been to hide the weaknesses of his whole nature, it may be, as far as we know, that he has come pretty near to understanding himself; we only wonder why a man has to be ill before he can be accessible to a truth of this kind. For there can be no doubt if anyone holds and expresses to others an opinion of himself such as this (an opinion which Hamlet held both of himself and of everyone else), he is ill, whether he is speaking the truth or whether he is being more or less unfair to himself. (Freud, 1957, pp. 255–257)

This could be a model of the confessional talk of addicts. Thus, it is not what is said in terms of its honesty or intelligibility that is at stake but what saying anything as such is seen by the theorist to be doing and how it is revealing what it stands for and to what it looks up as worth emulating or pursuing and what it says about itself under such conditions. The body can then serve as an image that centers our attention on automation and redemption in speaking practices, perhaps in the same way that theorizing itself needs to maintain its own singular response to automation reflected in its submission to the repetitious manner sanctioned by the canon. This provokes us to begin to formulate the struggle in the subject to develop an inventive relation to her conditions.

Freud wants us to appreciate the relation of theorizing to whatever content it theorizes as an exchange of hallucinations always permitting us to grasp how we are nothing rather than something without the *object a*. In such cases of Freud, it is not automation directly that is the problem but the failure to engage this automated talk dialectically. The patient uses a formula not malevolently but as a way of revealing something she finds inexpressible almost as a sign of intellectual fatigue that discloses her not wanting to think about something. Here, it is as if the commonplace is used to disfigure some matter of value and in its way inadvertently expresses and masks the singularity of the patient.

> The symbolic provides a form into which the subject is inserted at the level of his being. It's on the basis of the signifier that the subject recognizes himself as being this or that [...] [yet] [t]here is, in effect, something radically unassimilable to the signifier. It's quite simply the subject's singular experience. Why is he here? Where has he come from? What is he doing here? Why is he going to disappear? The signifier is incapable of providing him with the answer, for the good reason that it places him beyond death. The signifier already considers him dead, by nature it immortalizes him. (Lacan, 1997, pp. 179–180)

That is, the theorist recognizes himself as nothing rather than something as he comes to see how the signifier "considers him dead" by exposing the thin line between mortification and vitality.

Commonplaces

As a method, I propose that we try to locate in any commonplace the point of tension in its automated relationship to its own speaking practices as if it strives to step over or cross the boundaries of what seems to limit it. Here we begin to search out the imaginary as the place where the subject tries to envision more for and of himself, for and of the other, and for and of their joint world than he can put into words, while making use of these very words to do revelation as such. Unpacking any commonplace should in its way be a methodical revelation of a world imagined as relevant for the subject, as a matter requiring clarification, as a site of ambiguity and frustration, as a problem-solving situation for oneself and other and as a focus of mutually oriented action and collectivization. It is as if the commonplace establishes the related character of those touched by it, those speaking under its auspices. What is important is how the commonplace expresses what is inexpressible, which means by and large the experience of singularity in speech, the experience that seems to escape signification and yet can only be signified and expressed by virtue of what it exceeds, the materiality of language.

If we are to capture the spirit of the commonplace and its imaginary, then theorizing must playfully use and subvert its own commonplace linguistic temptations in an experimental rather than transgressive spirit. The recently released letters of Samuel Beckett (Josopovici, 2009) are instructive for the ways in which they lay out different relationships to the materiality of speaking practices. First, as a young man in his twenties, Beckett comments on his father's reaction to a publisher's rejection of his first novel (Frank is his father):

> Frank came back from his 10 days in Donegal last Tuesday [...] When he heard Heinemann had turned down (Murphy) he said: "Why can't you write the way people want," and when I replied that I could only write one way, i.e., as best I could (not the right answer by the way, not at all the right answer), he said it was a good thing for him he did not feel obliged to implement such a spirit at [...] his office. (Beckett, cited in Josopovici, 2009, p. 7)

Assuming language as a medium between minded beings with expectations of one another, he identifies the father's position as one favoring "writing the way people want" and in contrast to this, his position which abuses readers' expectations (presumably) in order to make them learn. Yet, Beckett finds his opposition immature, not because he feels it correct to be governed by the urge in order to satisfy others' satisfactions, but for the reason that his simple transgression seems to him unformulated. Thus the first distinction models an ego-alter transaction divided between pandering and self-indulgence, between one's wants and other's wants as if a zero-sum game, much like a master-slave transaction. If we give the other satisfaction we have none ourselves and we indulge ourselves, we give the other no satisfaction. Both his and the father's positions seem rigid and untenable as the mature Beckett of many years later recognizes. Thus, Beckett might surmise that his position in no way meant that he was abusing the reader, but playfully subverting language; that is, he was proposing to analyze the commonplace that gives people (readers) satisfaction in order to discover what gives satisfaction. Instead of taking the commonplace at face value or even trying to translate it into a more parsimonious and operational idiom, we try to rethink and calculate about what it is conflicted. He is interested in exploring how desire works itself out through the medium of language, and the commonplace seems the place to begin, neither by confirming it mechanically nor by abusing it mechanically, but through analysis, i.e., a dialectical engagement. The method proposed is to analyze the way in which the mechanization of self-feeling is disguised and worked out in language. His mature reflection overcomes the transference relation between writer and reader (between father and son).

> And more and more my language appears to me like a veil that one has to tear apart in order to get to those things (or the nothingness) lying behind it. Grammar and style! To me they seem to have become as irrelevant as a Biedermeier bathing suit or the imperturbability of a gentleman. A mask. It is to be hoped the time will come, thank god in some circles it already has, when language is best used when most efficiently abused [...] Or is literature alone to be left behind on that old, foul road long ago abandoned by music and painting? Is there something paralysingly sacred contained within the unnature of the word that does not belong to the elements of the other arts? Is there any reason why the terrifyingly arbitrary materiality of the word surface should not be dissolved, as, for example, the sound surface of Beethoven's Seventh Symphony is devoured by huge black pauses, so that for pages on end we cannot perceive it as other than a dizzying path of sounds connecting unfathomable chasms of silence? An answer is requested. (Beckett, cited in Josopovici, 2009, p. 7)

Here, the mind-body problem is recast as the analysis of the mechanization of self-feeling disclosed in any commonplace and its binding character, revealed in the material practices of speaking. The question Beckett poses of relating to habituation in thought and action by maintaining a space between self as other (giving undiluted satisfaction as if a slave to the other) and other as self (indulging oneself by treating the other as if a slave to one's lordship) is not resolved either by a resigned sense of fatal incommensurability between self and other. Rather, one treats oneself and the other as both the same and the other. This overcomes the limited solution of market value where satisfying the other (becoming an object of desire in such a limited way) dissolves oneself by diminishing the other's respect for one, or by achieving satisfaction for oneself without regard for the other (as if the disrespect of mastery as such). Here are some thought experiments I devised on this matter.

Stress

> A man wakes in the morning and cannot find the pen he left out on the
> table the night before. He has a mild condition of psoriasis that seems to
> get aggravated with stress. He begins scratching at his leg furiously until
> it bleeds while rummaging about for his lost pen and thinking about how
> he could have lost it. His daughter discovers his pen under a pile of papers
> and he stops scratching. Test question he poses to himself: how could the
> lost pen cause his outbreak? Is this what they mean by "stress?"

This is a good example of the imaginary. It is not the lost object that causes the
problem but the regime in which the object functions. Here is what this person knows
about himself: that the loss of the object reawakens him to the recognition that his ideal
of self-mastery includes organizing himself and his environment in ways that will permit
him to handle such contingencies so as to live a harmonious well-ordered life which
he controls and over which he has command. The imaginary here is a figure for the
anticipation and expectation of mastery as an ideal internal to him to which he never can
live up successfully and so, which always exists as if a foreign object or part inseparable
and yet separate with which his "real" part always struggles. The constant struggle in his
psyche is constructed by him as an encounter between his two parts, the part he aspires
to be but never can and the part he is, depicting the terrain of the imaginary idealized as
oriented to a solution he anticipates "right around the corner" (Žižek, 1997). If the pen is
what Benjamin would call a stage prop for pointing to larger matters, and the scratching
what Freud would call a symptom, then the trauma could be the loss of the innocent
sense of absolutism that organizes this fantasy of self-mastery, the loss of the idea that
one is in control and the terrifying recognition that one is in the hands of Other and
that Other will not answer, will not give reassurance, meaning that the subjectivity of
Other is always in question. The singularity of the commonplace signifier "stress" always
escapes determination for even as completely as we might describe it here as a symptom
of desire, this never can give satisfaction on why it takes the specific shape it does, i.e.,
why psoriasis rather than anything else. This means that the singularity of the agent also
escapes signification because, even if he has such a symptom, how it comes to belong to
him as more than external or accidental remains unresolved.

Representations of stress typically misrecognize an external condition as the cause of the
distress, such as the pen, whereas the cause seemed to be the imaginary relationship to self-
mastery. But note that when a trauma such as this is posited as the cause of the illness, it can
only be posited by virtue of its effects and through the signifying structure that makes it
what it already was. If we have no trouble rejecting the lost pen as a cause, then the trauma
can only be the cause by virtue of an elaborate interpretive structure that empowers us to
create associations and resemblances between these various effects in the first place. That

the relation between the trauma and psoriasis is produced through interpretations that make such connections coherent means that what is first, what is prior, is ambiguity and its unsettling character. In this way, the commonplace notion of stress recovers cause as a figure of speech for the enigma of ambiguity as intrinsic and irresolute.

The body has a mind of its own

We shall now speak of the recurrence of the body as an omnipresent feature of discourse struggling to put its world into words. Medical discussions of disease inadvertently permit us to grasp the ways in which the body is given voice through the depiction of disease and its workings. For example, in confronting physicians about conditions such as chronic lung disease, I have often been told that the body has a mind of its own. That the body is minded can suggest that it is oriented and so, that it could be an interlocutor. The cliché always raises the problem of what kind of interlocutor this minded body is, friendly or an adversary. The cliché avoids raising this problem, satisfied that noting the fact is sufficient: that the body has a mind of its own also means that it could keep this mind to itself as if a secret and so, seems privatized in ways that might surprise us. What medicine says here is that it is ignorant about what is happening with the disease, and its anthropomorphic reply is designed to give us reassurance by normalizing the body and showing that its resemblance (as minded) might make it approachable and accessible as one to be befriended.

The difficulty here is that if medicine says that it is ignorant of how the body acts in the case of disease, then by endowing the body with a mind of its own it pushes the problem back because nothing is known about the mind that the body has or about the kind of mind this is. That the body has a mind of its own sustains a vision of the body as Other in a way that makes it incalculable. As Mead (1967) reminds us, if the body does have a mind of its own it is because of the human self that conjures up such an image for itself and its use, disclosing such talk as an index of the imaginary. Let us see how this mind of the body is reputed to do its work.

In the most commonly discussed case that we can call *subversion*, the body seems a theater in which the intended antidotes to disease, whether in response to the multiplication of cancer cells or other infections of various kinds, instead of being arrested by these drugs or antibiotics, become absorbed, converting them through a mimetic process in which the disease overcomes its enemy by virtue of the immunity it develops as if in learning its ways, it repels the attacker through an *aufheben* in which its neutralization of the antidote strengthens the disease in its turn. This mimetic process of subversion-conversion is a familiar example of the way the body can be said to co-opt the mind by robbing its systematic interventionist strategies of any strength, turning them back with even greater force upon the creator. When the connection between the antidote and disease becomes a basis of solidarity, this can eliminate enmity as in films where the agent intending to attack the evil becomes co-opted, overpowered or converted to the cause of the evil because of the charm of evil or the vulnerability of good. Examples include corruption and law, giving an offer you can't refuse, or contagion where the antidote becomes infected (or when we come to take pleasure in what had given us pain).

This is a familiar model of problem-solving when the problem solved becomes a greater problem after its solution or when the antidote to something bad becomes even worse. In a way reminiscent of Deleuze's (1991, pp. 9–138) illustration of masochism that revealed the masochist as subverting the intended punishment by coming to take pleasure in it (as in the tendency to enjoy the whip, the force of the punishment is not simply discounted but annulled by virtue of its conversion into its opposite, into pleasure rather than pain, becoming the pleasure of the pain), we could say that disease learns from the corrective measures directed against it, becoming stronger and more skilled at reducing and limiting the agency of mind.

That the body has a mind of its own could be an occasion for calculation (by figuring what the body needs and desires we can give it what it wants) or military maneuvering, as in the adversarial relation to cancer, but in any and every case it raises the problem of the subjectivity of Other. This poses the problem of whether Other is friendly as Plato (1949b) had Timaeus assume in the dialogue of that name and as many religions believe, or instead as indifferent in ways maintained in the canon from Lucretius to Lacan. Here is Russell on the *jouissance* of Other.

> Brief and powerless is Man's life; on him and all his race doom falls pitiless and dark. Blind to good and evil, reckless of destruction, omnipotent matter rolls on its restless way; for Man condemned today to lose his dearest, to-morrow himself to pass through the gate of darkness, it remains only to cherish, ere yet the blow falls, the lofty thoughts that ennoble his little day. (Russell, cited in Burtt, 2003, p. 23)

If the body has a mind of its own, then the question of what it is to which the mind of this body is oriented must always leave us without a firm conclusion; on the one hand, we want to reject illusion and superstition in the name of intellectual virility, and yet we need some antidote, some prescription to carry on. In this sense, if this is not an empirical question since the subjectivity of Other is unknowable, then it can be a question of what is best for us, what it is healthy to believe, but this typically gives anything other than obsessive skepticism a bad name. In response to skepticism, the notion of the friendliness of the body can only be seen as fool's gold.

Mind over matter

This commonplace is usually an injunction advising us to exercise a degree of self-control in the expectation that calculating the body and its mechanics is a prelude to exercising command in much the way Bacon (1960) urged us to observe nature in order to control and predict its workings. That this is not simply the advice of biomedical expertise is shown in the naturopathic counsel to scrutinize our body systematically, discovering its needs and requirements in order to proceed with equanimity. For example, corporeal imbalances are inventoried to give the user a corpus of knowledge to navigate in monitoring oneself in everyday life through information about nutrition, digestion, toxins and various plans for purification. In such cases, the user is treated much like the Cartesian subject whose lack of knowledge was regarded as the most important source of human error and fallibility.

That the body is constructed along the lines of a table of organization, listing assorted sensitivities, propensities, lacks, imbalances and deficiencies, always modeling it after the machine and the subject after the operator of the machine, seems to make the inarguable assumption that self-management is the only efficient path for realizing a degree of equilibrium imagined as an ideal, the perfect connection between knowledge and its application that inheres in the imaginary construal of enlightenment, expecting mind to best exercise its causal force if it is undisturbed by sloth or the lack of information. Here, there seems to be more optimism regarding the body as Other since it is viewed as amenable to scrutiny, intervention and manipulation.

Yet, in recognition that the best intentions are limited in this way is the conception of somatic incapacities as requiring the kind of relief that can only be provided by external agencies. This routine scenario for pharmaceutical and prosthetic initiatives of all kinds amounts in its way to a plan for stimulating the body to defend oneself from its own deleterious effects now as if the body is not so amenable but a self-destructive lout within (e.g., a bad teenager in the family) or because the mind seems to lose its interest in managing the body, wanting to escape administration much like a fatigued corporate executive, politician or even academic who wants to get away from it all. Examples such as Prozac, Viagra and other stimulants recommend that we can no longer overcome conditions such as listlessness, fatigue, sexual impotence and the like and, so, that our self-sufficiency is limited to the extent that we need to rely on external help to supplement our diminished means and self-determining capacities, compelled by such deficiencies to seek external aid in order to help us regain our strength. This is similar to enlisting hired armies or mercenaries to do our own work, suggesting in its way that our limits force a dependency upon a lower order that we must now treat as necessary, creating a relaxation of standard (the necessary evil) on which we risk becoming dependent (addicted) in ways that can transform us permanently; that our so-called ends or higher purposes pale in impact because of our increasing dependency upon the means to pursue them, leading to these means coming to replace the ends in value for us. The idea that we need stimulation to live through a day, or to study, or to be sexual, says that our mental capacities cannot function powerfully in such activities in unaided ways, requiring help from outsiders. Because this image reminds us of the slogan of ends justifying means as when unsavory alliances or conduct done for higher purposes are viewed as infecting the subject with the same unsavory characteristics despite his protestations, we can identify this movement as a kind of dependency (that the means become the end suggests that the subject is co-opted by dependency to treat his means as his ends as in addiction). This movement of the body as an image of recurrence functions pervasively in collective life as when government or law has to adopt criminal methods to fight crime or one's enemies and is reflected in the warning about being reduced to the level of one's enemy. The idea of agency losing its powers and having to accept the assistance of amoral or indifferent forces always makes problematic the question of the authorship of any action as such (showing the pervasiveness of disavowal in seemingly contrasting cases—"it wasn't me who succeeded at that act, it was the drug"—is commensurate with the attribution of responsibility for any act, good or bad, to medication or to one's lower part as if analogous to not-guilty by reason of insanity attributions). That we come to depend upon what we do not respect is typically registered in the genre of the Hollywood western where the bourgeoisie of the city forfeit their sanctimonious ethics to use and misuse anyone in order to achieve their ends (for example, in *High Noon* and *The Black Knight*) showing how desperation is viewed as trumping integrity when push comes to shove.

Is a person more than a body?

> A man has a four-year-old daughter. The man has an injured leg due to a car accident that immobilizes him. The daughter asks: wouldn't you rather be Kenneth? No, answers the man, why do you ask? Because he doesn't have an injured leg, she answers. But I like who I am, he says. But do you like having an injured leg? No, I would rather not have an injured leg, but I want to be the same as I am. She says: Oh, I want you to stay as you are too.

Being is not a predicate. What one is must exceed any such conditions or characteristics and even if they add up to form a composite set of features, they will not provide a picture of what philosophers call "who" rather than "what" someone is (Kripke, 1977, on Nixon). The father and daughter's exchange is organized around the notion that what happens to the body or to its characterization still does not provide for the singularity of the father; in addition, there is a difference between being possessed by the condition as if it was all one is and being self-possessive in relation to it.

Nevertheless, the singularity of the father in excess of the injured leg lacks the tangibility and visibility of the characteristic in ways that always make the claim of singularity an occasion for the mockery of the many. To paraphrase Socrates (Plato, 1945), the many mock any claim to singularity, rejecting it as intangible, invisible and elitist in a way that requires any such claim to stand up to mockery (see the *Republic* on the difficulty of educating keen-witted youth in the face of this enmity). It seems as if this singularity is not assimilated to and by the signifier. This means that in some way the signifier must be used against itself, perhaps in the way we must disfigure the usage, the body of speech, by looking through it to its beyond, a beyond that is intrinsic to it and "interior."

Note also that the child could use any condition to raise such questions, for example, appearance, color or gender, always asking whether or not such conditions can or should be exchanged for Being and if Being is simply an aggregate of conditions such as these. Note also that the father is in no position to offer divine guidance and to unequivocally resolve the problem raised by the child, the problem of Being as Heidegger (1961) posed it in *An introduction to metaphysics*, because if Being is not a predicate and if it escapes signification in that way, then the father is in no position to say what it is with such finality, only that he maintains a relation to his body that needs to be measured by the way he imagines himself. The father cannot answer the child because Other does not answer the father, the father's mastery residing only in posing the question.

This scenario provides for more than can be determined by the signifier, seeing it not only as free association but as almost hallucinatory, showing the singularity of the talk to reside in some way in the manner in which parent and child cooperate to discuss the body and its status in relation to the being of each, as a way of bonding, as an incipient show of compassion and most important, as ways and means of representing distinction and of providing for it as such and of showing discernible interest in what gives satisfaction and with the limits of this. Here the relation to the injured leg is imagined as a relationship to nothing, as the leg becomes absorbed as an image in a web of associations and juxtapositions that use the relation to the body and to the injury as a pretext for searching out and discovering many other matters.

I discussed this problem in two papers in relation to stigma and disability (Blum 1982, 1985), the difference between being absorbed by the condition as if one is nothing other and having a relationship to it that makes a space between oneself and the condition. In some sense, there must be a relationship to the condition that begins to respect this interpretive space or gap, which is one way we might speak of the divided subject. That the subject is divided means that the representation of the body is part of a relationship, that the relationship is not indivisible, and that the different solutions might include the suggestion that the injury is of no import or that it is all-consuming to the point that there is nothing other.

Habitualization

A pervasive commonplace is evoked in the usage of gesture and its ritual in which the body's most prosaic activities and work, whether as expressions, extensions, reflexes or mundane efforts such as in grasping, clenching, tightening muscles, favoring different bodily parts, signifying and the like, become habits in Hegel's (1968) sense (as the mechanization of self-feeling), which, as such, function as if a second nature, displays of self-feeling at one remove (which Freud [Freud and Breuer, 1952] of course exploited and considerably developed through his notion of the symptom). Here as one describes oneself in unique and singular ways, ways that condense and displace self-feeling, any of the instabilities and tensions marked by the intimate and ambiguous history of self-feeling for a subject return in the shape of the posture assumed by an illness or disease. In these cases, we can suggest that the mind enters into an alliance with the body, using it (in the parlance) as a compensatory mechanism, and so essentially making a contract that cannot be broken, since enlisting the body to help the mind ward off dangers (trauma) can only take its toll in the mechanization of this negative self-feeling, a mechanization burdening the body in unique and inflexible ways. The mind repays the body by allowing it to mechanize its self-feeling in the shape of one of its functions; if the mind gives the body license in such a way it is in repayment for the body's assistance in helping mind defend itself against the contingent trauma. That the body always returns to demand repayment reminds us of the myth of the devil and the unbreakable pact one accepts when entering into such a relationship.

Just as when one feels unattractive and forced to use clothing or to favor selective manipulation of posture or body function to disguise this (as in concealing scars, limps, deformities, visual irregularities and the like with clothing items or by favoring other gestures that are designed to distract), the new emphasis puts strain on the mechanism that can weaken it. In related ways, posture and its dramatization in modes such as slouching, squinting, stooping and the range of such related indications can point to a line of descent (Nietzsche's comment on one who is heir to a family of accountants) or to some contingent moment or requirement of self-vigilance when a response becomes embraced and made mechanical because the danger envisioned at the time demanded such immediacy. In these cases, the imaginary rule of mind is only maintained intact by concealing the way the symptom can be read as a text that begins to tell a story of the subject having to pay homage to the body for helping it out of a difficult situation. This recognition is blurred by protests against "psychosomatic explanations" and "new age thinking" that always threaten to undermine the imaginary of self-composure.

Expression

Taking the body as an example, I have tried to provoke reflection by asking how we might use the signifier in a way against itself, for the signifier cannot exceed its own determination, cannot jump over its own shadow (so to speak). If language seems to deaden by removing us from intimate rapport with the experience that the name names, then it is still only language that might redeem the experience from which it seems alien, i.e., it is only language through which such vitality can be rediscovered. I have tried to show that we might begin to discern the signifier's relation to the limits of its own signification in the ways in which ordinary language tries to describe what escapes its determination and seems forced into catecheses in which speech uses its resources in ways that exceed its capacities, creating mixed metaphors and figurative moves that are always capable of revealing to theorizing a rich imaginative structure disclosed as inhabiting any commonplace almost as if an unthought surfeit of connotation.

The collision this prepares us for is between ordinary language or the material conditions of co-speaking, of usage and *doxa*, and the inexorable desire to measure the experience of such a domain by an aesthetic drive that seems to require its surpassing and its irresolution. This tension was anticipated in the language of Plato (1984) whose distinction between two types of image, likenesses and resemblances, built into the conception of resemblance the elements of phantasm and distortion necessary to empower an actor to act against or to resist his limits and in this space of desire, to suffer the frustration of the relationship of healing rather than the expectation of cure. Yet we resist ourselves, our formulaic grasp of what we do and say, not only with speech ad infinitum but by adding to such words and deeds a manner investing them with energy, with zest, a manner meant to bring our words and deeds out in ways reminiscent of spice, of accentuating their quality and tastefulness in ways meant to overcome the rude and unadorned approach to the word.

The idea of expression as the mundane grasp of an aesthetic relationship to speaking recurs in collective life as part of the desire to enhance what risks being automated, through embellishment, registered most typically in poise, grace and sex, and in writing and speech, a degree of eloquence. Yet if we think of gesture, posture, movement, the pose and the kind of experimentation with the body that forms the basis of all of the arts such as dance and singing, dramatized in pantomime but activities that require dexterity, we can appreciate these abilities as ways of making the body speak, but also as ways that are compromised in illness and disease. Thus, one aspect of illness and disease must relate to how the limit upon expressiveness is a silencing of the voice of the body. If taking a perspective on oneself must include giving voice as such to the body, enhancing its expressiveness as part of what the self seems to be as singular and incomparable, then the potential of expressiveness and the fear for its extinction must haunt both health and illness. How can expressiveness be factored into healing?

Symptom, trauma

We should appreciate that the tension between self and body that Mead (1967) first identified, ostensibly locating the relation between the same and the other (our unity in corporeality as a species and our difference that resides in being able to take a perspective on this and everything else), makes reference to nothing other than the desire to overstep our corporeality as a recurrent hope and the correlative fear for this impossibility. This is the tension anticipated in the preface between the use of the body as a standard of corporeality that speaking seeks to emulate and the desire to put the body into words and to give it voice. While it might seem now as if the body is the weaker party, dependent upon the mind to give it voice and to take a perspective on it as everything else, and this would certainly be in accord with Mead's proposition, the idea that the body is a paradigm of resemblance might give us pause since we wonder how a paradigm can be the weaker party.

Perhaps what is meant is that the corporeal model of the either/or is the standard of commonplace speaking (Mead's generalized other) and in this sense is always the empty beginning from which theorizing must develop, but then its weakness is a kind of strength, for like the actual body, it limits us and provides the conditions in terms of which our freedom is exercised. As a limit, corporeality is a condition that we inherit (the body, the commonplace formula, the generalized other, the symbolic order) and in terms of which we develop. The weakness of the body, more apparent than real, is spurious, for it is like the duck-rabbit, both weak and strong. And then the self, so imperious and aggrandizing in its ability to take a perspective on anything and everything, must be limited in its way by the very body in contrast to which it imagines its superiority, causing us to question whether self (and mind) is strong or weak or both like the duck-rabbit, making it difficult to distinguish weakness from strength.

If what recurs is the question of who is the weaker party, the body or the mind or both, then we can now revisit this recurrence as if a question that must ask for we who suffer the constant affliction of illness and disease, just who is the perpetrator and who is the victim, or as a question that both medicine and the interested parties touched by it always need to reflect upon, what of the body, is it one or the other or both? Freud tried to break the conventional tie of corporeality to language by redeeming this question as worth asking.

If the body materializes in the symptom as its visible mark, then we can then ask if the symptom is perpetrator or victim. Freud posed this question of the symptom as part of his desire to give the body voice, to make it speak. Freud's model in *Hysteria* (Freud and Breuer, 1952) seems to begin with the symptom (body) as the enigma to be formulated by trying to grasp its course as a condensed and displaced response to excitation introduced by unwelcome affect in response to a threat. Thus, an incompatible idea elicits a response that defends against it by driving the idea out, but preserves its trace in memory. The unwelcome thought always produces an affect that is both expelled and preserved in memory. Thus, resistance like the duck-rabbit is two-sided, expelling and preserving what it rejects in a trace that persists in disguised form in memory.

For Freud, the mechanization of self-feeling exceeds determination, investing the self with the aura of a machine that always makes the desire to take a perspective seem corporeal as if the effects of the mute and incorrigible body cannot be expelled. Influences of history, social structure and culture take many shapes in representations, and it is the Real that permits us to make visible this invisible machinery. So the relation of self to body, the power to take a perspective, cannot escape corporeality because such a singular human capacity cannot take a perspective without a remainder that is incalculable. Basically, the trauma as a painful affect and the correlative memory of it that becomes a persistent symptom can be content whose particularity consists in being only whatever elicits such a response and so insignificant in particular except as the source of such a threat, as the event. As a figure, the trauma can only stand as the image of that sum of excitation arousing threat, defense and memory, as the material for conversion to somatic symptom. Affectivity that is unresolved becomes displaced in the symptom in ways that make the body an occasion to calculate the *jouissance* created by unfulfilled desire, the fundamental and primordial frustration.

Thus, if the body seems the weaker party in relation to mind and the trauma it makes possible through its vulnerability, then it might be the mind that is the weaker party because of this vulnerability and the body that has the strength to rescue mind from itself to defer the threat. But if the trauma initiates this interaction, then it might have the strength that both mind and body lack. Then again, trauma seems to depend upon the seeing-as that makes its whatever into a source of unwelcome excitation (that is, makes its content a medium and not the message). In this three-cornered relationship, neither the body nor the mind nor the trauma can be the end, but it must always remain the position of the body to be the beginning, and so weak in that sense. In asking how we are to make sense of this without depending upon the resources of mind or trauma, Freud must remind us of the primordial force of seeing-as as the empty speech in terms of which we must develop. What we become aware of is the enigma of what remains after this three-cornered relationship.

To paraphrase Derrida, who somewhere is reputed to have said, "Behind every righteous presence there is a murder in progress" (cited in Dean 1986, p. 57), we can say that behind any and every disease there is an incompatible idea in the shape of an unresolved contradiction, the unfulfilled satisfaction named trauma as the trace of the incomparability of the person as unique as the footprint. That is, the trauma must be prepared by the unconscious meaning in a way that is perhaps Lacanian, that the trauma is an object that substitutes for the idiosyncratic instability of the unconscious, selected by it so to speak as its surrogate love object and so false because of such displacement. The exclusion of this eventful scene from the present means that it cannot be re-experienced as if a direct encounter (and so, cannot be cured), but it can be encountered as part of the work of taking a perspective, as a healing touch that must engage over and again the obscurity of the symptom as if a matter of life and death, constantly monitoring the body as such an interlocutor, seducing the body to gain its confidence, cajoling the mind to lay down its arms, trying forever to elicit from the trauma its secret, like the sphinx.

12

MOODS OF BEING

Introduction

Heidegger (1962) uses the trope of *dasein* to stand for the divided subject and its inheritance of circularity as his translation of the notion of *en medias res* that we have sustained throughout this narrative as his means of exploring the Grey Zone. For Heidegger, ambiguity is connected to the fateful existence of the subject in time, situated between the incalculable past and unforeseeable future, knowing only that the present *is* the past (the transference revealing the inexhaustible influence of any what-has-been upon us at present), and the present *is* the future (the unforeseeable what-will-be revealing that we are now what will be made of us then). Thus, the temporality of existence, best understood through the figure of action in the most mundane sense, identifies the space of ambiguity between influences and consequences as both the site of ambiguity and of anxiety. The anxiety of the actor, given by temporality and intermediacy, *is* not only by virtue of the space between transference and death (between fate, since our particularity exceeds and marks us repetitively, and destiny, since the life of such distinctiveness is in the hands of "a people yet to come," or in Laplanche [1999] as the unforeseeable remains of our message, what remains of our remains, its destination) but through the tension of being-in-the-world that makes anxiety an aspect of fundamental ambiguity, conferring anxiety upon *dasein* and its being as essential, and stamping the human as one for whom Being is an issue as we noted especially in our discussion of Mead. This issue of Being for its subject includes the unsettling, uncanny aspect of its ambiguity and the need and desire to care for and collect this experience. In these ways, we have rescued the notion of the Grey Zone from its burial place in near-at-hand notions as the lack of definition, of uncertainty in inference, in calculations of probability and the like, not because they are worthless, but rather because they are rudimentary efforts to objectify the Grey Zone by such thematizing (Heidegger, 1962, p. 414).

Typification

Heidegger (1962) adds to the specification of such an actor the need to formulate the aura of *das Ding* (the tension between the external and the intimate) as if correlative with the experience of discordance between mineness and the everyday (between incomparability and averageness) that marks the mundane relation of the social actor and, in this way, the desire to establish a thoughtful relation to readiness-at-hand, to the collective representation of whatever matters. In this way, Heidegger locates what we have called the intersubjectivity of mutually oriented action (Parson's [1951: 10, 48, 94] double contingency, the master-slave relation) as the relationship of the subject he calls, in the best sense, care or the capacity to take a perspective in the fullest sense as the "ownmost" aspect of the human that can elevate him for his best. If the human is distinctively the one for whom Being is an issue and is attached to this issue through the orientation to being oriented to, is attached to this very capacity to take a perspective on oneself and on everything else in ways that include being an object as such for any other one, then care is nothing else than the capacity to be oriented to being oriented to in ways that make the social (double contingency, mutually oriented action, recognition) the foundation of representation as such.

In this way, being human, as we have discussed, is both unsettling in its uncanny register and an incentive for understanding how its condition is "fallen" through its ownmost desire to grasp the manner in which such distinctiveness seems two-in-one, both present and absent, possessed as present at hand and, at the same time, experienced as lost. The idea of loss or falling that Heidegger introduces is a modern phenomenological way of reiterating the distinction of Plato between having and possessing knowledge (and, of course, self).

If it is necessary to negotiate the border between averageness and mineness in this lingo, it is because, as we discussed throughout for the notion of *dasein* and its application to the case of the patient, being typified as patient or as carrier of a particular disease seems to force the patient into a formulaic script that risks obliterating that sense of intimacy marked particularly in her self-understanding as an individual, a tension always being worked out in orienting to ways in which the apartness of a person from the category must or need exceed her togetherness with others so labeled, just as medicine is often viewed as trying to bring them back to the recognition of the primacy of their typicality. This struggle, often seen as the imposition of a biomedical reduction upon the patient, must also operate conversely when patients have to typify practitioners as simply doctors, nurses and others without respect to the person filling the category. This collision—its potential for conflict as well as for unctuous unreflective deference and brutal callousness—shows the relevance of the Grey Zone for this field of application, working to create the potential both for an adversarial aura and for the positive transference of medical cooperativeness. The relation to health and illness colored by this version of the mood of *dasein* tends to mask the opportunity for a genuine political engagement that could overcome the opposition while yet respecting the differences as in the Hegelian *aufheben* that addresses the relation between opposition and difference (the Same and the Other, togetherness and apartness) in ways reformulated by Rancière [2009b] as pedagogical incentives. What begins to matter in the encounter at this level is the capacity to represent the experience of this border (of togetherness and apartness) as conversational rather than by absorbing it in ways that petrify voice, a contrast of representational practices that correlate with melancholy (incorporation) and mourning (introjection) as developed by Abraham and Torok (1994) after Freud.

Covering up (aka: repression)

Heidegger is introduced at this point and in this way because he makes explicit, without acknowledgment of course, the unsettling power of temporality and loss that both Simmel and Freud introduced after Plato and his successors and that Lacan among others was to develop. Thus Heidegger tries to formulate Freud's unconscious as the kind of tragedy Simmel discusses as the tension between life and the need to give it form, as the seat of the desire to put the body into words by overcoming the standard of the word as a body (the desire to overcome the "they" of the generalized other or the either/or). Similarly, Heidegger invests Freud's unconscious with the desire for a conscience, the sense of being aroused by the lure of self-knowledge and its call (to *dasein*) to reclaim (what he calls again) its "ownmost possibilities." Heidegger talks as follows:

> The entity which in every case we ourselves are, is ontologically that which is farthest...Dasein's kind of Being thus demands that any ontological Interpretation which sets itself the goal of exhibiting the phenomena in their primordiality, should capture the Being of this entity, in spite of this entity's own tendency to cover things up. (Heidegger, 1962, p. 359)

Heidegger's various comments on the need of *dasein* to heed and to be "all ears" means to be responsive to the guilty knowledge of his own limits. Here the theorist comes to view at the fluid border between near and far that marks *en medias res* as the starting point of inquiry, Socrates' second sailing reiterated as the Wittgensteinian sense of indistinction between the familiar and its oddity, between having and possessing some notion as close as the self, now taking dramatic shape in the normal tendency to cover things up that Freud confronted in his efforts to come to terms with the behavior of his patients. Here Heidegger restates Freud's question for psychoanalysis: "And what if the entity which becomes the theme of the existential analytic, hides the Being that belongs to it, and does so in its very way of being?" (Heidegger, 1962, p. 359). After Freud and many others, Heidegger brings to view the Grey Zone as a way of thinking through the self-disguising character of the human subject but, further, the sense that covering up must include both subject and theorist (exemplified and exaggerated in the division of *dasein*) and all and sundry who reflect upon the actor, forcing upon us the need to acknowledge our togetherness (considering theorizing as one of the disguises of *dasein*) and our apartness with respect to what we here share.

Measuring up and/or not

If the relation of theorist to patient and to medicine, or theorist to the content of health and illness, is as a relationship of inquiry to whatever the representation of health and illness covers up, and if theorizing is its own manner of covering up, then we must put on the agenda the question of what is covered up.

Covering up, concealment and disguise point to the problem of the divided self, divided in and for itself, at best trying to redeem what is in some sense alien and other. Since desire itself cannot stand as an unmoved mover and must in some inexplicable way be prepared or grounded, i.e., desired, and the desire to desire (much like Heidegger's call of conscience) is both a necessity and enigmatic as such, the loss is always of one self for one self and so, essential to the division as its experience per se.

This is why Heidegger seems correct in formulating the desire for a conscience as primordial, akin in its way to the desire to be at home with oneself, to hear and see oneself in a manner that is intimate (integral, indivisible) and not external. The desire for conscience is something like the desire to relate to oneself as if in dialogue, what Arendt (1971) calls thinking. It is Freud who best allows us to appreciate this struggle in thinking due to its self-concealing character, the way the mind must interrupt itself to impede thinking. This desire for conscience as desire for thinking (its "interior monologue," thought thinking itself) can only be pleasurable because chasing the enigma is pleasurable in its way and not simply painful. Thus, Heidegger after Hegel identifies thought thinking itself, the thinking study of thought, as a primordial demand of *dasein*, but does not, unlike Freud, try to ground this as desire. Even Arendt's notion of analogy strives to show the work of thought suffering its need to objectify itself as part of a desire to come to view, to be recognized, to orient to being oriented to (see Hegel, 1968, especially Chapter 1 on the "thinking study of things"). Heidegger's strategy is to appropriate Hegel's "thinking study of thought" as a locus of collectivization in everyday life for anyman and so as a problem for *dasein* of sorting out its relations of topicality and resourcefulness, of mixing and matching these propensities in many and varied ways, alternatively treating thought as resource (circumspection, near-at-hand) and as topic (by aspiring to unravel the existential-analytic of the "they").

Thus, thinking always drives to recover what is lost, its command and sense of mastery, an effort forever foiled by those incalculable and indecipherable influences often created by thought itself. In defending against unwelcome affect, thinking must establish a line of defense against those influences that, in its becoming habituated as if second nature, are seen as fortification against any effort to rethink them. Rethinking that aspires to redeem and recover what is lost must come up against its own resistances in ways that seem to mark rethinking as self-destructive, tending to view the pleasure taken in such thought as masochistic or as infantile in the words of Callicles' condemnation of Socrates' penchant for theorizing. In this way, the circumspection of *dasein* and its absorption in the near-at-hand can be implicitly prized as a realistic or practical gesture instead of a melancholic response to the Grey Zone because the desire of *dasein* to think its ownmost limits seems fated to fail when measured against its own near-at-hand standard of circumspection, seeming in a curious way to pit *dasein* against himself, divided in that way and so, vulnerable to guilt and fated to such accusation, often seeming to the other to take (surplus) pleasure in a self-indulgent (because) self-defeating gesture. How this occurs is attributed to the work of the unconscious. Humans are then called by the demand of conscience to think about what is covered up and in the best sense this means that we are called to think the unconscious as the source of covering up as we are called to recover what we conceal. If the conscience is what calls us, then the desire for a conscience is the desire to be called to clarify our division and the enigma of how we are played upon almost as if the ventriloquist's puppet (Blum, 2001a).

Freud's scenario

Freud's (Freud and Breuer, 1952) writings sustain various notions of loss as, for example, the sense of loss in the *Hysteria* papers and studies that focus upon the relation of symptom to trauma. Here, what is lost for the subject is any sense of being in position to interpretively master one's past, making of any present a gap in knowing its past (but only for one exercised by such an interest). The majority, then, could not only remain unmindful but revel in this since the desire for such repossession can only introduce frustration. *Dasein*, the human subject at its best, is desirous in such a way and so essentially implicated in anxiety, the anxiety aroused by the condition of the one who is essentially attached to such an impossible concern as a necessary feature of being human.

Note that the loss here, based on the relation of visible symptom to the remains of the trauma that one can desire to recover at best under the influence of an intervention, is an important emblem of the loss of self-knowledge in one guise, a loss that remains invisible or only visible in and through its remains. This is because the configuration of specific and contingent influences upon a person that come to mark her as unique or special in some way are as if a collection of foreign influences, forming, as Laplanche (1999) says, an alien presence in the soul whose remains or traces, though displaced, are persistent. The past is the present in the sense that the person *is* her history insofar as the person is a unique upshot of externals, accidents and contingencies (named history) that exceed self-determination and that must recur constantly through its traces. The symptom shows how each and every attempt to rationalize the incomparable influences of the alien presence that is mine and mine alone within can only confirm the way the accidental must remain exterior and alien as both an intimate presence and an externality whose mineness reveals the persistent shadow of *das Ding*. In this model of loss, the remains of the remainder both exceed and mark the life that in its innermost fateful strivings must seek impossibly to rationalize. Here, then, the trauma seems to mark that hypothetical time of any concept (the eventful loss of the sense of innocent absolutism that sustains the signifier as self-evident and so the indivisibility of self as such and the assurance this supports) as the eventful emergence of haunting traces of the remains of particularity that seem to continue and recur as if a surfeit in excess of whatever can be determined and so, by implication, as an image of what seems to be lost.

Thus it seems not the trauma that is the origin of anxiety (the unwelcome affect and the response to it that displaces it in the symptom) but the stylized and habituated orientation to threat that presupposes a ground laid in an anterior social condition. What Freud seems to cover over is an awareness that the trauma does not begin anything but is more like a symptom of another beginning that serves as if its template. That is, if the symptom translates the trauma (converts it in Freud's idiom) then just what does the trauma convert, what kind of elementary problem does it seem to represent? This is to suggest that all are equal before the trauma, everyone having their own, that is, their own way of being attached to their trauma, everyone having their idiosyncratic attachment to the imaginary invasion of unwelcome affect and their own way of working it out (and here we refer to that incomparability of the unconscious as the source of the drive for apartness within the context of togetherness).

In the *Transference* papers and the studies that bear upon therapy, Freud (1963, pp. 105–117; Lacan, 1988, pp. 38–51, 237–246) stresses how the past plays upon any present as the sense of history that time must erase in ways that make any present appear determined by virtue of the repetitiousness of the past to and for a subject in the present, also functioning as an occasion for grasping one's historicality in this very sense by working through such influences in seeking to imagine how they must have been created at their present as unsettling. More than this, the transference identifies a present to which past influences are generalized and applied as if a transfer of what was originally an unselfconscious adaptation to conditions at that time to demands of sociality, displaced in any present in the shape of automated habits and stylized modes of self-presentation that enter into one's taking a perspective on oneself in each and every relationship and to each and every other; in this way, one's past functions as both a powerful resource for trust and affection that is necessary for learning and simultaneously as a negative remembrance that can retard any positive process.

Transference as trust, affection and the capacity for patience that is reflective is a requirement of teaching and therapy, just as its reduction to adversarial transactions and exchanges is an impediment. Thus, transference can be both or either positive and/or negative in the same way that the self as a love object in narcissism might be a necessity for survival and a self-protective gesture. Freud only hints at the alternative to self-indulgent narcissism as glimpsed in the ways in which he differentiates self-love in its various shapes ranging from megalomania and paranoia to normal self-regard. Parallel to these relations between positive and negative transference, good and bad narcissism and discourse that works through its resistances (abreaction) rather than fortifies itself against such talk defensively, Freud's use of the mourning and melancholia polarity dramatically establishes two different (positive and negative) relationships to loss. Here, we can begin to formulate the landscape of loss as a love object in ways that include not simply other persons and even selves, but ideas as well, and most important, that sense of mastery and indivisible and unassailable integrity that Lacan (1988) identified as the mirror image, both as an incentive for aspiring to something more and as a continuous source of frustration and aggression against which *dasein* is fated to measure itself as both fallen and guilty, desirous of conscience.

First Freud identifies pathological sadness as melancholia and suggests for any pathological expression of the human subject that the inquirer search for a "normal prototype." The normal prototype is the translation of such a phenomenon into its normal experience, searching for the collective treatment of loss as present at hand, a ready-to-hand object of circumspection as in grief. Freud advises to find a normal prototype for the experience of loss (of losing the love object), and he offers such a solution in the case of grieving the loss of a loved one as in mourning. Thus, the pathological relation to loss (melancholia) that can be ascribed to any sense of being fallen or of suffering finitude is best understood through its "translation" to the mundane situation in which a person to whom we are attached dies (and by extension even here, can apply to abandonment, rejection as well). For Freud then, the primordial example of such abandonment might be Oedipus, but it makes reference to castration and the different ways in which the loss of the penis is oriented to. What is important is that if the human actor is marked by temporality and the correlative experience of falling, guilt and anxiety, then the actor is exercised by a sense of losing what must be repossessed and of needing and desiring to care for such redemption. Like the mirror image, the Grey Zone of loss is two-sided, both fatality and incentive, both unfulfilled desire and death drive, stimulating in a manner that produces extremes and moderation. If Heidegger intends his theorizing to stand as a positive relationship to loss for *dasein* instead of the inauthentic relation of *multis* (of the "they," the generalized other), then this desire must always begin and end under the auspices of the very symbolic order to which we are subject, bringing to mind again Baudrillard's (2006) "objective irony." More specifically, for Freud, the *two* relations of melancholia (pathology) and mourning (abreaction or working it out) stand as two attempts to address and formulate for oneself our relation to language and our sense of losing its unambiguous support: melancholia arrested by a vision of speech as if a body, tends to absorb or bury the sense of loss in a way that renders it harmless through denial and its formulaic solutions, whereas mourning, accepting the loss of ambiguity for what it is, heals rather than cures loss by recognizing the need to give voice to the body (like the inanimate word), to make it speak.

Tongue-tied and talkative

Abraham and Torok (1994) develop this distinction between mourning and melancholia as two relationships to loss, modeled after the normal prototype as grief and the action of grieving, distinguishing loss of the love object (in our case, perhaps, the unambiguous sense of self-regard) in one case as melancholy, which incorporates this experience of loss so completely that it leaves no space for reflection, literally absorbing the lost object in a way that renders one mute, in contrast to the action of mourning that introjects the lost object as if externalizing it by making it topical and conversational, an object of and for representation. Prosaically, mourning as introjection makes loss conversational while incorporation paralyzes the actor by identifying her so completely with the loss that her petrification renders her mute, preventing her from objectifying her grief (and pain). In its way, the subject of loss in melancholy cannot initiate a relationship to the experience of grief because the identification is so complete that it seems as if she has lost herself, become dead. On the other hand, while experiencing the import of the loss, mourning recognizes how this gesture represents a change that must be worked through as part of maintaining vitality. What is essential to melancholy according to Abraham and Torok is that it resists change, defends the status quo protectively because mortification can only be inert.

To appreciate mourning as a course of action that is embodied and suffered, they identify its two shapes in one case as "demetaphorization," when the symbolic is treated literally as if the death of a love object is so total that it overwhelms representation, causing only inaction as if one cannot influence the condition through symbolization. For example, in this sense of normal grief, the death of a loved one is as if one's own death, making life impossible because one finalizes her life (as if the living dead) since her relationship to loss is treated as immune to influence. In contrast is the notion that even in grief one needs to find desire as the revival of vitality under such new conditions, signaling the demand of change and its responsibility. In melancholy, the subject treats the loss as so powerful that its appearance of ending two lives protects the status quo under the illusion that action can make no difference, that nothing can be done. Thus, here, the Grey Zone, acknowledging the ambiguity of the border between subject and lost object (the togetherness and apartness), is simply buried as a recognition in a way (incorporated) that makes inaction seem the only apparent alternative because nothing has appeared to change since the end of everything makes survival and resignation immune to influence, meaning that after the loss it seems as if nothing will or can change, the subject has nothing to do but accept the loss as an end.

In the other example of melancholy, the loss is objectified but in such an external way that the subject acts as if it does not apply to him, or since it happens to everyone as in the cliché, he must adjust to it as if it has no effect. Thus, the demand to survive a significant loss operates by externalizing demand and loss in a way that denies the decisiveness of the loss by treating it as incidental rather than essential. If this seems to improve upon demetaphorization by at least recognizing the loss, it can only do so by the subject denying his togetherness with the love object as reciprocal influences of import upon one another. In this case too, the denial of change occurs in a manner where one can say of the loss that its import is still not a decisive influence (as if it does not apply to me), allowing life to go on as usual.

The relation to the Grey Zone and to speech is important if we treat this as an illustration of measuring up to the loss of an unambiguous standard: in one case melancholy can live in denial, speaking as if the idealization of the either/or as a standard is not a loss because as an ideal, it is so much a part of the speaker that it cannot be objectified as topic, as conversational, since for all practical purposes it has never occurred and nothing needs to be done. This accounts for the desultory speaking practices of melancholic empiricism. For example, many inquirers who profess to recognize ambiguity as the Grey Zone continue to act as if such a recognition is so final (fatal) that nothing should/could be done or can change (language is just like that!) in much the same way that many talk about distress in the world or in organizations and social relations (nothing can be done fails to see the recognition as itself a representation that can be acted upon). In the other case of melancholia, the loss is recognized as a problem that one can be immunized against as if it is not allowed to affect one's actions, as when the speaker exempts himself from the ambiguity he finds pervasive and universal by declarations that always show how he conceives of himself as different by virtue of being knowledgeable about that and so as immune to the influence of the Grey Zone even as he speaks of it, as if he somehow miraculously escapes the ambiguity he finds everywhere and which seems to empower him to lead those who do not know to recognize it.

In the best sense, this is a precedent for survival offered by classical stoicism and epicureanism as a defense against unruly emotions following from great disappointment, and in the worst sense it is probably shown in someone's refusal (like Heidegger) to take action with respect to oneself (for example, if the Grey Zone is as a universal that must include the one who affirms it, it can serve as a pretext for avoiding responsibility for any action as if in some inexplicable sense his being part of it also is a way of standing apart). Thus, in relation to his concrete decision with respect to his Nazism, Heidegger could argue that because the Grey Zone applies to everyone in a way that must include him, he remains powerless to influence action and is thus innocent, implying that *dasein* is a victim of ambiguity and so exempt from guilt or innocence. This raises the interesting question of the place of truth and falsity, of right and wrong in the world of *dasein*, i.e., the need to differentiate between different ways and means of relating to our division.

In material I have collected dealing with persons being caught red-handed and charged for conflicts of interest, corruption and the like, it has been interesting to note how they negotiate the line between agency and determinism in evading responsibility when culpability seems obvious. For example, an architect, who was on the board that selected the firm that later hired him, apparently influencing the choice of them over others in a competition, claimed with his political chums that personnel selection was a private matter and not a public (political) concern, treating the literal symbolically as if the fact of the conflict is discounted because of the category as in the generic legalistic argument that can deny agency because wrongdoing does not coincide with the classification. In another case, a confessed Nazi war criminal claimed exemption because "it was another time, other rules," as if this condition made him another person, as if he was apart from the action and it was not he, the same person, who did the act. The melancholic character of such gestures lies in their resignation exhibited towards themselves, their taking a perspective as an example of inaction because, in defending the status quo, they tend to remain the same. In contrast, the recollection would need to mourn the integrity that was lost by acting on the remains in a way that risks creating a new situation (vis-à-vis the relation of one to himself) instead of trying to remain unchanged and untouched by denying what was done as not what it was because it could be classified otherwise or as "not me" because it is incidental to who I am at present. Guilt that is melancholic appears to use the wrong not to mourn the loss of a standard but to resist changing one's relationship, that is, to survive without alteration.

Anxiety

The basic condition of anxiety relates to loss only in the sense of the lost connection between what is called the aim of the object or its intention and the cause or grounds of this aim. In this sense, Lacan (1981b, pp. 67–78; 2006, 206–268) can speak of two objects after the convention of differentiating action in terms of its manifest appearances and tacit connecting tissue (the *object a*) that brings together what seems apart. This is dramatized particularly well in the case of attraction to commodities that are basically means of satisfying other interests and in any case where the relation of want to desire is unhinged, not wanting what is desired or not desiring what is wanted. Anxiety here is productive insofar as it orients the subject to this gap and the need on the one hand to ground want in a reflection on the desire it represents or conversely to deliberate on the implications of what is desired. In such cases, anxiety is coeval with the *aporia* and is productive on this account or else remains diffuse and possibly hysterical.

If, in Freud, any unwelcome affect has to be handled, solved or dealt with in a way that makes the relief of anxiety a perennial project for *dasein*, then such relief takes the form of problem-solving that uses objects of desire (as sanctioned by the code, the generalized other, the symbolic order) as a means for solving the problem caused by the "true" object, that imaginary self-understanding of mastery and its realization that marks the surplus pleasure of any acquisition (the "what it is really after and trying to say") that this objectification both conceals and can exhibit to a discerning eye. It is this gap that itself guarantees how the problem of anxiety is never resolved since even the acquisition of the object leaves desire unfulfilled (not only in accord with Durkheim's *anomie* [1961] in which the solution to a problem becomes a new problem ad infinitum) because the object pursued is only one of many ways (means) for realizing desire as such and must always leave the trace of such equivocality as a haunting and inconclusive remainder.

Anxiety is structured by the symbolic order, just as expectations guarantee success and failure, and so moods of elation and disappointment in ways originally recognized by stoicism and the philosophy of Epictetus, urging the withdrawal of attachment to expectations as a means of producing tranquility and harmony. Yet the symbolic order cannot be escaped since tranquility and the moderation of attachment simply become a new regime. Thus unpleasant affect, relieved in many ways through various means and actions, can only surface as the unwelcome affect registered in any reconciliation. Both obsession and hysteria can be grasped as attempts to solve this problem of the symbolic order, in one case by excelling at doing exactly and literally whatever the expectation requires (prosaically called "overconformity") as a means of self-defense against what is imagined as unruly forces, and in the other case, of seeking to escape from requirements through an overcoming that submits to its own new requirements as in the rebellious gesture of fashion that still must conform to its own expectations of style. That the symbolic order cannot be escaped grounds Heidegger's conception of the anxiety of *dasein* as normal (in Durkheim [1938b], as a social fact external and coercive).

For Lacan, if the substitute object or object pursued as an aim of acquisition is for the neurotic a lure of the fantastic structure (Miller, 2006a, p. 18), then this simply means that, for example, the commodity pursued is a fantasy because it substitutes for the "true" and invisible object, the *object a*, and so is the object that remains in the place of the demands of the Other. If these demands are "authentic" by virtue of being emblematic of the normal everyday life of the subject in the way that the unconscious and the *object a* of its fantasy must be as they are, then what always becomes "inauthentic" or false is the typical misrecognition of *dasein* concerning what he wants and desires, a misrecognition registered in a range of examples of normal and pathological types of problem-solving in the recurrent shapes of misrecognition and adaptation structured by the interplay between imaginary and symbolic order.

Excursus on disfigurement

The recognition that the aim depends upon the symbolic order does not make that connection false or inauthentic in ways that require renunciation of such aims, but this relation itself between aim and its grounds, this recognition of the relation or not in ways creating action or melancholia, in ways that can be a productive *aporia* or moment of resignation, is where the divide resides. Thus when Miller rightly talks of the neurotic attempt to make the *object a*, the invisible connection, visible in the aimed for object, it is not the relation itself that is inauthentic but the pursuit based on this recognition (the pursuit called "neurotic"). Therefore, where Miller (2006a, p. 18) quotes Lacan as saying "the demand of the Other takes on the function of object in its fantasy and in this way the falsified petit objet a becomes bait for the other and it passes into the field of the Other," he is trying to imagine the notion of fascination that Heidegger (1962, p. 105) mentions as *dasein*'s tendency "to lose itself in what it encounters within the world and be fascinated by it," except that Heidegger rehabilitates the productivity of anxiety by treating the "fantasy" as *aporetic* rather than a clinical malady. This comes alive in his notion of the way "breaks in the referential totality in which circumspection operates" can be treated as part of the "productivity" of *dasein* in relation to his care for being as such.

Note as a similar but different inflection how Heidegger seeks to provide a phenomenological ground for the connection of anxiety to the *aporia*, in a way less complicated than Lacan's topography of inner life and more detailed than Wittgenstein's glosses on finding the routine odd or queer. Heidegger's conception of the productive anxiety of the *aporia* seems to hover between its identity as an uncanny moment and a reversal.

> Similarly when something ready-to-hand is found missing, though its everyday presence has been so obvious that we have never taken any notice of it, this makes a *break* in those referential contexts which circumspection discovers. Our circumspection comes up against emptiness, and now sees for the first time *what* the missing article was ready-to-hand *with*, and what it was ready-to-hand *for*. The environment announces itself afresh. (Heidegger, 1962, p. 105)

Where Lacan focuses upon this "break" and its correlative anxiety as productive, just as Wittgenstein would, its productivity is based upon a fantasy or misrecognition that substitutes an aimed-for object falsely for the real desire in a way that sees the "break" as a course of action that attempts to master the phenomenon by making a signifier out of it as the word can be said to master the thought by condensing it and reducing it. In contrast, Heidegger's break does not seem oriented in the same way, not grounded in an imaginary of mastery or in desire as such, but stimulated by an encounter that forces adaptation as if the *aporia* is an external condition impinging upon the subject.

If Heidegger's anxiety is seen to produce the move to inquiry (the break breaks the connection to the "they"), Lacan's break (and anxiety) does not mediate in this way, is not a result of the lost connection with the object and an attempt to relieve the lack, because it precedes the lack as the fundamental anxiety that is displaced and replayed in different guises, emergent in its time as a defense against the enigma of birth.

The capacity of *dasein* to be normal must exist as part of the range of solutions we imagine as its discourse, such as those named neurotic, hysteric and obsessive, because adaptation is a normal means of solving the problem of the symbolic order and the anxiety remaining from such irresolution. The use of "misrecognition" and "fantasy" can itself lead to misrecognizing the unconscious as simply a seat of error, making distortion pathological and external to the discourse rather than one of its shapes (in the way Plato [1984] treats distortion as an inescapable aspect of perspective in the *Sophist*). That the anxiety of *dasein has* to be distorted means that it has to be represented in ways that can be both productive and inauthentic. This is to say that the usage of "fantasy" often suggests that the *object a* or the unconscious itself is the source of error whereas such a universal is best conceived, despite its singularity, as a problem to be solved, a problem whose attempted reconciliations lead to the fantastic and distorted solutions typically inventoried. Note some of the examples.

In general, the Symbolic can be treated as real as in the excesses of celebrity worship, parasocial interaction with media figures as if they are known and friends, terrorism that treats murder as if gesture, all making what Whitehead called the fallacy of misplaced concreteness (confusing the idea with its enactment). While we have noted that the symbolic must be oriented to actualization and its measurement by life and that the pedagogical aim here inspires travesty and surrealism at its best, these are examples where the attempt to make the desire into the aimed-for object seems to equate them in ways that are not reflective towards the relation itself, tending in its way to confuse substitution with translation, equating with analogizing, neutralizing the relation of the Same to the Other.

Alternatively, the Real is equated with the Symbolic in all cases that use classification to deny the action ("it wasn't me"), including some of the distortions of holocaust denial, reasonable doubt or legalism (denying what happened because the category of "proof" cannot be proven, making anything the same as the other). All seem to rest upon the premise of the causal priority of mind or image because anything that is, has to be thought as what is. This adaptation, the extreme or deformed position of the notion of representation and of the symbolic order as necessary, used in the opposite but related way the other distortion, can at its worst commit the error Lacan mentions of substituting aimed-for object for its desire, treating what is aimed for as if it is a ground.

This is all to show the Grey Zone reflected in the anxiety of *dasein* in normal and distorted ways as a discourse of problem-solving and a scene of many adaptations in which distorted relations to normal prototypes can be explored as cases or productive occasions. Even further, it implies that empiricism and idealism are the generic academic formats for representing the Grey Zone in ways that disfigure its ambiguity, solutions that are extreme because they are bent on eliminating the remainder. Thus, in cases such as these, the distortions appear to result from misrecognizing the collectivization invited by the relation of togetherness to apartness in the discourse itself, imagining the connection of parts and whole, one and the other, as one of substitution rather than a more violent transformation out of a desire to reconcile ambiguity and the anxiety that remains.

Primal scene/discourse without speech

We can now appreciate the tension between fascination and seduction that Baudrillard (1990) made so much of, not as a relation of pathological to normal in some sense, but, as he implied, part of a discourse on being moved, where in one case fascination risks being arrested at the level of the substitution and its glorification unless there is a "productive" *aporia* that unsettles this tendency, inviting it to ask more of itself. What we need to realize too is that this capacity itself, the desire to be moved and to overcome the stasis of the arrested position (prosaically registered in the distinction of melancholy and mourning) cannot simply emerge by itself as if the unmoved mover, needing in its way to reference a history or an elementary situation where its ground for such receptivity (or not) might (could) have been laid. In contrast to melancholic relations to the loss of a love object, now as an object to love, to be in love with, to be committed to, the loss of the power of seduction, Freud (Freud and Breuer, 1952) depicts abreaction as his strategy of working through the loss in *Hysteria*. In this study, I have used healing as a figure for this desire for desire, the need for the self-arousal of seductiveness as the way that inquiry imagines, at its best, neutralizing the commonplace, the formulaic, with a violence that mixes aesthetic and ethical propensities differing from hysteria or obsession, a violence still respectful of the content or signifier in the way we that have tried to treat health and illness, but not deferential, a capacity to navigate the relation between the togetherness and apartness of multitudinous views (here of health and illness).

Pathos begins to describe the inability of the subject to comprehend what is happening, the incapacity to speak, represent and narrate in ways that can introject the experience of loss and so that might reflectively represent the experience of the pain of Being. At the most pacific level, the pain of Being can make reference to the anxiety of *dasein* and suffering as the desire to make some sense of this, the story of this desire and its convolutions. Here we can say that Being needs to be suffered wordlessly as both mine and average and everyday (in Heidegger's idiom), as what Plato called a mix, and as a relationship of togetherness to apartness (in Rancière). Simmel's (1971) conception of the tragedy of the human subject makes of this the desire of *dasein* to mourn Being and so to suffer the border between melancholic incorporation (fateful mortality) and mournful introjection (desiring to represent this). As Simmel saw, a mournful relationship to Being makes extraordinary demands, demands for what Lacan calls "a discourse without speech" (see Miller, 2006b), a discourse that in exceeding aesthetics and ethics still leaves a remainder.

Laplanche (1999) formulates the suffering of Being as the pursuit of the enigma represented in Freud's description of the primal scene as the hypothetical eventful and elemental time of the social and the fundamental ambiguity of the message it delivers to the helpless child, first through the spectacle it offers of the insularity of the parents and their mutually oriented satisfaction in their sexuality and its exclusiveness that seems to appear for the child as both private and public, as a lure and a rebuff, an experience that separates child from adult, and simultaneously in the togetherness of such action as if performance, strangely meant to exhibit this separation as both pleasurable and mysterious, making a demand to understand and to act that must remain mysterious. If adults seem to reflect the first materialization of Other and its separation and demand for participation, then they are simply the visible form standing for the force of the relationship (its togetherness and apartness as such) and the question that must remain regarding the place of the child in this. We could say that the parents or the interaction is what is aimed at in a way that misrecognizes this substitution as Other instead of the relationship itself and the connective tissue of these who are apart in their togetherness as if a silent and demanding question. Why should this discourse without speech not be the problem to be solved that leaves its mark of irresolution in any and every action as if remains that are enigmatic traces of Other? As a story, it has all of the ingredients of authority and dependency, representation as re-presenting, inclusion and exclusion, organization and membership, that any story of the social requires.

> There is not only the reality of the other "in itself," forever unattainable (the parents and their enjoyment) together with the other "for me" existing only in my imagination; there is also—primordially—the other who addresses me, the other who "wants" something of me […]. (Laplanche, 1999, p. 78)

Is *dasein's* suffering of Being in part not a continuous quest to find out what is wanted of one, what is wanted of me? We can begin to formulate the Grey Zone in this respect as a figure for an elemental social situation that is inscribed in the soul of *dasein* as if a template to be repeated and reiterated in various and heterogeneous settings as if (what Plato might call) the original writing on the soul. This is the sense of Lacan's "dying without pain" (Miller, 2006c, p. 14).

If we divest this hypothesis of the elementary situation of its unnecessary connection to the primal scene of sexuality (witnessing the sexual act and its violence, cathecting the mother's breast), then we can approach it as the foundation of the social insofar as it distinguishes both separation and unity as apartness and togetherness reflected in child and parents, each complete unto themselves and yet parts of a whole in relation to a kind of unity (that each is separate in itself and together in relation to the whole that includes them). Here, the separateness dramatized by the insularity of the parental couple in relation to the child, a gesture that simultaneously bans and invites the participation of the child, can be seen as both internal (for any subject as such) and external (with respect to the mystery of authority), a paradigm for the tension between two inflections of otherness that inevitably must enter into the "discourse without speech" because its fundamental silence applies both to the mute and helpless child and to the parents who cannot account articulately for their exhibitionism or entertainment, i.e., cannot ground the social.

Elementary situation

The elementary situation contains the border (generation) separating what is together and implying the togetherness of what is apart (see Gans [1982] for a different but related vision of the elementary situation). The situation includes the interdiction that prohibits and yet invites mixing, suggesting on the one hand the pleasure of each keeping to its own and on the other hand the pleasure of their togetherness as both reprimand and invitation. The message offered of each to the other concerns what it is and what it is not to measure up and must raise as the implicit question, what is it, this measuring up? The silence of the participants, the members, refers to the mute child and to the adults who cannot ground the interdiction, who cannot put into words the reason for the interdiction as anything more than conventional. Blum and McHugh (1984) discussed this in relation to Piaget's child Jacqueline, who was told not to spoil the towel because mother would not like it. Here the reason given is arbitrary, because focusing on such consequences is a weak lesson, not only inviting conformist behavior in other contexts but also reversible if the child was to say the same, e.g., that she spoils the towel because she likes it. Short of saying, "Because I said so!" in a preemptory manner, the adult cannot ground the interdiction as anything other than an appeal to convention. Basically, the child should not spoil the towel because that is not the way we do things, thus appealing to a notion of collective purpose and joint action that makes observable not only the convention of agreements that bind this collective but the way it sacrifices disagreement or apartness, raising the question of what kind of balance should be represented as a conversational topic (Rancière's uncounted part). This enigma refers to the unstated and unanswered question of what is and is not a family, such that the members who vary stand for different relations to it, and how are these variations to be related to this unity as required or obligatory and as limits or opportunities for discretion? This question makes reference to the enigma of the social bond in reference to what we mean to and for one another and to the whole and what it means for us (a version of the canonical concern of political theory and of the social order problem). That there has to be silence in reference to the convention in this sense makes of this question an enigma, evoking the trace of its undecidability for all parties. The Grey Zone appears in the elementary situation in the two-sidedness of the enigma and the message it delivers, that it can be treated as an obscenity (unthought and unspoken) or taken up and topicalized, incorporated or introjected.

A first grasp of the imprint of the elementary situation makes reference to what message this enigma delivers, at first concerning the grounds and reason of and for the interdiction separating parent from child, then in the idea of measuring up and the child's failure to do so or not, the implication of a distribution of knowledge as something adult parents have and child lacks, needing to be disseminated in such a way as to elevate the child, instead of recognizing as Rancière (2009b) says in other contexts that everyone is an ignoramus as if confronting in common a text (the rule, the convention) and seeking together and apart to figure out how it stands in relation to this commonplace. Thus the enigma of the code (in miniature here) imagined as the adult demand and its interpellation (what is wanted of me?) suggests that this ignorance cannot be cured because no one really knows the ground of the code or the source of the interdiction (also see Bonner, 1998).

Not measuring up can then be fantasized by the child in ways that misrecognize her lack as such a failure, treated with resignation as if something unchangeable, or detached and displaced in a symptom as if not part of her. The enigma of the code can stimulate such imagining in ways that might lead to compulsive attempts to excel at what is taken as the rule (do not spoil…) as in obsession or as hysterical attempts to replace the code with another (flaunt spoiling or, as in fashion, adopting new styles to replace old in ways that are still coded and stylized). Here then, we might have Jacqueline either as the precocious premature adult (the obsessive, the little goodie two-shoes) or as the rebellious adolescent (the hysteric, the rebel without a cause).

Equality and its demands

That the enigma cannot be cured means that everyone is equal and comes together (parent and child), despite their apartness, to address the enigma of what is meant as if innocent, as if it is a text rather than a context of knowledge transfer where a superior produces knowledge for an inferior. That situation is based upon the model of transmitting information (for example, about boiling water, walking in traffic, location of parks, etc.) and not about "concepts." In this way, the message delivered by the elementary situation is not that the enigma is the solution, answer, resolution or cure but that it is the curious problem of how to represent the enigmatic, i.e., what remains is the enigma of representation, how to represent the enigmatic. The message of the enigma is that its representation is what is essential and not its cure. In this sense, the imprint of the elementary scene is the message that introjecting and topicalizing the interdiction (the code, the rule or the symbolic) rather than burying it (incorporation) is what needs to be done (Bonner, 1998).

The elementary situation creates a blueprint for what comes after by inflicting upon the mute body the conditions in terms of which it imagines receiving and returning influence and acting upon events, institutionalizing (in the idiom of sociology) extreme and mean relations to the representation of togetherness and apartness that constitutes the dynamic of social life as a dialectical force. What is first present is not the absence of meaning or its loss but the enigma and the desire to orient to it, to see-as, marking the primacy of the aesthetic in ways that will stamp all other relations. What is also first present is the relationship of stronger to weaker party inflected in the border between inclusion and exclusion, authority and dependency, marking the primacy of the ethical in ways that will stamp all other relations (Bonner, 1998). Such remains become visible and sometimes operational in the transference, in symptoms and in the plurality of actions done and undone throughout the course of a life. The remainder as the imprint of such a scene on each and every one equally, as the remains that persist as indelible throughout a life, is the mixture needing to be matched, the apartness needing to come together, the recurrent action of translating the message of enigma per se, of coming to terms with the message as itself the enigma, the message that there is nothing to it but its enigma, that the enigma is what there is (and so that we heal ourselves not by proposing to solve the enigma but by representing it as a condition that remains).

Now, Lacan's (1981b; 2006, pp.575–584) "Other does not answer" resonates as the enigmatic message of the unconscious, the message each and every life receives, that "foreign presence" that must lure *dasein* to be in continuous pursuit, displacing itself in many guises, the enticing feint of mastery that it is two-sided (master and slave, lure and quarry), undecipherable and life-affirming by virtue of this. Thus, all are equal with respect to the enigmatic nature of Other (Heidegger's Being) that *dasein* invests with both authority and distance, inexplicable in itself as a kind of separation, and all are equal in imagining being called and in needing and desiring to reenact the seduction of the message, the enigma of Other, performing the as-if of being seduced by a demanding Other who, apart and together, entertains, exhibits and yet excludes, inviting *dasein* to treat such a pursuit of the enigma as its matter of life and death because it is the enigma that must remain.

What remains as the capacity to be stimulated by the desire for desire means that life and death are correlative with circulation and its extinction (McHugh, 2010) in ways that mark the absence of desire as living death and the imaginary of death as the end of circulation. In this way, castration in the deepest sense makes reference to being abandoned by desire and, if healing ambiguity is possible beyond aesthetics and ethics (beyond inquiry and its discursive irresolution), this suggests that the pursuit of desire itself must be possible neither as illusory nor false consciousness but as the uncanny *jouissance* of seduction, the capacity to influence and be influenced, to remain in circulation. This begins to identify mourning as something other than melancholia, applying not only to the loss of objects who are gone but, as in the case of our own impending death, or for the love object we grieve as lost, or for the vanished ideal, as persisting effects in circulation. In this way, melancholic loss, abandoned by desire, abandons both self and Other, for in making the death of the Other one's own death, it can only fetishize togetherness, and in making the death of the other inessential to self it can only fetishize apartness. In contrast, mourning resists treating loss as an affliction that makes inaction the only course and that deprives us of the capacity to improvise inventively, proposing that action upon such conditions in pursuit of their implications for us and all others is action that always remains to be done. What all of this suggests is that loss only figures as an animating aspect of human desire if we formulate it in relation to the enigma and its primordial ground, for the enigma relieves us of the fantasy of loss, showing in its way that nothing was possessed in the first place to be lost, and if the message signifies loss it is simply because it is in its nature to be oriented to, in Kenneth Burke's (1957) words, to be a mystery.

The mystery that there is a lack (that the enigma marks a lack of a conclusion, a resolution, that what is aimed for is what is lacked) covers over the recognition that this notion of lack lacks, which is how Lacan talks about the trace and the remains as such (Miller, 2006a, p. 26); it is not a solution that is lacked but the idea that a conclusion is lacked is what is lacking (that is, is what is in need). What any conclusion lacks is the absence of desire to resist its remains, making what is lacked a way of orienting to desire as such. In this case, what is lacked is a means of grasping the relief of anxiety as lacking this recognition, that this expectation (imaginary) of relieving anxiety is what is to be found lacking (deficient, in need). The impossible relief of anxiety is an enigma whose uncanniness can only become "productive" as an *aporia* when it is experienced as the very anxiety that produces any object of desire, any aimed-for object. What is seen and felt as strange is that the love for the object falsifies (in the idiom of Lacan) or displaces the *object a* (the enigmatic relation of what is desired to what is wanted, the connection) by making it show up in the aimed-for object (Miller, 2006a, pp. 11, 18, 21). Love for the object substitutes for the drive that animates this pursuit, making that drive manifest itself in the object. Or in terms of my narrative, love for the object is a way of making seeing-as show up in the object since our love for the object is caused by the process, enabling us to see (it) as the whatever that we see it as, the aimed-for object as one of many means of expressing what we see it as, our ground and cause. The enigmatic remains of this relationship (what remains of this inability to be self-grounding as the anxiety it releases) produces the object by making what is aimed for (the object of desire) a substitute for this connection that seems to lack visibility and so is falsely treated as absent (because its effects are visible). The cause of inspiration (the object grounding the action as the dream of surplus pleasure, mastery) is falsified through the choice of a misrecognized tangible near-at-hand object as its substitute. Productive anxiety, the uncanny, as an *aporia*, is produced in this space where lack is anticipated as preceding and producing anxiety as if a cause in a way that is challenged when the remains come "as in a detour to manifest itself as a visible effect that does not conform to the expectation of visibility" (Miller 2006a, pp. 33–44, 49). Lacan joins the *aporia* and the uncanny as the experience of estrangement in which orienting to being oriented to is dramatized as an engagement with the reversibility of outside and inside of oneself as if the inside that is seen and the outside that is unseen leads one to feel the gaze, experiencing the unseen as cause of seeing-as, and what is seen in seeing-as as if leaving a remainder that cannot be seen. Thus, the uncanny is formulated as "taking a perspective on oneself," duck and rabbit, the subject experiencing her own strangeness, seeing oneself and seeing oneself as unseen, not completely knowing what she sees and not completely seeing what she knows.

The mystery of birth

Birth is the most accidental and external event, not in the sense of being unplanned or fortuitous, but in the remains it must leave as the question of what we mean to one and each other. If no one knows what will result from the birth, then what remains after birth is not only the question of our satisfactions together and apart, but also whether our togetherness is an artifact of chance or conditions that we inherit rather than choose. Any response to this question must remain enigmatic in the way that enthusiasm for any result can be seen as loyalty or as a gesture that must rationalize the event and its particularity, seeing either the best that can be made or an open question, who are we to and for each other, we who mysteriously expect, demand and seek to measure up? Note that this question can never be answered no matter the volubility of respondent, for any answer, whether a pretext or true in its heart of hearts, can and must be a misrecognition whose effects can only remain. Thus, Other never answers and silence is the law of the scene. That is, even the unconditional affirmation of love misrecognizes the object it praises for the surplus pleasure it reflects (the need and desire to be in love with love) and the subject, whether satisfied or not, can only "translate" the ambiguity of any protestation into the enigma forever to be engaged and suffered.

What do we mean severally as apart and as together? If the grounds for the Grey Zone are laid in this elementary situation as our hypothesis imagines, then the grounds of the social must be prepared here as the need and desire to connect apartness and togetherness, the relation of each to one another and to the family as a whole, and of the family to the others, to them each and to the whole (Bonner, 1998). The elementary situation of the primal scene identifies its fundamental problem as that of the polity, the need to come to terms with the irrational and incoherent differences that a subject inherits as her fate, the problem of the mystery of togetherness and apartness.

The primal scene hypothesizes, then, the problem of exploring ambiguity and the place of the subject in relation to its remains as the name of the Grey Zone as a social phenomenon, the eventful engagement with the social as the problem of collectivization. The relation connecting difference and unity, variations and their apartness to togetherness, recognizes the silence of the scene, not as an emptiness vacated by meaning as in the void, but as an abundance of ways of seeing, so many possible ways of seeing-as (so many ways of relating to or translating the event of birth and the so-called primal scene), that anxiety can only be correlative with the enigma of what we mean to and for one another and how the whole stands in relation to its parts (and vice versa). Rancière's emancipated spectator imagines the subject of anxiety desiring to treat the lack of a conclusion and this irresolution that must remain, pointing to the *aporia* of recognizing how what we think we lack (the resolution) is what is eternally lacking (in the way Lacan says, that the lack lacks).

13

CONCLUSION

Introduction

I have used the idea of the split or division in the subject as the inevitable starting point of reflexivity that needs to be assumed as a condition of the human subject, the subject imagined as thought-thinking-itself, making the *object a* the relationship that, as Žižek (2007, pp. 130–141) says, lacks a mirror image, and so, that stands for any beginning as both empty and full, inevitably oriented to supplying coherence to and for itself by bringing together what seems apart, being empty in this way and full enough to know this as in Plato's *Khora* (and as in the figure of Hegel's *becoming*). In this narrative, the notion of mediation and intermediacy implies the *object a* in the sense that there can be no other to mediation (and so no original) because mediation cannot meditate upon itself as if its relation to itself is mediated by an Other. Thus, the throwness of the human subject refers to anyone's inheritance of the problem of the relation of Same to Other as a fateful condition and as a problem to work through. The uncanny nature of any origin, as if a result, follows from this starting point, making the Grey Zone correlative to speaking. In the idiom of Lacan, *en medias res* translates into a formulation of the *object a* as a fundamental non-specular "object" that materializes in the visible effects of seeing-as, in ways that make the Grey Zone a practice, the necessary and desirable relationship to ambiguity that haunts life as the remainder, leaving its traces in many ways.

If the Grey Zone makes reference to our abandonment by the ideal of the either/or and its standard of unambiguous indivisibility, then the figure of castration making reference to this loss can provide for different forms of adaptation as postures that we described at various points, whether as fearful orientations to dispossession and accumulation or as compensatory attempts to rectify what is lacked, or various conversions and translations of loss to lack and back again. The pervasive notion of loss, whether Heidegger's falling (1962, pp. 346, 399–400), Lacan's alienation (1981b) or Arendt's conditions (1958), all replay or translate *en medias res* under the sign making possible all of these figures.

235

The hole in Being, beginning with the divided subject and with loss, can only ground theorizing as a possibility if the imaginary of the human subject is grasped in its way as aesthetic. What seems necessary is a view of theorizing that negates and collects in a way that must provide for the relation of theorist to collective as both together and apart, that provides for this ambiguity, forever rendered decisive by Plato in the figure of the Divided Line. This togetherness must be recognized in the need to conceive of the participation of theorizing in what it theorizes in ways that risk obliterating the possibility of theorizing itself if it is simply absorbed by the symbolic order or code (the generalized other) as a difference in degree and not kind. In providing for the distinctiveness of theorizing in relation to the collective of which it is part, the temptation to inflate the difference in order to give form to theorizing risks cutting it apart from the very usage upon which it depends. In this narrative, I have tried to show different relations to this Grey Zone (of the relation between the Same and the Other) as a dialectic dramatized variously in Baudrillard's notion of "objective irony," and in travesty.

In conceiving of any starting point as inheriting the problematic relation of togetherness and apartness registered, for example, in Rancière's translation of *en medias res* as the implicit equality imposed upon all whose relatedness is established by the signifier, we can anticipate collectivization as potentially political in the best sense as a pedagogical occasion. If thought uses the signifier as a condensation and displacement of its desire, as a falsification of the surplus pleasure it seeks, then the collective is equal by virtue of this signifier that functions totemistically to establish a relatedness among all who are touched by it. Following this logic, we can say that the signifier mediates to and among those touched by it not because it produces anxiety (the anxious member who lacks its meaning) but because it (the signifier) is produced by the anxiety that separates each and every subject who desires impossibly to condense it in the word. Anxiety is not equivalent to the uncertainty of the signifier (that health is not definable, etc.) as if correlative with the loss of such a definition (the lost object), but when this lack (of a definition) is itself seen to be lacking, that the expectation of definition as relief of anxiety is what is lacking, then this expectation and its impossibility is the experience of anxiety. Anxiety, part of the death drive and its insistence, is beyond the pleasure principle and its homeostatic expectation of the relief of anxiety in this sense, that it is this expectation of relief that is Real and irresolute.

Equality established by the totemic force of the commonplace (the word, signification) that, received in a multitude of ways by those marked differently, makes possible the dialogical encounter of those who are separate and equal as an occasion of talking together, of mutually oriented action that can and does experiment with discursive means of influencing oneself and the other. Thus among those who equally confront the problem of ambiguity within the context of their differences with respect to roles, positions, history and all of the influences summed up both in the figures of inequality and in the conception of an unconscious, we assume as a common need an equalizing force for any beginning. First, it appears as the aesthetic desire to connect and link (to see-as) as the grounds of any and every translation and transformation, and second, it appears as the ethical desire to be accountable to the face of the other, the façade of vulnerability of the weaker part(y) disclosed as the unformedness and undeveloped nature of any beginning. Yet, if togetherness is constantly renovated through the desire to explore common speech in ways true to varied and individual capacities to see-as, then such togetherness is always seen-as grounded in something other, as visionary in its own way, as represented in a manner always open to accusation; such apartness must be limited by the capacity to give voice to the commonplace by restoring its powers and listening to the relation of its wants to its desire, in the way any translation of common speech must hold itself accountable for the violence it exercises upon the defenseless material it works over (Levinas, 1969, pp. 187–220). Still, above and beyond such good-heartedness and its imaginary commitment to negation (or, as Plato says, to truth and knowledge) and the surplus pleasure implied by mastery as such, the functional pursuit of what remains must persist as if a drive in circulation for self-maintaining *jouissance*; in other words, what must remain is the remainder and the relentless recurrence of its drive to live beyond the pleasure of hermeneutic irresolution, the pursuit called the death drive.

Negations

To develop Žižek's grammar, we might note how the narrative in this study formulates what he calls, after Hegel, the four negations or, in Lacanian, the passage of the *object a*, as if different ways of registering the presence of the "foreign intruder" or alien element in speech and in the experience of division or *das Ding*, different ways of "working it out," first as representation itself (the symbolic order and the disturbing effect of mediation on the sense of indivisible immediacy that this intuition releases), then successively as usage (the disturbing plurality reflected in the intrusion of signification in the apprehension of the signifier), discourse (the disturbing effect of the notion of relatedness, the relation of symptom to trauma, form, elementary problem, Same and Other) and the likely story (the disturbing effect of inconclusive irresolution, the remains of its rationalization of accident).

In this respect, the inescapability of mediation, stipulated as a beginning on faith, can only be demonstrated by narrating such a passage in a way that must measure the story by its application to life (its consequences for living) in a manner that has to leave a remainder. This is what I believee Jacques-Alain Miller to mean when he speaks as follows: "The unconscious means that thought is caused by the non-thought that one cannot capture in the present, except by capturing it in its consequences" (Miller, 2006c, p. 23). Further, the distinction between symptom and *sinthome* that he develops from Lacan makes reference to the limits of the symbolic order and the hole in Being that this limit discloses as the inconsistent consistency of its artifice, exposed both and at once as a necessity for counteracting a naïve essentialism and as a necessity for embodiment in and as an essentialism of action that it seems to deny, thus both duck and rabbit.

To Miller, the truth of the symbolic order as a relationship of subject modeled after the problematic affinity of symptom to its ground is "laughable" (Miller, 2006c, pp. 10–11) as a standard for life (in a way similar to our discussion of travesty) because it is automated in a manner that confuses the symbolic with the Real; it ignores the demand of what remains as needing to be acted upon definitively rather than equivocally, it disregards the need of the symbolic to be tested by an essentialism of action that is necessary and yet irresolute (see his distinction between the interpretation of dreams and the dream of interpretation in "Detached pieces" [Miller, 2006b, pp. 38–39]). Miller's comment that man has a body acknowledges *object a* as the embodiment of *jouissance* in action. In this sense, if the body is a paradigm of representation, then we can say that embodiment is a standard of actualization in the way that language needs to have the effect of truth (not in derivations or operational consequences in the conventional sense but in the implications we have discussed as Plato's notion of the effects of writing upon the soul).

I have tried to develop this sense in the narrative by dramatizing the symbolic order as construction (artifice, architectonic) both necessary and desirable and simultaneously by trying to develop a strategy of travesty that essentializes any such representation by provocatively reading it as an automated master plan for living in ways that can only expose its limits and the suppressed work of negotiating ambiguity that it must leave unthought. What Freud teaches us is that if representation is necessary insofar as imagination needs to be represented, then what comes after (the symbolic order) is necessary to understand what is before. If construction is the law of the land (artifice), then it takes a variety of normal and pathological forms and is tied not to veracity but to influence, in the way any construction is not immune to influence (as teaching, therapy and dialogue can confirm) and any construction can have an influence. This means that the symbolic need be made actual and that this gap, though a zone of indeterminacy, is the measure of the Real, making inaction always seem a melancholy choice. In this way education, like therapy, depends upon the possibility for seducing the subject to desire desire.

Narrative and the Divided Line

If each negation functions as if an *aporia*, then the succession of negations imagines the narrative of theorizing as the graph of desire represented in and for any content, making each negation a moment of productive anxiety and the trajectory as a whole as if an infusion of alterity, a progressive estrangement intended as provocative, as enabling. The content itself mirrors the movement of the ideal speaker, the *dasein*, playfully encountering and clarifying to and for herself her automated tendencies within by working to give form to the commonplace as itself a collective discourse of problem-solving. Thus at one and the same time, the collectivization of the discourse as a social formation animated by an unspoken problem is both the object that is represented (the content, e.g., health and illness) and the means and method of representation (i.e., the trajectory itself imitates the formation of a dialogue or conversation as a social formation rather than as an aggregate of views). The relation of Same to Other, of togetherness and apartness as a problem to negotiate, applies at one and the same time to the representation of the content to which inquiry makes reference and to the movement of representation itself and its making reference to making reference. Even more, the relation of theorizing to the content it formulates is in its way an instance of the relation of what is apart (representation and its content) to what is together (representation and its content) embodied in the ideal speaker as the bearer of such ambiguity, the subject of and for the Grey Zone. It is in this sense that Jacques Rancière can be seen to engage narrative in the spirit of Plato's Divided Line.

Rancière (1999, 2009b) tries to formulate conversation, the dialogue over a content, as if a relationship between equal parties and a third, a content, commonplace, usage, image or text, that can be understood in my terms (following Durkheim) as if a totem that establishes, by virtue of its status as beginning (topic, *topos*), a relatedness among those touched by it. He tries to show any relationship to the signifier that we understand as inquiry or theorizing, as posing for its participants the problem, at one and the same time, of reaching an accord of sorts with respect to the content and as exhibiting over the course of this engagement an increasingly refined sociality, i.e., a relationship true to the notion of the social in the best sense. Such a relationship need be more than a display of interdependencies, transactions and exchanges, or of discrete narratives or confessions as in a cycle of stories told and retold, inviting recourse to the additional assumption that its being "mutually oriented action" (Weber, 1947) is animated by an ambiguous sense of collective purpose (Swanson, 1992, for the best sociological treatment) and, in this way, by the need to solve the enigma of the social.

As a model of conversation, the social requires more than similarity, interdependence, sharing and even common interests, more than mutually oriented action; it requires the demand that it orient to some sense of its existence in time, to its perpetuity and productivity. Whether specific conditions remain arguable or not over this and that, it is implied that a dialogue overcomes its character as an aggregate or common association, as a heap of opinions, an exchange of positions or doctrines or a collection of views and expressive affirmations, by imitating in some shape this desire for shared being (Nancy, 1991; McHugh, 2005). Thus Rancière converts inquiry itself into a formulation of the conditions necessary for a good conversation or, in the idiom of sociology, conditions enabling the transformation of an aggregate into a collective or of a heap of discrete and externally related speakers into a social relationship. Here is a version of the sociological conception.

> The participants in a collectivity have a dual status. All of them try to use the collective relationship for their own private—special—interests. But at the same time, they find that to use the collectivity they must maintain and serve as its agents: they must be sensitive to its requirements and must support its interests. In the first capacity, these participants are constituent bodies. In the second, they are agents. (Swanson, 1971, p. 607)

This sociological vision of the divided self, the split in the subject, resurrects it in a way that coordinates the trajectory formulating the graph of desire with the formation of a collective. In this sense, the subject, divided between being a constituent body of the collective and being an agent, seems split by two different relationships to the collective, but the difference is only made explicit in a formulation of Simmel that identifies the division as internal in the way of *das Ding*, as the tension between being part of the whole (as if an agent vis-à-vis the external generalized other) and being a totality or whole in her own right (as a constituent body). This tension between absolutism or one's sense of being apart and complete unto oneself always must coexist, coincide and be comprised by one's sacrifice to and for the totality or code of the collective (Simmel, 1956, especially pp. 30–39).

In terms of conversation, such sacrifice requires the movement of the subject from absolutism towards some sense of commitment to the joint action of conversation as if it makes demands upon the subject for constant readjustment in ways that are always problematic. This conflict animates the conventional canon of political theory, especially in the shape inflected by Locke, Hobbes and Rousseau, as the need for an antidote to unregulated subjectivity and, in its epistemological analogue, to unregulated linguistic excess. But in this convention, collectivization is always measured by a generic notion of the code and of the subject that tends to treat the end of dialogue or joint action as if privative, both the collective and its subject envisioned as needing to compromise their best capacities in order to coexist and live together. (We can think of this as the vision of the social animated by Anglo-American academic philosophy and its circumspect relation to ambiguity, always suspicious of the conception of an ideal speaker whether for individual or collective.) The question raised by a stronger conception, a conception of the social that might strengthen the idea of the bond and of the subject, invites seeing the relation of togetherness to apartness as reciprocally fertilizing each as a means to a conception of shared Being. Thus if Rancière repositions the collective as equal participants, what he does is reformulate the asymmetry integral to any beginning (that someone must define the terms and conditions of the beginning) as a function both necessary and desirable (the function of leadership as mastery, for example, teacher or therapist), as the force of initiation that is required, and as a force whose dissemination must be self-liquidating if it is not to maintain itself as domination, becoming through the mutation of conversation into collective action a shared focus stimulated by the totemic force of the topic or third.

First and second speaker

Some time ago, with colleagues (McHugh et al., 1974), we sought to use the rudimentary or first exchange between student writer and teacher reader as the starting point for developing a pedagogical orientation to the writing of theoretical papers, papers intending to exemplify reflective practice in writing on topics, the expectation not only that theorizing could be practiced in writing but that the teaching of such writing was itself theoretical. We imagined exposition as both collective in ways we have discussed and as a reflective movement in process of becoming mutually oriented and communal. Despite the beginning as an asymmetrical association of teacher and student, we sought to reposition writing and reading as a relation between participants, conceived as reciprocally pursuing a notion of revision as joint action.

At that time, we used the vocabulary of ego and alter to identify first and second speakers in a process designed to be exemplified in the writing of a paper as if an exchange of offers and replies characterizing a revision, where the first draft is "deepened" through a continuous engagement with its decisive terms of reference (what we called its auspices or grounds). Between members of a team working together, that process was described in stages of writing, replying and editing, in which each stage was said to be oriented towards moving the narrative along, not through criticism of its omissions, but by reformulating the original in ways intended to develop its strength. Each draft was thought to amplify what was implicit in the previous one.

Thus, the problem of speaking first (concretely of course) raises the question of responsibility for the speech that precedes and follows. The intervention in the writing of the first speaker to invite her to reflect upon the grounds of writing initiated, and to perform as if a respondent to herself in the actual practice of her writing, is an instance of mastery in the way any pedagogical initiative must be, but the initiative had the aim of both enforcing a standard and disseminating over the course of the exposition to the point where the standard could be transformed in the hands of the writer to be used and "translated" in ways particular to her. The canon speaks about this as self-reflection and, in the current case, it is meant to suggest that self-reflection can be treated as conduct in which the author's participation in her very own writing is reflectively intensified in ways that are demonstrable in practice. Such a first speaker does not at the beginning await correction, rebuttal or even assent, but a gesture that invites her to rethink her question. Such gestures, given through the responses of others, encourage the writer to intervene more decisively in the text she is producing.

It is the first speaker who must suffer the risk of thinking about what beginning implies. In this sense, if we might read any paper and its evolutionary *poeisis* as such a sequence, as a revision in this sense, then we can also read any collective engagement with the content as if, at first, a collection of first speeches, designed not only to attract collaborating readers but readers committed to stimulate and sustain the responsive powers and editing discipline of each and all and to help them collect themselves in and through their writing practices, the collective narrative itself becoming a work in revision as the first speeches become recollected and refashioned in ways that point to a discursive center.

In this way, using writing as a model, reading, interpreting and translating, centered by a totemic locus, display collectivization among those whose co-presence is mediated by the content or commonplace as a process whereby an aggregate or heap of individual speakers, who happen to be proximal or addressing the same, can form themselves as if interdependent, mutually oriented and possibly communal, as the case may be. In this way, the representation of any matter (content, commonplace, signifier or text) can at the same time be self-organizing as a discourse or conversation about its "object," objectifying the content as if a discourse as its way of objectifying itself as if a discourse, each using the other as a means for this purpose.

If papers in their way show the unfinished character of any piece of writing, then this suggests that they show how any paper remains an occasion to initiate replies and editing that orients to sustain its original vitality in the shape of dialogue. Writing is incomplete because dialogue is unfinished. The ambiguity of such writing gives us another opportunity to recognize, engage and refine the temporal dimension of our productivity (that our writing exists as something for others to make use of). This is one way of grasping the discourse of mastery, the inequity of any beginning, as a function of leadership destined to be dissolved and resuscitated as if remains through the reciprocal care invested in one another as equally engaged by the same task and fated to realize different relationships to this common bond.

The discourse of mastery

Thus Rancière's (2009b) figure of the ignorant schoolmaster is meant to demonstrate the travesty of the corruption of the initial asymmetry in its image of teaching that refuses to relinquish its grip, that confuses mastery with hierarchic command of material, continuing to dominate the student through pedantry and its model of knowledge transfer instead of desiring to convert such inequity through the reciprocity of teaching and learning inaugurated in Plato's conception of the mathematical as preparation for the Academy and to use its initial advantage as means for a positive transference rather than impediment. Such a powerful conversion animates capacities to see one as the other and the other as one, to reflect upon the togetherness and apartness of teacher and learner. In recovering this difference and its collision as a replay of the tension between positive and negative senses of transference, we can appreciate the ambiguous border that distinguishes the enabling from stultifying resonances of leadership and its imaginary. Just as initial specialization and leadership undergoes mutation in the course of collectivization, so must conversation put aside by putting into question its source in the authority of commonplace distinctions sanctified by the generalized other. In this way, Rancière must impersonate the teacher-as-leader in order to put into question that model of knowledge translation supported by the pedant, reinventing the pedant as the alter for the ignorant schoolmaster whose very sacrifice must demonstrate the travesty of the bad conversation.

In this way, the discourse of mastery, the need for an asymmetrical beginning and its conversion through dissemination, can be understood as both necessary and desirable in the way of the paternal function in Lacan, the necessity of a beginning and the investment of the name, the need for emplacement as necessary in the way representation is, conferring upon the speaker a legitimate order of regime and expectation that the subject both inherits and is driven to put into question. As Miller says:

> He designs a new figure of the father, the one who knows that the object a is irreducible to the symbol. A father who would not be the dupe of the paternal metaphor, who would not believe that it could accomplish an integral symbolization, and who would know on the contrary how to relate desire to the object petit a as its cause. (Miller, 2006a, p. 42)

The figure of the ignorant schoolmaster is one way of contributing to the redesign of the paternal function by challenging the misrecognition of the discourse of mastery in ways that put it into question, not as a means of realizing power as a way of relieving anxiety, but as an occasion for rethinking how the anxiety of the social causes relentless hallucinations in representations of power.

This imaginary trajectory of collective behavior, mimicking the sociological vision of a mass transformed into public and then community, is correlative with the image of the transformation of an aggregate of views into a discourse and an analysis in a way that relates exposition and collectivization as both together (the Same) and apart (the Other). In this process, he depicts what we have called the ideal speaker as the trajectory of an "emancipated spectator," moving from an external relation to observing and doing as if they are related but basically apart as two different functions (as the either/or) or towards some grasp of their opaque connectedness, being represented as if one moving socially through an encounter with the ambiguity of the border between individual and member, from orienting to oneself and others as if inflecting intersecting and indeterminate senses as types, positions, roles and identities.

The assumed equality of the participants before the content, in disarming any scholarly advantage or external inequity, is meant to impose an innocence leading to the disengagement necessary for heeding the particular contribution of any other (their voice) in a way that can engage what is said without interference, forcing upon them all a mutually oriented relationship to their reciprocity. What equality means here is that any social relationship in this sense must repossess in the relationship of each to the other, equality as a condition. The assumption of equality as anything else in this model is not an empirical description of what exists (as Socrates says, "down to the last detail") but a formulation of the conditions required of a social relationship or conversation on a content in the best sense (a good version of what social policy means to call "best practices"), capable of identifying in its way how an emancipated relation *to* the symbolic order is both together and apart, is neither a passive nor pedantic embrace (the schoolmaster) nor an escape (the "politico") but an innovative relation to the missing part, to the uncountable irresolution that unsettles any order. What the emancipated speaker knows is that the failure of the conversation to reach an accord over the question of the signifier is not a lack of the signifier itself but of the expectation that accord can relieve anxiety, that the symbolic order is fated to structure expectations that must leave as remains the primordial anxiety of ambiguity, the Grey Zone. This can be called a modernization of Plato's figure of the Divided Line because the moment of emancipation as the *aporia*, or negation that seems different in kind and not in degree from the other negations, is that inescapable apprehension of our own uncanny participation, that we appear for ourselves as both part and whole in relation to the social, both absolute in our eyes (apart) and together to Other (relative), startled, as Lacan might say, by this striking fusion of inside and outside that makes us seem to ourselves as if the lining or glove, both the Same and Other.

The remainder

If the aesthetics of theorizing is discernible in the need and desire to imagine and transform one's apartness and togetherness in relation to such an imaginary trajectory, then each stage, negation and receptiveness to the *aporia* must depend upon the capacity of *dasein* to move itself, to animate itself to and for such movement. This necessity, first glimpsed in the figure of Socrates' daemon or Aristotle's notion of wonder, or in the primordial example of Hesiod's shepherd and his need to be inspired in the wilds by the song of the muses, shows theorizing as grounded in drive and devotion, accidental as reflected in Socrates' story of being singled out by the oracle for this vocation, as a desire inheriting the fateful potential to be inventive and/or to devolve into hysteria.

Similarly, the ethics of theorizing must be discernible not simply in seeing-as but in the use of this art as such to mix and match the dissimilar and heterogeneous voices of the collective as reflected in the plurality of views inhabiting any content as the weaker part of discourse, that undeveloped mix that must exceed the signifier as its remains and beginning to develop that stimulating and self-disguising enigma that can only be seen-as the same and the other, as together and apart, by first listening to the different views, hearing voice by giving face, as varying attempts to reconcile the anxiety of the object, the relation between the conclusion as aimed-for object and the grounds of the pursuit as such, its imaginative structure. This drive to strengthen weakness marking the ethical, reflected in Levinas' conception of the vulnerability of the Other and of the defenselessness of the unformed as such, and in Plato's conception of the mathematical as grounding the reciprocity of teaching and learning in the mutually oriented care and concern that can devolve into the obsessive fixation on survival, must show shared being as the materialization of this interplay, the scene where aesthetics and ethics must coexist socially. This means that the relation of aesthetics to ethics is not self-evident and simple but is itself a relation of what is apart to what is together, both imaginative and symbolic, mediated by the drive for disengagement and then again, always and only a preface to what remains.

Mead's self, Heidegger's conception of care, and the *object a* each and all reflect this trajectory as a course of problem solving that McHugh and I (1984, pp. 113–151) translated into the graph of desire of an oriented actor, conceived as passing through such stages as if an ideal speaker, orienting to the Grey Zone in different ways (also see my various studies in 1982, 1991a, 1996, 2003).

The unspoken trajectory of the ideal speaker for this work, imagining the one who must strive impossibly to solve the Grey Zone as a problem, identifies this subject as one who heals ambiguity rather than cures it: because ambiguity is not a disease, what must be healed before all else is this very notion that ambiguity is a sickness. Healing oneself in the classic sense is then the problem for the oriented actor and her better half, the ideal speaker. What the trajectory reveals is that at any and every point, the vexatious character of what remains after determination, of the remainder that exceeds symbolization, left over in excess of the word, needs to be construed as path and incentive, as simulating enigma rather than as a catastrophe. In part, this suggests that ambiguity and its intractability needs to be introjected rather than incorporated (in the idiom of Freud) or talked over rather than buried alive within in the idiom of Abraham and Torok. This is partly due to the remains being a remainder and so a trace of what is thought lost.

What necessarily must remain is desire itself, if not to be taken for granted as self-evident, that source of energy necessary to animate the dead word, even more, to arouse oneself to that point. In this way, we follow Lacan in saying that desire, never fulfilled, is still not found wanting as if its present is always unfinished business vis-à-vis a future that it can envision as some final solution (according to the model of paradigmatic succession and progress, which defines any present as lacking in that sense), but rather for the reason that any end is necessarily a beginning and so is always open to *amplification*. Thus here it is not the imperfection of representation as incomplete that is at stake but a tension at its core that reveals how what is explicit must always have implications. The reversibility between beginning and end makes space for desire as the constancy of pursuing the implication of what is explicit, the trace of unthought, unstated remains always inviting specification in ways that mark any result.

Similar to the remains of desire, the finality of any discourse, supposedly clinched by an interpretation, must be *irresolute*, for even if reasons must come to an end, as Wittgenstein says, the interpretation, always *sui generis*, must be more than a synthesis or sum of the views and positions it reviews and collects, but it must be an implicit reply to a problem. In a manner memorialized in Meno's paradox (Plato, 1949c), if any speech is both knowledgeable and innocent at the same time, innocent enough to begin and knowledgeable enough to end, then we can always ask of it for what and why it speaks. Here we might follow Plato (1949b) in identifying what remains as *Khora*, the space that, both duck and rabbit, must be imagined before as the ground but can only be seen as such, after in its effects, in the talk that follows and is seen-as related to what comes before.

It is the unconscious, standing for the alien or foreign presence within, that identifies the influence of accidental conditions of whatever content, the idiosyncratic stamp of the person as a repository of incoherent effects we call history, as the extraneous and intimate presence within of the "whatever" that recurs as the message of the particular to the universal, the message of the unconscious that the symptom must deliver in ways that always disturb the personal façade of equanimity. (Laplanche, 1999, pp. 64–80, 114, 173–74, 256). What the recurrence of the symptom confirms is the accidental remains of alien exteriority, always disclosing throughout a life the instabilities in every attempt to rationalize particularity. Thus what remains in action is *estrangement* as the excess that can only be healed in the way the signature or bias persists throughout its dissemination as the circulation of a life (Blum, 2003).

If unfulfilled desire stimulates the death drive, and incomplete discourse stimulates the remains of any signifier as its many senses (as in Being has many senses), then the remains of desire *and* discourse can only conjure up an image of the pursuit of truth as equipment for living (constantly beginning, constantly driving to remove contradiction and inconsistency, constantly trying to find reassurance) where such a pursuit can only depend in its way upon the uncanny capacity to be moved, the capacity to be inspired by the strangest conditions within, the "whatever," in ways that are fortuitous. Thus what must remain in excess of both desire and discourse, the capacity to be inspired by division, by *das Ding*, is the capacity to be moved by estrangement, to be moved to influence and be influenced, and so, in its way, to be in passage as the constancy of reanimation whose circulation must be coeval with life. If, as Derrida suggests, life is correlative with the *aporia* and death with the imaginary of its extinction, then life is commensurate with the recurrent desire for seduction, to seduce and be seduced by desire itself.

For the *aporia* means to be moved, to be turned around in that sense, and what must circulate is this capacity itself. Theorizing then stages this being turned around, this continuous estrangement as such, and any reflection upon theorizing as a practice must show the convolutions in such a graph of desire, its course of action, its best and worst shapes, its mixture of aesthetics and ethics, its devolution in postures of hysteria and obsession, and its normal and persistent negotiation of instabilities.

The relation of theorizing to its content, always beginning in the midst of sociality and limited by and participating in the very terms and conditions governing and guiding the collective life upon which it reflects, compelled to impossibly desire to master its own servitude (its own *multis* within), must fertilize a range of relationships to its beginning with any content or signifier as such. Lacan's discourse of the master (2007, pp. 11–87, 197–205), identified prematurely with philosophy as if one of four alternative discourses differing in kind from one another, simply imagines the unthought and unstated ground of any and all representation in the social relationship per se in ways that make explicit the systemic character of whatever order is implicit in varied relations to the signifier, an order whose resonances reveal the discourse of the master as a way of reinstating the generalized other or the "they" as if a regime that any speaker must inherit *en medias res*.

The discourse of mastery sensitizes us to the notions of mastery and the surplus pleasure it seems to evoke and satisfy in the speaking situation, showing how any regime (normative order in sociology, or "apparatus" as it is called by some) can only gloss this order that it must be seen to assume and to idealize, the subject, courses of action and knowledge it both typifies and relates as the mosaic of interpretations emblematic of the social world it takes for granted. In this respect, we appreciate how Jacques-Alain Miller can call the unconscious the discourse of the master insofar as the condition of intermediacy that the subject must inherit includes as this legacy the past, its accidental externality and the habituated ruses and strategies of accommodation (including rules, grammar, generalized other, identity, roles, positions and stock of knowledge) and the excess that must remain, exceed determination and persist recurrently through any life, that excess typified by Freud as the unconscious.

When we begin in the midst of the common speech, the commonplace or "they" of Heidegger, we encounter the talk *as* its representation as what we see and hear, of what is "there" both aesthetically and ethically, aesthetic as we see-as, seeing the talk as what it is by virtue of whatever unspoken resources enable us to connect in this way, always neutralizing the commonplace as such, seeing it as oriented to something other, to an image of mastery or pleasure. Here the capacity to see-as must depend upon our being moved to see-as, to take hold in this way, making the passage of inquiry aesthetic through and through by virtue of its desire to elevate itself and the other. Yet inquiry must be more than analogizing insofar as seeing-as has to be grounded in the desire for more of oneself and the other, imagining that giving face to the other (in seeing-as) arouses self in the strongest sense of self-regard, both mine and average, ennobling and enabling the "we" to stay in circulation, to maintain the life of what remains ethically.

Seeing-as must be limited by the defenselessness of the face it interprets and so by its accountability to the weaker party whether the other person, oneself, and always the unformed and undeveloped empty signifier, the part whose vulnerability to interpretation demands of any construction that it be accountable for its application. In this way, the seeing-as of aesthetics and the listening of ethics seem like normal prototypes, necessary but insufficient because what exceeds aesthetics and ethics as the ambiguity that remains after desire, fails to bring to realization anything other than the irresolute trace that needs to be converted into a lure and object of pursuit, the enigma upon which the life of theorizing depends. The death drive as a figure for this compulsion to strive to bring together what is apart functions much like a principle of "logical consistency," driving this pursuit of life "almost as if a function of the body" (Miller, 2006b, p. 38). Thus the foreign presence within both begins and ends the story.

Similarly, the so-called discourses of hysteria and obsession sensitize us to the aesthetic and ethical elements of such relations by starting with their disfigured shapes as such postures (and their exemplary distortions in identity politics [hysteria] and university corporatism [obsession]). What we see is that the relationship of theorizing to its content (in this study, the Grey Zone of health and illness) is a relationship of inquiry to an imaginative structure and symbolic order that serves as an environment of knowledge and problem-solving, assuming a range of shapes and guises.

The body as remains

In some way, as anxiety precedes the symptom rather than follows from it, this means that the primal scene, the birth trauma, and the need for reassurance that remains from the irresolution of its enigma, can be seen as displaced in the symptom in the way that makes a symptom, such as an illness, a defense against anxiety. This identifies the unconscious as the domain of the message communicated (the medium that is the message in the idiom of McLuhan [1964]), the message of the symptom that it is a defense. This message cannot be reassuring, and yet, in its way, it is stimulating because it makes necessary the need to pursue accounts of the relation of symptom to its history, etiology and, at best, to the imaginary trauma it appears to recall. Anxiety, imagined as the result of the symptom, the illness, is treated as the lack (unexplained or lost object) to be relieved through representations that can range from hallucinations of genetic conditions, to confessions of survivors, to abortive attempts to "put into words" the symptomatology and history as if telling, revealing narratives themselves as symptoms of anxiety, as distorted attempts to translate anxiety into speech, into accounts.

Thus if the defensive work of the symptom identifies the unconscious (as if the symptom or illness defends against the enigma), then the defense against the enigma (of the symptom) can be seen as a fortification against the enigma of its representation. Here the representation of the symptom seems to reinvent symptom as something else, perhaps as what Lacan called the *sinthome* (1976–1977). There is a difference between representing the body as a symptom of anxiety and orienting to the representation of this (this connection itself) as a reflection of anxiety. If in one case the lack of an account produces anxiety, then in the other case anxiety produces the need for and expectation of an account.

So instead of saying that anxiety is caused by the symptom, as if having the unexplained illness causes anxiety over that, leading to the need for its explanation, expecting that such an account will relieve the anxiety of this lack, we see that the distress over ambiguity causes various condensations and displacements, primordial anxiety producing the need for its condensation in speech, for the word, for the symbolic order, causing the many and varied attempts to represent the word as if an image of an original, a relation of symptom to its causes. In other words, anxiety and not the symptom causes the desire for its relief, in contrast to the notion that the grounds of anxiety lie in some anterior obfuscation of the meaning that causes the symptom, as if the perplexity about the symptom makes the anxiety happen; instead the symptom displaces anxiety and does not relieve it, the anxiety remaining to cause the representations and to cause the anxiety that must remain after the explanations themselves fail to relieve anxiety, showing the accounts to be lacking. It is anxiety over representation, its ambiguity and so essential lack that causes fantastic narratives and accounts of illness.

Therefore, (1) the anxiety of the Grey Zone creates (produces or causes) the unconscious and its symptom (illness), and (2) the anxiety of the Grey Zone of representation (of the symptom and of illness), the ambiguity of representation, creates the automated responses that materialize in formulaic relations to word and deed, to action as such. The solution posed of (3) seeing the representation of the illness as if a dialogical trajectory, reflecting mutually oriented action between speakers imagined as equal with respect to a totemic signifier, usage or third, hypothesizes as the objective of the co-speaking a shared but not identical recognition of the difference between the expectation of relief of anxiety through an account of the illness and healing the anxiety that knows how any such hermeneutic relief must lack or leave remains (but not anxiety that must inevitably remain). If analysis progresses it is in this way, from expecting the relief of anxiety through the cure of interpretation, hermeneutics, construction, and the contrasting need to heal oneself through the acknowledgment of the necessity of remains as such.

Remains as such

The remains of the primal scene, nothing less than the primordial anxiety of the Grey Zone and its inheritance, are converted into a symptom repetitiously enacted as if an impersonal force throughout a life. Healing, relating to the Grey Zone in the best sense as a materialization of Arendt's stages of thinking, will, and judgment (1971), inevitably finds its place in the stages of medicalized discourse as diagnosis (thinking), prescription (will) and testing (judgment). Often in tension with medical advice, what thought needs to think is how the symptom is structured by the symbolic order, making the hole in Being the ambiguity integral to the conversion of the symptom, the everlasting remains of the primal scene. This is the object of diagnosis in the strongest sense. If the mechanism or process of conversion is figuratively grasped as the *object a*, as the image that supplies coherence or orderliness, then prescribing, in the strongest sense as thought thinking this out, always must orient at its best to the impossible task of changing this relationship (the self-knowledge of the Greeks that remains beyond the reaches of willfulness). The judgment that enters into health, and what is called its self-monitoring or testing, always has to engage itself (taking a perspective as such) with the question of how the failure to change is good-hearted or a pretext to sustain the symptom, a question always remaining because Other does not answer. What remains is figuring out who one is and how it stands.

Life and death

This border dramatizes the Grey Zone as what Hegel might call "the real matter," for life might be understood as seducing us or tricking us to think that we go on forever. This is reflected in the insistence of the drive beyond pleasure and its disruption, the drive to continue that remains beyond the pleasure principle, revealing how we live almost as if automatically and compulsively, as if for continuation itself above and in excess of pleasure, as if the otherness of the seduction is inspired, as Baudrillard might suggest, by a sorcerer, not one malevolent, litigious or sadistic (the sophist or the devil), but one who wants us to continue or as an employer who wants us to return to work even though we know termination is our fate. In this way, the relation of Melville's character Bartleby to his employer makes sense as the absurdist version of the Grey Zone in the relation of subject to Other, here travestied as the relation of a strange man to his employer, bringing us to an awareness of the limits of our passion in this narrative for the dialogical itself and its healing touch as a relief of anxiety, grounded as it is in the imaginary of conversation, what I think of as the anxiety of theorizing.

Given the necessity of the self and its doubling that we have maintained throughout, we can acknowledge an affinity between birth and death, that we must exist in and be oriented to, seeking assurance that we are something rather than nothing, a pursuit that always remains unresolved. If the need for self-assurance created by birth never dissolves, then it is death that might begin to teach us that self-assurance as such just makes no difference. If in this way the gift of life might seem the gift of anxiety and its remains (to the wide awake rather than the sleepwalkers), then we still might see that life cannot exist "only in the mind" as some say, but "realistically" in effects and remains and in remaining as such. If birth marks the depersonalization of a beginning and the origin of being acted upon as the seat of fantasy and imagination, of the unconscious, then being acted upon in death, seemingly different as the most extreme image of depersonalization, still might produce before the fact productive anxiety over the remains that will remain, making this enigma unknown in the deepest sense, not as in inference, probability or gambling and *fortuna*, but in prayerful practice as yet unfathomable. The Grey Zone would gather strength as an aid to weakness if it might so insistently force itself upon life that we could engage it resourcefully and with light-hearted levity to measure ourselves in word, deed and action, to elevate ourselves at any present for its present.

Abraham, N. and Torok, M., 1994. *The shell and the kernel, volume 1*. Translated from French by N.T. Rand. Chicago: University of Chicago Press.

Agamben, G., 1998. *Homo sacer: sovereign power and bare life*. Translated from Italian by D. Heller-Roazen. Stanford: Stanford University Press.

— 2000. *Remnants of Auschwitz: the witness and the archive*. Translated from Italian by D. Heller-Roazen. New York: Zone Books.

— 2009. *What is an apparatus? and other essays*. Translated from Italian by D. Kishik and S. Pedatella. Stanford: Stanford University Press.

Ambuel, D., 2007. *Image and paradigm in Plato's* Sophist. Las Vegas: Parmenides Publishing.

Anderson, S., 1996. *Winesburg, Ohio*. C.E. Modlin and R.L. White, eds. New York: Norton.

Arendt, H., 1951. *Totalitarianism: part three of the origins of totalitarianism*. San Diego: Harcourt Brace Jovanovich.

— 1954. *Between past and future*. New York: Penguin.

— 1958. *The human condition*. Chicago: University of Chicago Press.

— 1971. *The life of the mind*. New York: Harcourt Brace Jovanovich.

— 2005. *The promise of politics*. J. Kohn, ed. New York: Schocken Books.

Aristotle, 1966. *Metaphysics.* Translated from Greek by H.G. Apostole. Bloomington: Indiana University Press.

Bacon, F., 1960. *The new organon and related writings.* F.H. Anderson, ed. New York: Bobbs-Merrill.

Bataille, G., 1985. The big toe. In: A. Stoekl, ed. *Visions of excess: selected writings 1927–1939.* Translated from French by A. Stoekl with C.R. Lovitt and D.M. Leslie, Jr. Minneapolis: University of Minnesota Press, pp. 2–23.

Baudelaire, C., 1972. *Selected writings on art and artists.* Translated from French by P.E. Charvet. Harmondsworth, UK: Penguin.

Baudrillard, J., 1983a. *In the shadow of the silent minorities, or The end of the social.* Translated from French by P. Foss. New York: Semiotexte.

— 1983b. *Simulations.* S. Lotringer, ed. Translated from French by P. Foss, P. Patton and P. Beitchman. New York: Semiotexte.

— 1990. *Seduction.* Translated from French by B. Singer. New York: St. Martin's Press.

— 1993. *The transparency of evil: essays on extreme phenomena.* Translated from French by J. Benedict. London: Verso.

— 1998. *The consumer society: myths and structures.* Translated from French by C. Turner. London: Sage.

— 2006. *The evil demon of images.* Translated from French by P. Patton and P. Foss. Sydney: Power Institute Publications.

Benardete, S., 1989. *Socrates' second sailing: on Plato's Republic.* Chicago: University of Chicago Press.

Benjamin, W., 1971. *Illuminations.* H. Arendt, ed. Translated from German by H. Zohn. London: Jonathan Cape.

— 1978. *Reflections: essays, aphorisms, biographical writings.* P. Demetz, ed. Translated from German by E. Jephcott. New York: Schocken Books.

— 1998. *The origin of German tragic drama*. Translated from German by J. Osbourne. London: Verso.

— 1999. *The arcades project*. R. Tiedemann, ed. Translated from Germany by H. Eiland and K. McLaughlin. New York: Belknap Press.

Bennett, J., 1995. *The act itself*. Oxford: Clarendon.

Bergson, H., 1956. Laughter. In: W. Sypher, ed., 1980. *Comedy*. Baltimore: Johns Hopkins University Press, pp. 44–68.

Beun-Chown, J., 2007. How to spot a psychopath. *Canadian Living*, November. http://juliewrite.omcsocial.com/article/lifestylefamily/relationships/the-psychopath-next-door/2586. Accessed 29 April 2010.

Birchall, B.C., 1981. Hegel's notion of aufheben. *Inquiry* 24(1), pp. 75–103.

Blanchot, M., 1982. *The space of literature*. Translated from French by A. Smock. Lincoln: University of Nebraska Press.

Blum, A., 1970. The sociology of mental illness. In: J. Douglas, ed. *Deviance and respectability: the social construction of moral meanings*. New York: Basic Books, pp. 31–61.

— 1973. Reading Marx. *Sociological Inquiry* 43(1), pp. 23–34.

— 1974. *Theorizing*. London: Heinemann.

— 1982. Victim, patient, client, pariah: steps in the self-understanding of the experience of suffering an affliction. *Reflections: Canadian Journal of Visual Impairment* 1, pp. 64–82.

— 1985. The collective representation of affliction: some reflections on disability and disease as social facts. *Theoretical Medicine and Bioethics* 6(2), pp. 221–232.

— 1991a. The melancholy life world of the university. *Dianoia* 2(1), pp. 16–42.

— 1991b. On the problematic nature of the everyday: the example of still life painting. In: *Section on the Sociology of Art: Meetings of the American Sociological Association*. Cincinnati, OH, 23–27 August. Unpublished.

— 1993. Travesty. *Studies in Symbolic Interaction: A Research Annual* 15, pp. 83–101.

— 1996. Panic and fear: on the phenomenology of despair. *The Sociological Quarterly* 37(4), pp. 673–698.

— 2001a. Voice and its appropriation: the ventriloquist and the dummy. *Poiesis* 3, pp. 114–125.

— 2001b. Scenes. *Public* 22/23, pp. 7–35.

— 2003. *The imaginative structure of the city.* Montreal: McGill-Queen's University Press.

— 2005. Ground Zero comme spectacle. Translated from English by G. Perreault. *Sociologie et Sociétés* 37(1), pp. 87–108.

— 2007. Comparing cities: on the mutual honouring of peculiarities. In: J. Sloan, ed. *Urban enigmas: Montreal, Toronto, and the problem of comparing cities.* Montreal: McGill-Queen's University Press, pp. 115–151.

— 2010a (forthcoming). Life, death, and the in-between: the duck-rabbit/the face of the clown. In: T. Connolly, ed., 2010. *Spectacular death: interdisciplinary perspectives on mortality and (un)representability.* Bristol, UK: Intellect Press.

— 2010b (forthcoming). Born again: why two births are better than one. In: E. Grenzer and J. Plecash, eds. *Of indeterminate birth: studies in the culture of origins, fertility, and creation.* Bristol, UK: Intellect Press.

Blum, A. and McHugh, P., 1980. Irony, the absolute, and the notion. *Maieutics* 1(1), pp. 136–144.

— 1984. *Self-reflection in the arts and sciences.* Atlantic Highlands, NJ: Humanities Press.

Boltanski, L., 1999. *Distant suffering.* Translated from French by G. Burchell. Cambridge: Cambridge University Press.

Bonner, K., 1998. *Power and parenting: a hermeneutic of the human condition.* New York: St. Martin's Press.

— 2007a. Health, well-being and intoxication. In: Inter-Disciplinary.Net: *Sixth Global Conference Making Sense of: Health, Illness and Disease*. Oxford, UK, 9–12 July. Inter-Disciplinary.Net: Oxfordshire, UK. http://www.inter-disciplinary.net/ptb/mso/hid/hid6/bonner%20paper.pdf. Accessed 11 May, 2010.

— 2007b. A fry-up and an espresso: Bewley's Café and the cosmopolitan Dublin. *New Hibernia Review* 11(2), pp. 9–20.

— 2008. Politics, principles, and death in *Antigone*. In: *Who Are We? Old, New, and Timeless Questions from Old Texts: Fourteenth Annual Conference of the Association for Core Texts and Courses*. Plymouth, MA, 3–6 April.

— 2009a. A dialogical exploration of the grey zone of health and illness: medical science, anthropology, and Plato on alcohol consumption. *Theoretical Medicine and Bioethics* 30(2), pp. 81–103.

— 2009b. Temple Bar, density and circulation: the city as a terrain of many voices. In: W. Straw and A. Boutras, eds. *Circulation*. Montreal: McGill-Queen's University Press.

Burke, K., 1957. *The philosophy of literary form*. New York: Vintage.

— 1965. *Permanence and change: an anatomy of purpose*. Indianapolis: Bobbs-Merrill.

— 1969. *A grammar of motives*. Berkeley: University of California Press.

Burtt, E.A., 2003. *The metaphysical foundations of modern science*. New York: Dover.

Connolly, T., 2002. *William Blake and the body*. Houndmills, UK: Palgrave Macmillan.

— 2009. Anna Barbauld's "To a little invisible being…" In: T. Connolly and S. Clark, eds. *Liberating medicine 1720–1835*. London: Pickering & Chatto, pp. 209–224.

— 2010a (forthcoming). "Mother of unworthy woe": infant death and sentimental maternity in women's poetry. In: T. Connolly, ed. *Spectacular death: interdisciplinary perspectives on mortality and (un)representability*. Bristol, UK: Intellect Press.

— 2010b (forthcoming). "Fear not / to unfold your dark visions of torment": Blake and Emin's bad sex aesthetic. In: T. Connolly and H. Bruder, eds. *Queer Blake*. Houndmills, UK: Palgrave Macmillan.

Dalby, P., 2007. He just got it…they all have it…are you next? *The Toronto Star*, 1 Nov. pp. Y1, Y10.

Dean, C., 1986. "Law and Sacrifice: Bataille, Lacan, and the Critique of the Subject." *Representations*, 13, pp. 42-62.

De Certeau, M., 1984. *The practice of everyday life*. Translated from French by S. Rendall. Berkeley: University of California Press.

De Coulanges, F., 1955. *The ancient city: a study on the religion, laws, and institutions of Greece and Rome*. Translated from French by W. Small. Garden City, NY: Doubleday Anchor Books.

Deleuze, G., 2002. *Pure immanence: essays on a life*. Translated from French by A. Boyman. New York: Zone Books.

Deleuze, G. and Guattari, F., 1994. *What is philosophy?*. Translated from French by H. Tomlinson and G. Burchell. New York: Columbia University Press.

Deleuze, G. and von Sacher-Masoch, L., 1991. *Masochism: Coldness and cruelty & Venus in furs*. Translated from French and German by J. McNeil. New York: Zone Books.

De Montaigne, M., 1943. *Selected essays*. Translated from French by D.M. Frame. New York: Walter J. Black.

Derrida, J., 1982. "Ousia and Gramme": note on a note from *Being and time*. *Margins of Philosophy*. Translated from French by A. Bass. Chicago: University of Chicago Press, pp. 29–67.

— 1993. *Aporias*. Translated from French by T. Dutoit. Stanford: Stanford University Press.

— 2002. *Without alibi*. Translated from French by P. Kamuf. Stanford: Stanford University Press.

Descartes, R., 1960. *Discourse on method*. Translated from French by A. Wollaston. Baltimore: Penguin.

Didi-Huberman, G., 2005. *Confronting images: questioning the ends of a certain history of art*. Translated from French by J. Goodman. University Park, PA: Pennsylvania State University Press.

References

Dorter, K., 1977. The dialectic of Plato's method of hypothesis. *Philosophical Forum* 7, pp. 159–187.

Durkheim, E., 1938a. Division of labor in society. *American Journal of Sociology* 4, pp. 319–328.

— 1938b. *The rules of sociological method*. Glencoe, NY: The Free Press.

— 1961. *The elementary forms of the religious life*. New York: Collier Books.

Elias, N., 1978–1982. *The civilizing process*. Translated from German by E. Jephcott. New York: Urizen Books.

Felman, S., 2002. *The scandal of the speaking body: Don Juan with J.L. Austin, or Seduction in two languages*. Translated from French by C. Porter. Stanford: Stanford University Press.

Fink, B., 2004. *Lacan to the letter: reading Écrits closely*. Minneapolis: University of Minnesota Press.

Florida, R., 2002. *The rise of the creative class*. New York: Basic Books.

Foucault, M., 1965. *Madness and civilization: a history of insanity in the age of reason*. Translated from French by R. Howard. New York: Pantheon Books.

— 1973. *The birth of the clinic: an archeology of medical perception*. Translated from French by A.M. Sheridan Smith. New York: Pantheon Books.

— 1977. *Language, counter-memory, practice*. D. Beauchard, ed. Translated from French by D.F. Bouchard and S. Simon. Ithaca: Cornell University Press.

Freidson, E. 1988. *Profession of medicine: a study of the sociology of applied knowledge*. Chicago: University of Chicago Press.

Freud, S., 1957. *Mourning and melancholia, Volume 11, on metapsychology: the theory of psychoanalysis*. Translated from German by J. Strachey. London: Penguin.

— 1961. *Beyond the pleasure principle*. Translated from German by J. Strachey. New York: Norton.

— 1963. *Therapy and technique*. P. Rieff, ed. New York: Collier Books.

— 2003. *The uncanny*. Translated from German by D. McLintock. New York: Penguin Classics.

Freud, S. and Breuer, J., 1952. *Studies in hysteria*. New York: Penguin.

Gadamer, H.G., 1986. *The ideal of the good in Platonic-Aristotelian philosophy*. Translated from German by C. Smith. New Haven: Yale University Press.

— 1996. *The enigma of health*. Translated from German by J. Gaigea and N. Walker. Stanford: Stanford University Press.

Gans, E., 1982. Beckett and the problem of modern culture. *SubStance* 11(2), pp. 3–15.

Garfinkel, H., 1967. *Studies in ethnomethodology*. Englewood Cliffs, NJ: Prentice Hall.

Girard, R., 1977. *Violence and the sacred*. Translated from French by P. Gregory. Baltimore: Johns Hopkins University Press.

Goffman, E., 1961a. *Asylums: essays on the social situation of mental patients and other inmates*. Garden City, NY: Anchor.

— 1961b. *The presentation of self in everyday life*. Garden City, NY: Anchor.

— 1963. *Behavior in public places*. Glencoe, IL: The Free Press.

Gordon, A., 2007. Party's over: most students don't drink heavily but the problem is, they think everyone else does. *The Toronto Star*, 27 Oct. LexisNexis Academic, http://academic.lexisnexis.com. Accessed 23 September 2009.

Greene, T., 1982. "Erasmus's 'Festina lente': vulnerabilities of the humanist text." In: J.D Lyons and S.G. Nichols, Jr., eds. *Mimesis from mirror to method, Augustine to Descartes*. Hanover, NH: University Press of New England, pp. 132–148.

Hegel, G.W.F., 1967. *The phenomenology of mind*. Translated from German by J.B. Baillie. New York: Harper Torch Books.

— 1968. *The logic of Hegel, 2nd edition*. Translated from German by W. Wallace. London: Oxford University Press.

— 1970. *Hegel's Philosophy of nature, being part two of the Encyclopedia of the philosophical sciences*. Translated from German by A.V. Miller. Oxford: Clarendon Press.

Heidegger, M., 1961. *An introduction to metaphysics*. Translated from German by R. Manheim. Garden City, NY: Doubleday Anchor Books.

— 1962. *Being and time*. Translated from German by J. Macquarrie and E. Robinson. London: SCM Press.

— 1982. *The question concerning technology and other essays*. Translated from German by W. Lovitt. New York: Harper Perennial.

Henry, R., 2009. States consider cutting drug help for seniors. *The Associated Press*, 27 May. http://www.msnbc.msn.com/id/30966094/. Accessed 25 September 2009.

Hesiod. 1953. *Theogony*. Translated from Greek by N.O. Brown. Indianapolis: Library of Liberal Arts.

Hobbes, T., 1994. *Leviathan*. E. Curley, ed. Indianapolis: Hackett Publishing Company.

Hume, D., 1956. *An enquiry concerning human understanding*. Los Angeles: Gateway Editions, Inc.

Jain, S.S., 1999. The prosthetic imagination: enabling and disabling the prosthesis trope. *Science, Technology, and Human Values* 24(1), pp. 31–54.

Johnson, B., 2008. *Persons and things*. Boston: Harvard University Press.

Josopivici, G., 2009. Voice test. *The Times Literary Supplement*, 13 March, p. 7.

Kant, I., 1929. *Critique of pure reason*. Translated from German by K.Smith. New York: St. Martin's Press.

— 2007. *Critique of judgement*. N. Walker, ed. Translated from German by J.C. Meredith. Oxford: Oxford University Press.

Kierkegaard, S., 1955. *Fear and trembling and The sickness unto death*. Translated from Danish by W. Lowrie. Garden City, NY: Doubleday Anchor Books.

— 1962. *The present age*. Translated from Danish by A. Dru. New York: Harper Perennial.

Kripke, S.A., 1977. Identity and necessity. In S.P. Schwartz, ed. *Naming, necessity, and natural kinds*. Ithaca: Cornell University Press, pp. 66–101.

Lacan, J., 1976–1977. Le sinthome. In: *Jacques Lacan's Seminar XXIII*. J.A. Miller, ed. Translated from French by L. Thurston. *Ornicar?* 6–11. http://www.sduk.us/ beaver/PDF/Lacan-Seminar23_Sinthome_English.pdf. Accessed 10 May, 2010.

— 1981a. *Speech and language in psychoanalysis*. Translated from French by A. Wilden. Baltimore: Johns Hopkins University Press.

— 1981b. *The seminar of Jacques Lacan, Book XI: The four fundamental concepts of psychoanalysis*. Translated by A. Sheridan. New York: Norton.

— 1988. *The seminar of Jacques Lacan, Book I: Freud's papers on technique 1953–1954*. Translated from French by S. Tomaselli. New York: Norton.

— 1991. *The seminar of Jacques Lacan, Book II: The ego in Freud's theory and in the technique of psychoanalysis 1954–1955*. Translated from French by S. Tomaselli. New York: Norton.

— 1992. *The seminar of Jacques Lacan, Book VII: The ethics of psychoanalysis 1959–1960*. Translated from French by D. Porter. New York: Norton.

— 1997. *The seminar of Jacques Lacan, Book III: The psychoses 1955–1956*. Translated from French by R. Grigg. New York: Norton.

— 2006. *Écrits*. Translated from French by B. Fink. New York: Norton.

— 2007. *The seminar of Jacques Lacan, Book XVII: The other side of psychoanalysis*. Translated from French by R. Grigg. New York: Norton.

Laplanche, J., 1976. *Life and death in psychoanalysis*. Translated from French by J. Mehlman. Baltimore: Johns Hopkins University Press.

— 1989. *New foundations for psychoanalysis*. Translated from French by D. Macey. Oxford: Basil Blackwell.

— 1999. *Essays on otherness*. Translated from French by J. Fletcher. London: Routledge.

Levi, P., 1988. *The drowned and the saved.* Translated from Italian by R. Rosenthal. New York: Summit Books.

Levinas, E., 1969. *Totality and infinity: an essay on exteriority.* Translated from French by A. Lingis. Pittsburgh: Duquesne University Press.

— 1978. *Existence and existents.* Translated from French by A. Lingis. The Hague: Martinus Nijhoff.

— 1987. *Time and the other and additional essays.* Translated from French by R. Cohen. Pittsburgh: Duquesne University Press.

Leys, R., 2007. *From guilt to shame.* Princeton: Princeton University Press.

Locke, J., 1947. *An essay concerning human understanding.* London: JM Dent.

Lyon, J.B., 2005. "You can kill, but you cannot bring to life": aesthetic education and the instrumentalization of pain in Schiller and Hölderlin. *Literature and Medicine* 24(1), pp. 31–50.

Malinowski, B., 1955. *Magic, science, and religion and other essays.* Garden City, NY: Doubleday Anchor Books.

Marcuse, H., 1964. *One dimensional man.* Boston: Beacon Press.

Marx, K., 1964. *Selected writings in sociology and social philosophy.* T. B. Bottomore and M. Rubel, eds. Translated from German by T. B. Bottomore. New York: McGraw-Hill.

Marx, K. and Engels, F., 1960. *The German ideology, parts I and III.* Pascal, R., ed. New York: International Publishers.

McHugh, P., 1968. *Defining the situation.* Minneapolis: Bobbs-Merill.

— 2005. Shared being, old promises, and the joint of necessity of affirmative action. *Human studies* 28, pp. 129–156.

— 2010 (forthcoming). How the dead circulate (in life). In: T. Connolly, ed. *Spectacular death: interdisciplinary perspectives on mortality and (un)representability.* Bristol, UK: Intellect Press.

McHugh, P., Raffel, S., Foss, D.C. and Blum, A., 1974. *On the beginning of social inquiry.* London: Routledge & Kegan Paul.

McLuhan, M., 1964. *Understanding media: the extensions of man.* New York: McGraw-Hill.

Mead, G.H., 1967. *Mind, self, and society: from the standpoint of a social behaviorist.* In: C.W. Morris, ed. *Works of George Herbert Mead, Volume 1.* Chicago: University of Chicago Press.

Melville, H., 1951. *Billy Budd and other stories.* London: J. Lehmann.

Miller, B. and Scoffield, H., 2009. Aging: the growing cost. *The Globe and Mail*, 9 July. LexisNexis Academic, http://academic.lexisnexis.com. Accessed 25 September 2009.

Miller, J.A., 2006a. Introduction to reading Jacques Lacan's seminar on *Anxiety* II. Translated from French by B.P. Fulks. *lacanian ink* 27, pp. 8–63.

— 2006b. Detached pieces. Translated from French by B.P. Fulks. *lacanian ink* 28, pp. 26–41.

— 2006c. Profane illuminations. Translated from French by B.P. Fulks. *lacanian ink* 28, pp. 8–25.

— 2007. A reading from Jacques Lacan's seminar *From an other to the other* II. Translated from French by B.P. Fulks. *lacanian ink* 30, pp. 8–63.

Monsebraaten, L. and Daly, R., 2007. Diabetes lurks in urban sprawl; Ailing Toronto neighbourhoods. *The Toronto Star*, 1 Nov. pp. A1, A11.

Nancy, J.L., 1991. *The inoperative community.* Translated from French by P. Connor and L. Garbus. Minneapolis: University of Minnesota Press.

Nietzsche, F., 1956. *The birth of tragedy and The genealogy of morals.* Translated from German by F. Golffing. Garden City, NY: Doubleday Anchor Books.

Park, R.E., 1926. The urban community as a special pattern and a moral order. In: E.W. Burgess, ed. *The urban community.* Chicago: University of Chicago Press, pp. 3–18.

Parsons, T., 1937. *Structure of social action*. New York: McGraw-Hill.

— 1951. *The social system*. Glencoe, IL: The Free Press.

—1964. *Social structure and personality*. Glencoe, IL: The Free Press.

Plato, 1945. *The republic of Plato*. Translated from Greek by F.M. Cornford. London: Oxford University Press.

—1949a. *Theaetetus*. Translated from Greek by B. Jowett. Indianapolis: Library of the Liberal Arts/Bobbs-Merrill.

— 1949b. *Timaeus*. Translated from Greek by B. Jowett. Indianapolis: Library of the Liberal Arts/Bobbs-Merrill.

— 1949c. *Plato's Meno*. Translated from Greek by F. Cornford. Indianapolis: Library of the Liberal Arts/Bobbs-Merrill.

— 1955. *Plato's Phaedo*. Translated from Greek by R.S. Bluck. Indianapolis: Library of the Liberal Arts/Bobbs-Merrill.

— 1956. *Phaedrus*. Translated from Greek by W.C. Helmbold and W.G. Rabinowitz. Indianapolis: Library of the Liberal Arts/Bobbs-Merrill.

— 1960. *Plato's examination of the pleasure (The Philebus)*. Translated from Greek by R. Hackforth. Indianapolis: Library of the Liberal Arts/Bobbs-Merrill.

—1984. *Sophist*. In: S. Benardete, ed. Translated from Greek by S. Benardete. *The being of the beautiful: Plato's* Theaetetus, Sophist *and* Statesman. Chicago: University of Chicago Press.

Popper, K.R., 1971. *The open society and its enemies, volume 1: the spell of Plato*. Princeton: Princeton University Press.

Radley, A., 1999. The aesthetics of illness: narrative, horror, and the sublime. *Sociology of Health and Illness* 21(6), pp. 778–796.

Raffel, S., 1985. Health and life. *Theoretical Medicine and Bioethics* 6(2), pp. 153–165.

Rancière, J., 1992. Politics, identification, and subjectivization. *October* 61, pp. 58–64.

— 1994. Discovering new worlds: politics of travel and metaphor. In: G. Robertson et al., eds. *Travellers' tales: narratives of home and displacement.* London: Routledge, pp. 29–37.

— 1999. *Disagreement: politics and philosophy.* Translated from French by J. Rose. Minneapolis: University of Minnesota Press.

— 2004. *The politics of aesthetics: the distribution of the sensible.* Translated from French by G. Rockhill. London: Continuum.

— 2006. Thinking between disciplines: an aesthetics of knowledge. Translated from French by J. Roffe. *Parrhesia* 1, pp. 1–12.

— 2007. *The future of the image.* Translated from French by G. Elliott. London: Verso.

— 2009a. *Aesthetics and its discontents.* Translated from French by S. Corcoran. Malden, MA: Polity Press.

— 2009b. *The emancipated spectator.* Translated from French by G. Elliott. London: Verso.

Rodwin, V.G., 2001. Urban health: is the city infected? In: M. Marinker, ed. *Medicine and humanity.* London: King's Fund, pp. 141–152.

Rosen, S., 1980. *The limits of analysis.* New York: Basic Books.

Rosset, C., 1989. Of a real that has yet to come. *SubStance* 18(3), pp. 5–21.

Russell, B., 1949. *The problems of philosophy.* Oxford: Oxford University Press.

Ryle, G., 1949. *The concept of mind.* Chicago: University of Chicago Press.

Sacks, H., 1992. *Lectures on conversation, Volumes 1 and 11.* G. Jefferson, ed. Oxford: Blackwell Publishers.

Santner, E.L., 2001. *On the psychotheology of everyday life: reflections on Freud and Rosenzweig.* Chicago: University Of Chicago Press.

Sartre, J.P., 1968. *Search for a method.* Translated from French by H.E. Barnes. New York: Vintage.

Scanlon, T.M., 1998. *What we owe to each other*. Cambridge, MA: Belknap Press of Harvard University Press.

Scarry, E., 1985. *The body in pain: the making and unmaking of the world*. New York: Oxford University Press.

Schumpeter, J.A., 1992. *Capitalism, socialism, and democracy*. London: Routledge.

Schutz A., 1973. Common sense and scientific interpretation. In: M.A. Natanson and H.L. van Breda, eds. *Collected papers, Volume 1: the problem of social reality*. The Hague: Martinus Nijhoff, pp. 7–34.

Schwenger, P., 2000. Corpsing the image. *Critical Inquiry* 26, pp. 395–413.

Scott, J. and Marshall, G., 2005. "Medicalization." *A dictionary of sociology*. http://www.enotes.com/oxsoc-encyclopedia/medicalization. Accessed 11 May, 2010.

Serres, M., 1982. *The parasite*. Translated from French by L.R. Schehr. Minneapolis: University of Minnesota Press.

— 2008a. *The five senses: a philosophy of mingled bodies (I)*. Translated from French by M. Sankey and P. Cowley. London: Continuum.

— 2008b. *The troubadour of knowledge*. Translated from French by S.F. Glaser with W. Paulson. Ann Arbor: University of Michigan Press.

Shils, E., 1981. *Tradition*. Chicago: University of Chicago Press.

Simmel, G., 1956. *The sociology of Georg Simmel*. K. Wolff, ed. Translated from German by K. Wolff. Glencoe, IL: The Free Press.

— 1959. *Georg Simmel, 1858–1918: a collection of essays*. Translated from German by R.H. Weingartner. Columbus: Ohio State University Press.

— 1971. *Georg Simmel on individuality and social forms*. D.N. Levine, ed. Chicago: University of Chicago Press.

— 1991. The problem of style. Translated from German by M. Ritter. *Theory, Culture and Society* 8(3), pp. 63–71.

Sontag, S., 1978. *Illness as metaphor*. New York: Farrar, Straus and Giroux.

Stanislavski, C., 1989. *Building a character*. Translated from Russian by E.R. Hapgood. New York: Routledge/Theatre Arts Book.

Starobinski, J., 1985. *Montaigne in motion*. Translated from French by A. Goldhammer. Chicago: University of Chicago Press.

Stengers, I., 1997. *Power and invention: situating science*. Translated from French by P. Bains. Minneapolis: University of Minnesota Press.

Stinchcombe, A., 1986. Reason and rationality. *Sociological Theory* 4, pp. 151–166.

Stoichita, V., 2008. *The Pygmalion effect: from Ovid to Hitchcock*. Translated from French by A. Anderson. Chicago: University of Chicago Press.

Swanson, G.E., 1971. An organizational analysis of collectivities. *American Sociological Review* 36(4), pp. 607–624.

— 1992. Doing things together: some basic forms of agency and structure in collective action and some explanations. *Social Psychology Quarterly* 55(2), pp. 94–117.

Teskey, G., 2006. *Delirious Milton: the fate of the poet in modernity*. Cambridge, MA: Harvard University Press.

Thrift, N., 2004a. Transurbanism. *Urban Geography* 25(8), pp. 724–734.

— 2004b. Intensities of feeling: towards a spatial politics of affect. *Geografiska Annaler* 86B(1), pp. 57–78.

Tiffany, D., 2008. Rhapsodic measures. *Critical Inquiry* 34(S2), pp. 147–169.

Van Haute, P., 1998. Death and sublimation in Lacan's reading of *Antigone*. In: S. Harasym, ed. *Levinas and Lacan: the missed encounter*. Albany: State University of New York Press, pp. 103–121.

Vischer, A.L., 1966. *On growing old*. Translated from French by G. Onn. London: George Allen & Unwin.

Weber, M., 1930. *The protestant work ethic and the spirit of capitalism*. Translated from German by T. Parsons. London: George Allen & Unwin.

— 1947. *The theory of social and economic organization*. Translated from German by A.M. Henderson and T. Parsons. New York: The Free Press.

— 1958. "Science as a vocation." *From Max Weber: essays in sociology*. H.H. Gerth and C.W. Mills, eds. Translated from German by H.H. Gerth and C.W. Mills. pp. 129–156.

Whitehead, A.N., 1967. *Adventures of ideas*. New York: The Free Press.

Wills, D., 1995. *Prosthesis*. Stanford: Stanford University Press.

Wittgenstein, L., 1953. *Philosophical investigations*. Translated from German by G.E.M. Anscombe. New York: Macmillan.

— 1965. "A lecture on ethics." *The Philosophical Review*, 7(1), pp. 3–12.

Wolin, R., 1990. *The politics of being: the political thought of Martin Heidegger*. New York: Columbia University Press.

Žižek, S., 1997. *The plague of fantasies*. London: Verso.

— 2007. From *objet a* to subtraction. *lacanian ink* 30, pp. 130–141.